MW00424479

CANARY

In a

COVID WORLD

HOW PROPAGANDA AND CENSORSHIP
CHANGED OUR (MY) WORLD

A COLLECTION OF ESSAYS FROM
34 CONTEMPORARY THOUGHT LEADERS.

Edited by C.H. Klotz

Canary House Publishing

Canary *In a* Covid World™
How Propaganda And Censorship Changed Our (My) World.

Published by: Canary House Publishing
ISBN: 978-1-7390525-0-8

Disclaimer: The information presented in this book is not a substitute for evaluation and treatment by a medical doctor. The information contained herein is for educational purposes only and each essay is independent of the others and reflects the views of the specific author. It is not intended to be a substitute for professional medical advice. The reader should always consult with his or her physician to determine the appropriateness of the information for his or her own medical situation and treatment plan. Reading this book does not constitute a physician-patient relationship.

This book is dedicated to all those courageous people who defied the propaganda, who researched the truth and who spoke out, loudly or quietly, to inform and warn others, against powerful authorities and the ill-advised public health measures which have caused more harm than good.

It is also dedicated to all those who lost their lives from COVID, those who have been injured and suffer, because they were denied the complete picture.

Three dollars from each book sold will be donated to React19 to support the vaccine-injured as well as to CHD and ICAN to support ongoing litigation against government censorship, overreach, propaganda and corruption.

Follow us on Substack: https://canaryinacovidworld.substack.com and Twitter/X https://twitter.com/canary_covid

Special thanks to these 34 authors who contributed to this book so others can learn the truth behind the censorship and propaganda which dominated the COVID era.

Colin McAdam *Internationally acclaimed novelist*

Brianne Dressen *Vaccine injured and co-founder of advocacy group React19*

Dr. George Fareed *Family Physician who successfully treated over 20,000 Covid patients*

UK MP Sir Christopher Chope *Conservative Member of the UK Parliament, Chair of the UK Parliament's All-Party Parliamentary Group on Covid-19 Vaccine Damage*

Dr. Pierre Kory *Lung, Pulmonary ICU Specialist and co-founder of the FLCCC*

Elizabeth Woodworth *Retired Health Science Librarian, BC Ministry of Health*

Dr. Michael Nevradakis *Journalist and senior reporter for The Defender and CHD TV host*

Edward Dowd *Former Wall Street analyst and Blackrock portfolio manager & author of "Cause Unknown."*

Dr. Jessica Rose *Researcher*

Dr. Joseph Fraiman *Emergency medicine physician and researcher*

Trish Wood *Journalist and former CBC Fifth Estate anchor, host of "Trish Wood is Critical" podcast*

Dr. Ryan Cole *Pathologist*

Dr. Aseem Malhotra *British Cardiologist*

Senator Ron Johnson *Senior US Senator from Wisconsin*

Dr. Peter A. McCullough *Practicing Internist and Cardiologist*

Dr. Norman Fenton *Professor of Risk, Queen Mary University of London*

Rodney Palmer *A 20-year veteran of Canadian journalism at the CBC & CTV*

Dr. Paul Marik *Pulmonary and Critical Care Specialist & co-founder of the FLCCC*

Dr. Jay Bhattacharya *Professor of Medicine, Economics, and Health Research Policy at Stanford University*

Dr. Joseph Ladapo *Florida Surgeon General and Professor of Medicine at the University of Florida*

Drs. Robert & Jill Malone *Scientist, physician and the original inventor of mRNA vaccination as a technology*

Lord Sumption *Retired Senior UK Supreme Court Judge*

Professor Bruce Pardy *Professor of law at Queen's University and Executive Director of Rights Probe*

Drs. James & Maggie Thorp *Board-certified in obstetrics and gynecology (OB/GYN) as well as a specialist in maternal-fetal medicine.*

Dr. Naomi Wolf *Author of 7 nonfiction bestsellers. Cofounder/CEO, DailyClout.io*

Steve Kirsch *Entrepreneur & founder of Vaccine Safety Research Foundation*

John Leake *Historian and co-author of "The Courage To Face Covid19"*

Dr. Mary O'Connor *Family physician*

Dr. Harvey Risch *Professor Emeritus of Epidemiology, Yale School of Public Health & Medicine*

Dr. Sam Dubé *Mathematician, physician, strength coach, and broadcaster*

Margaret Anna Alice *Writer who blogs about propaganda, mass control, psychology, politics, and health with a focus on COVID*

Dr. Michael Rectenwald *Author and fellow at Hillsdale College*

Dr. Peter & Ginger Breggin *Psychiatrist*

Professor Denis Rancourt *Scientist*

Contents

Introduction

The contributors to this collection of essays are courageous people.

They are critical thinkers who are prepared to put everything on the line to speak their truth. For as you will learn, they have been censored, they have been cancelled, they have been persecuted and they have been silenced across oceans. Yet still they strive to alert us all to what COVID was, and what may lie ahead.

They are community leaders. They are novelists, journalists, lawyers, judges, scientists, doctors, academics, politicians, researchers, vaccine-injured and data experts. Some shouted from the rooftops from the very beginning of the pandemic, others found their voices as the contradictions in public and health policy became undeniable.

What unites them is that they have given those looking for answers, factual evidence. They have alleviated fear and given us hope. They have shown us all that if our opinions fall outside those deemed acceptable by mainstream media, we are not alone.

The subject of COVID is often too sensitive to introduce into polite conversation. Battle lines are drawn and more often than not there's no amount of data, facts or opinion that will change perspectives. However, we believe that once people understand that their opinions have been formed based on information that has been heavily censored and that most legacy media are now instruments of propaganda, they will be more inclined to entertain the possibility that all is not what it seems.

The endeavour of this book is to bring thoughtful voices together to sing as one choir. The diversity of these voices that harmonise may allow others to hear the music. Over the last three years solo voices have too often been drowned out of the discourse.

For once you see it, you can't unsee it. You'll understand the power of censorship and propaganda to conceal the lies and dishonesty that now underpin our societal foundations.

Speak your truth. Be critical. Stay free.

CHAPTER 1

Where Your Fear Begins

Colin McAdam

Internationally acclaimed novelist

Colin McAdam has a PhD from Cambridge University and is an internationally acclaimed novelist. He has written for Harpers, Granta, Salon and Hazlitt, among other journals, and his books have won or been shortlisted for several prizes including the Amazon Best First Novel award, the Commonwealth Writers Prize, the Giller, GGs and the Rogers Writers Trust Fiction Prize. His most recent novel is *BLACK DOVE*, a story about genetic editing and the adventures of a grieving father and son.

My business is telling stories. I think, all the time, about the role of them in our lives, how much we need stories, how our need for them distinguishes us from other apes yet serves an ape function of protecting our groups: stories in the form of scripture, shared collections of tales that we can unite around or use to exclude others; fairy tales we can tell to prepare our children for their journeys in the woods.

Stories can warn us, scare us, light up the darkness, chase away boredom. And they can also make us brave.

I think the word 'narrative' has never been more commonly used than it has over the past three years – sometimes a substitute for 'spin', always a synonym of 'story'.

To some, the story of COVID goes like this: a virus of zoonotic origin jumped species and was spread in a wet market in Wuhan; it burned indiscriminately through populations in Iran and Italy, and carried on throughout the world; it is dangerous for old and young, causes long-term disabilities, and even though it is airborne it can be contained by locking down populations for certain periods of time and is mitigated if everyone wears a mask, gets vaccinated multiple times, and stays six feet apart in well-ventilated spaces if not apart completely.

To others the story starts with a lab in Wuhan, with gain-of-function research conducted either to develop bioweapons or to help understand theoretical pandemics; the virus's furin cleavage site and genome reveal it is man-made; it probably began spreading long before we realized; it is harmful only to the very ill and the very old, is not contracted by everyone, even within small settings, and is for the most part experienced as a cold or flu; and, like the flu, the vaccines given for it (which are mostly not vaccines but experimental gene therapies) are often not effective in reducing transmission or severity (and are sometimes dangerous themselves).

One of these stories is told by the mainstream media, and the other has largely been censored. The first brings benefits to pharmaceutical companies (in terms of selling vaccines and medications); it benefits technology providers (Zoom, Microsoft, telecommunications companies, anything that facilitates work from home, remote learning and online shopping); it benefits those who like controlling information (the media and politicians in power); and it benefits those who own the media and politicians (pharmaceutical companies and technology providers). It is also an appealing story to those who believe their government will look after them, that strangers are foolish and to be kept at arm's length, that it's easier to take medication than to be healthy and that those who make the medication could not possibly be so evil as to create a virus and market its cure.

Of the two COVID narratives, the second is based on fear of those in power and the first on fear of each other. Even though we were meant to be all in this together, to lock down and take our lumps, the purpose of that story, certainly its consequence, was to keep us apart. As that story came to dominate, we were kept from friends, from restaurants, from bars, movies, live music, gyms, stores, parks, beaches and playgrounds. We were told we might be sick without knowing it, that everyone was a vector of disease. We hid each other's faces and made children think they would kill their grandmothers by going to school.

I was not inclined to like that story. I didn't really want to hear it. If every day's a gift, given that we are mortal, should we really postpone its enjoyment? Can we presume we will have more days? If I love people, if people need love, how long should we be apart? Two weeks, a month, the school year, the summer. Wait for the winter to pass. Do it for the healthcare system, do it for the teachers, the front-line workers. It's not hard to wear a mask, everything can be bought or done online.

I've tried to remember all of the absurdities, tragedies and indignities that I witnessed or went through over those early years of COVID, but it occurs to me that none of it was unique to me. Millions of people, billions, could trump my stories or trot out examples of hideous things forced upon them by scared, power-hungry and incompetent bureaucrats. Children overdosing and hanging themselves because they were told they had no future, that the world was in fact finally burning and it was harmful to turn to each other for relief.

One difficult thing about our shared COVID experience is that it wasn't really shared, not just because of isolation but because vast numbers of people have had no voice. We've heard about the struggles of teachers and nurses, of government workers afraid to return to work, but what about the Vietnamese family who owned the dry cleaner in one of those shuttered office buildings? What about the 70-year-old crossing guard who suddenly had nothing to wake up for, or the drywaller who lost his business during the shutdown of construction? Where did we hear about their suicides and collapse, what happened to their families? What if those had been weighed against the actual experience of the majority who caught COVID?

I was never particularly distrustful of the media. Many of my friends have been journalists and I've written for magazines and papers. Of course I've been conscious of bias, but it wasn't until January 2022 that the way I looked at public discourse changed profoundly.

At the end of that month some truckers came to town.

I believe most thinking people grew a little tired of the mainstream presentation of this disease, after two years of fear-mongering. I had taken solace in as many hard facts as I could find – one useful source was simply Health Canada's website, where the curve of hospitalizations and deaths had always been thickest for those already at the end of life. Once I learned from the CDC's own reckoning that more than 96 per cent of COVID deaths occurred among people with *three* co-morbidities, I grew a little disdainful of my neighbours riding mountain bikes with masks on.

Two years of seeing other hard stats out of the UK and elsewhere, showing that children were predominantly unharmed by this virus, that COVID was, of course, a serious disease for a few, but was best considered a hastener not a killer. Two years of isolation from friends, of three school closures, two curfews, four levels of police leaning into my car window to ask me where I was going. Two years of not just statistics but of knowing friends, some in their eighties and nineties who had a hard time with COVID for a couple of weeks, some for months, who said the last thing they ever wanted was for the world to stop while they felt ill. Knowing other friends who lost their music careers, their coffee shops, their livelihoods and sense of purpose, because of this story we were told to believe.

My wife and I had taken our two vaccines almost a year prior to the trucks arriving. Our daughter's school had told us that unless we had her vaccinated she would not only be kept from her friends at lunch but she would not be allowed to attend the following year.

Here in Canada we continued to contemplate lockdowns while countries like the UK had been open for almost a year. Live music and sporting events came alive again elsewhere but here in Canada we continued to have our holiday gatherings monitored by neighbours and police. My wife saw two women fighting on a train because one had taken off her mask to do her make-up. We lined up to show vaccine passports at the liquor store. The media talked about wastewater signals and ostracized anyone who didn't continue to embrace the new orthodoxies, anyone who didn't wear a mask, never earnestly inquiring into whether these new phylacteries, these virtue-signalling impositions on our faces were ever more than suffocating, bacterial rags that denied us our beauty and communion.

By January 2022 I had had enough. I couldn't bear another word of it. It had been remarkable to me that no one in Canada with any mainstream voice – no political party, no media outlet, no public intellectual (to the extent that we have any) – had spoken out meaningfully against these years of lockdown and overreach. We have a Charter of Rights here, which is meant to stand above the meddling of politicians, to guarantee us freedom of movement, of assembly and speech, but it was clearly a meaningless document. Truly excellent research had come elsewhere from people like Matt Ridley, from Vanity Fair's Katherine Eban and later from Alex Washburne to show me that this virus was almost unquestionably man-made. And to consider it man-made was not an act of anti-Asian hatred but a recognition that some small group of sociopaths decided to heed their perverse curiosity and create a disease that had made a group of people (millions!) suffer and die in the name of preventing death and suffering. I had watched everyone learn to hate each other in the name of caring, everyone denying life in the name of living, compassionate artists wagging their fingers or screaming at people who didn't do as they did, and no one shouting at the people who deserved it most: the ones who created the disease, and the mother-fuckers who told us we should hide and hate each other but continue to buy what they sold.

I *loved* that the truckers were coming.

We had moved to a place in rural Quebec, just across the river from Ottawa, Canada's capital, which was where the convoy was heading, and I wanted to have a look at what they stood for. Misogynists, homophobes, transphobes, even Islamaphobes, according to our Prime Minister. An embarrassing and ragged group of grease-stained ignoramuses; "yobs," as one somehow eminent journalist described them.

Our media said the convoy was funded by Russia and was a vehicle for white supremacists, but what I had seen on social media from supporters of the convoy was, of course, something very different. These were the people we hadn't heard about, the ones who couldn't "pivot", the ones who either had no laptop to hide behind or didn't consider it a very full life to hide behind a laptop. Wanting to speak out, wanting to agitate because our politicians and media in Canada were, at best, feckless and inert.

I was aware of being depressed, how joyless this country had felt for two years. How depressed, I hadn't quite realized. I drove towards Ottawa and came to an overpass just as some bearded strangers unfurled a banner that read "Freedom", and I started crying.

That word "freedom" has since become a source of mockery, those opposed to the convoy finding it laughable that anyone should pursue it while we were meant to be cowering together. I'm reminded of the often compared ideal of the Canadian constitution, where we celebrate "peace, order and good government", and the ideal in the American Declaration of Independence of "life, liberty and the pursuit of happiness". I wonder who is more laughable, or to be pitied: the man celebrating the bars of his prison or the one trying to get out.

I arrived in Ottawa just as the trucks were coming in, in typically awful weather – minus 30, the wind blowing, the sun shining and all the usual signals that humans should never have tried to live here. I had a spring in my step. Pick-up trucks, semi-trailers, cars with flags, everyone honking and cheering. I ran a bit, partly to stay warm. I can see myself now without embarrassment: a bald guy with a broken knee, trying to run like a kid.

The convoy has been called an insurrection, an occupation, at best a protest, but for most of the people who were there with open eyes it was a celebration. Lots of Fuck Trudeau signs, of course, but a lot of love in the air. There was a giddiness to that day for one simple reason: we *wanted* to get together.

I shook hands with all kinds of people, hugged a big drunk in Carhartt overalls, wandered around and chatted. Met a mother whose son couldn't play hockey on his team without being vaccinated, who died the morning after inoculation. The gym owner who lost his business, his house, his income, deemed inessential by people who still enjoyed the novelty of working at home in their pyjamas. These people who should be heard, the mute and inglorious – they weren't there just out of bitterness, they were there to feel connection. They were protesting, they had complaints, but they were there to overcome. To be brave.

One of the things I learned over these years is how class-conscious, how insecure and unempathetic so much of my cohort truly is. We in the Arts community are meant to be the ones who look in the dark corners, the ones who care about the oppressed and sing the sorrows of those who have no time or strength to sing. We are meant to think critically, to challenge authority and champion the individual under the thumb of the man. Shortly before the truckers arrived I heard about Neil Young ("Rockin in the Free World") boycotting Spotify because it hosted Joe Rogan, a man who dared to interview a couple of scientists who, I'm guessing, knew more about vaccination and mRNA technology than Neil Young did. And I, as an artist, as a 'liberal', as someone who surely must care about other people more than other people do, was meant to boycott Spotify as well, to put my fingers in my ears and continue to believe that other story.

Ignorance and divisiveness have become virtues, as long as they align with looking liberal.

I wanted my wife and daughter to see this gathering so we went the following day. The crowd had become huge. Not just 'truckers' but families with strollers, Sikhs, indigenous singers, the young and old, everyone joyful, everyone friendly, fat dudes shouting 'I love you!' in a way that startled my daughter. We walked through the downtown mall to get to Parliament Hill and many people were unmasked, the first to dare in that building for two years. It feels unspeakably pathetic to remember how hesitant I was to take that goddamn thing off my face. Pathetic to think how beautiful it was to see smiles.

I've known Ottawa on and off for many years, and I had never seen it so lively, so friendly.

And how was the event covered in the news?

In that crowd of tens of thousands we saw one journalist, a woman with a microphone and a cameraman, and that night on CBC and CTV were stories of white supremacy, a Nazi flag spotted in the crowd, talk of truckers attacking a homeless shelter. Later in the "occupation" were claims of arson, rape, pissing on statues and anti-Semitism. There were winking and superior glances at bouncy castles and hot tubs, and under every story, good or bad, was a suggestion of indecency about this whole thing. We were all meant to be in this together, why were these grubby people protesting?

I was appalled. Gut-deep disappointed in what my supposed equals, fellow liberals and journalists were doing.

My house is fifteen minutes from Parliament Hill and I know of one other neighbour who bothered to go in person. The police soon made it next to impossible to visit, and my friends from elsewhere who dine on mainstream media continue to be certain that this was a gathering of foreign-funded reprobates, small minded and *infra dig*.

Darker days were ahead. Bank accounts frozen, crowds trampled, mandates continuing for months. In Canada, as elsewhere, the social contract has largely fallen apart. No sense of common cause, divided according to the stories that brought us here.

All-cause mortality numbers for that period of 2020-2022 are now becoming clearer, and among OECD countries Canada has been dreadful, one of the worst. If the stories of the people neglected by our policies will never appear in the media, they will at least sadly appear in statistics.

The country faring the best in this group, of course, is Sweden, where they believed it wasn't legal to lock people down. A clip from CNN comes to mind, from May 2020, where a Swedish woman is getting her hair done and saying, "sooner or later we will get corona, so ..." She shrugs.

Imagine if that had been the message: be brave.

When I think of propaganda, I think of story again. The familiar slogan "Keep calm and carry on," was a wartime sentiment created by Britain's Ministry of Information. A message to the citizens to be brave. During war a government must view its populace not only as citizens but as potential soldiery.

So what does a government want, that tells its people to be afraid?

Here we sit, behind our masks and laptops, locked in the cages of our bandwidth and Zoom meetings, Amazon packages giving us comfort all around. Neither citizens nor soldiers, but customers.

CHAPTER 2

The Collateral Damage of American Censorship; Desperate Messages, Lives Broken

Brianne Dressen

Vaccine injured and co-founder of advocacy group React19

Brianne Dressen was a previously healthy mother of two and a preschool teacher. Her life took a dramatic turn after her own injury in the AstraZeneca Covid vaccine clinical trial. Determined to change her negative reaction into positive action, she co-founded React19.org, a patient advocacy organization currently consisting of over 30,000 members. It was created by the Covid Vaccine injured, for the Covid vaccine injured.

"Sorry if this is too forward. Not sure if you can point me in the right direction. I have lost my hunger/fullness cues since v in October among other adverse reactions. I am scared and they keep pegging me as depressed and trying to give me high powered anti-depressants like ketamine. Husband and I are not speaking anymore because of how sick I am and he thinks it's depression and I won't take the meds. I can't find a doctor to help or even talk to me without thinking it's anxiety or depression. I don't want to live like this. Do you have any ideas? I'm so scared because I have to force myself to eat. I don't feel emotions anymore so I can't connect with my family. I have serious brain fog/concentration issues. All of my relationships are gone with my kids, hubby, and friends. I just sit and search my phone trying to find answers. A miracle if you will so that something will get better. I am basically disabled because my brain doesn't function. I can't work out because of my hr and not eating enough. It's heartbreaking. I have no life anymore. I am scared of the future. I need to heal for my family. And for my future. I can't see living like this for 40 more years."

January 2022, another desperate message. This time from Trish who was experiencing just what I had after my COVID vaccine in November

2020. The need for some sort of relief, the fear of the unknown, the abandonment, her cries for help were all too familiar.

As I was young and healthy, the "why" for me was to protect those around me, to do my part to help get us all out of the pandemic faster. My news source, NPR, was telling me this was the way back to normal life, that the vaccines were the only way. Being a lifetime vaccine taker with no issues, the call to roll up my sleeve to be a part of the solution was never something I had questioned. I didn't know there were other options, I didn't understand the importance of "natural immunity," or alternative therapies. The media, the government, and the drug companies, ensured that I didn't know about these other very important pieces of information in the COVID debate.

My days of working with my preschool class, taking my small children on little nature hikes, are now replaced with progressive neuropathy, severe food intolerances, limb weakness, and more than 20 other symptoms. My life now revolves entirely around my physical condition, which is best described by my fellow injured, as worse than death.

As a member of the clinical trial for AstraZeneca, I reached out to the drug company for help, only to be met with silence. No help, not even a phone call. After the clinical trial report was published in the New England Journal of Medicine, we noticed several inconsistencies; AstraZeneca states that they follow all adverse events for 730 days. I last heard from them on day 60. That is well over two years of critical safety data gone. AstraZeneca also states that the individuals who didn't get a second dose *chose* to forego getting the second dose. AstraZeneca instructed the test clinic that *I not* get a second dose.

Perplexed by these issues, I reached out to the New England Journal of Medicine and requested a revision, a rapid response, or an investigation. Dr. Eric Rubin, editor in chief at the NEJM and also on the FDA's COVID vaccine advisory committee, replied to let me know that my case would have "little to no effect," as I was just "one in a study with tens of thousands." This was just the first of many issues I saw that can now be defined as scientific censorship.

As I still wanted to be a part of the solution, I enrolled in a study at the National Institutes of Health, under Dr. Avindra Nath. I was one of several people flown out to the NIH for this study on neurological complications after COVID vaccination. The concepts of molecular mimicry, micro-clotting, and the near-identical presentation of Long-COVID were all being investigated while we were there. We received diagnostic testing, and therapies. Our progress was to be followed for months. By my final day at the NIH I lay in my hospital bed, optimistic about the improvements I was already experiencing from treatment. The lead researcher on the study came into my room and told me point blank not to talk about the research going on at the NIH. There were so many other research participants who had received this same instruction from the NIH. With the repeated promise that they would disclose their findings, we stopped talking about it in our support groups and removed posts about the research. We gladly complied with this form of self-censorship requested by our health agency.

The researchers at the NIH then experienced scientific censorship. This study from the NIH has yet to make it to peer-reviewed publication. After months and months of struggling to land any credible journal, the researchers finally put their study up on a pre-print server where it remains to this day, conveniently "out for public review." There's been no press release, no guidance to the medical community. We made multiple attempts to hold them to account, and saw one small article in ScienceMag.org. After more than a year, the NIH researchers released a small editorial in Neurology.org discussing the need for early intervention and immunotherapy, something that the NIH had shared with us privately more than a year prior. This is the extent to which the federal government has notified the medical community of these findings from their investigations into the COVID vaccine adverse reactions.

What would have happened had these respected researchers been able to share their findings openly? Had their clinical guidance been published in notable journals, press releases issued, and guidance provided via the CDC's COCA? Had their emergency care teams been equipped with the tools necessary to identify and treat these conditions urgently, would these mothers, fathers, sons, and daughters be back to work, and others still be alive? Where would all of those who were injured after me be today had this scientific censorship not taken place?

Science must be the final frontier for truth, regardless of how inconvenient that truth is. My participation in the scientific process was twisted into nothing more than propaganda, not just once, but twice. I can't help wondering where the truth really lies? If I can no longer trust these institutions and reputable journals to share all perspectives and findings, if I can no longer rely on these institutions to help navigate complex diseases, where can I go to find reliable and unbiased help?

Six months after my injury it became very apparent that all of the usual steps we were told to take to report to the government, to drug companies were going nowhere. Our experiences with severe and on-going adverse reactions were being ignored. We reached out to mainstream media reporters and were told time and time again that they could not report on COVID vaccine injuries. Given that the United States government issued PR contracts with news agencies totaling more than $1-billion to promote the COVID vaccines, it is no surprise that there has been a complete block on stories that contradict the "safe and effective" narrative. One reporter I worked with received a threatening letter from the state health department, telling her and her editor, essentially "to shut up or else." Media censorship, influenced heavily by the drug companies and the United States government is very much alive and well.

The importance of telling the truth, regardless of the cost, is not lost on Senator Ron Johnson. He provided us a platform to tell our stories for the first time on June 28, 2021. After seven months of living with my injury, after my trip to the NIH, and after meeting thousands of people like me who had no idea this could happen to them, I was one of six chosen to participate in this first press conference.

We crafted our short presentations, making every word count. We were determined to represent the injured population and also appeal to the public. Surely once they hear our stories they will begin to ask questions, we thought. We can then shift our focus from advocacy and go back to healing our own severely broken bodies. The media ran a few stories about the press conference, many of which blasted Senator Ron Johnson as a misinformation spreader. None of the stories showed our faces or shared our harrowing experiences. Our truths remained hidden from view, while a lie was then amplified by mainstream media about what occurred that summer day in Milwaukee.

Within 24 hours of this first press conference we experienced our first major censorship from big tech. Facebook shut down our first support group. Then, without notice Facebook shut down a second support group. We lost contact with close to 4,000 people injured by COVID vaccines in just one short week. The war against the injured had begun, merely because we finally spoke loud enough that someone might hear our cries for help.

Labelled as worthless by mainstream media, big tech, and the government, we were relegated to our sick beds, conditioned into shame and confusion, unsure why this was happening. Why would they need to do this? We were on their team. But now a blameless injury to a player meant dismissal from the team.

I later learned about a project funded by the Bill Gates foundation called the Virality Project. This project provided briefings to the White House on all information regarding COVID that may sway public opinion. Little did we know, the Virality Project was logging our every move after Senator Johnson's press conference. They specifically logged Senator Johnson's press conference, the media's response to the conference, and even my own involvement in a small news story that discussed my work with Senator Mike Lee, who was asking the FDA pointed questions about the clinical trials. This information was then used by the White House to craft demands to big tech companies to censor our "true stories that may drive vaccine hesitancy." Our right to free speech was not only tampered with, but all-out blocked by our own presidency.

Not only did these major companies abandon us, but they coerced and manipulated the public into abandoning us as well. Labels from big tech such as misinformation, not only discouraged us from reaching out for help, but it conditioned our communities and families to refrain from supporting us as well. These conversations then became something that could only be whispered carefully in the halls of hospitals, or even the grocery store.

The ever-changing censorship algorithms and unpredictable threats of shutting down accounts and support communities forced our support group administrators to spend more time managing the censorship algorithms than we actually did helping people. We had to use code words like "dancing" or "the v" instead of the words "vaccine reaction." It got so bad that we could no longer post the latest science articles that were not part of their narrative. Publications by the British Medical Journal were censored and labelled as misinformation by Facebook's "fact-checkers." We are forced to ask why Facebook's fact-checkers, at best writers with a degree in communications, are empowered to overrule the opinions and conclusions of experienced academics working through the BMJ?

A young mother of four who was injured by her COVID vaccine shared her injury on her Facebook profile; it was taken down as misinformation. Struggling with her medical teams, struggling to find any help whatsoever, she shared stories of her lived experience; more cries for help. Her lived experience was labelled as misinformation. She was notified that she was now shadow-banned (her posts would be put lower in the algorithm so people couldn't see them). Her crime? Crying out for help. Her posts were not seen and her direct message, the one that I included at the beginning of this essay, were blocked. Isolated, desperate, with nobody able to bear witness to her suffering, left with nowhere to turn for relief, she ended her life. Like so many others - your neighbour, your friend, your sister - she was a good person who deserved so much better.

This avoidable tragedy was a result of big tech's modern-day book-burning campaign. Where would this woman be today, had the NIH issued a press release and published their findings? Would her physicians have taken her seriously? Where would her children be today, had their mother been offered even a tiny shred of dignity?

Despite the many efforts to isolate and separate us, the injured have been able to gather, and we are determined to change our negative reactions into positive action. We have launched an advocacy organisation called React19.org, which represents 30,000+ vaccine injured people, that provides physical, emotional, and financial support to those suffering adverse reactions to the COVID vaccines. This allows us to gather, free to share our experiences, solutions, and even our disappointment with the failing government systems. However, because of censorship, the general public has yet to discover we exist, leaving many injured still lost and alone.

So true to who we are, we are now fighting through the U.S. Federal court system. I have joined Ernest Ramirez, Dr. Nikki Holland, Suzanna Newell, Kristi Dobbs, Shaun Barcavage NP, in a suit filed against the White House administration, President Joe Biden, CDC, U.S. Surgeon General, Stanford, et al. The purpose of this suit is to protect our constitutional rights of freedom to assemble and free speech. All plaintiffs have pages of censorship examples and stories that deserve to be told. The censorship in this lawsuit must be just the beginning of many more to come.

A friend once told me, "You might never touch a million people but you might touch that one, who will touch a million." Never underestimate the power of your voice. Never shut-up, never give up. Keep talking, keep sharing these stories, keep demanding better.

CHAPTER 3

No One Needs To Die From COVID

Dr. George Fareed

Family Physician who successfully treated over
20,000 Covid patients

Dr. George Fareed graduated with honors from Harvard Medical School in 1970. He pursued research work at the NIAID, and as faculty both at Harvard and UCLA. In 1991 he left the academic and biotechnology worlds to pursue his true calling in family medicine in an underserved region of California. In 1992, he created HIV services for Imperial Valley, after recognizing the need for early treatment with antivirals to alleviate the advancement of HIV to AIDS. His experience with antivirals would become critical thirty years later, when he created those services—but this time for treating COVID-19. Along with his colleague Brian Tyson, he published the book, *"Overcoming the COVID-19 Darkness: How Two Doctors Successfully Treated 7000 Patients."*

No one needs to die from COVID.

Over three years ago, in March 2020, I began administering early treatments for patients with COVID. Along with my colleague Brian Tyson, in the first year and a half of the pandemic, we successfully treated well over 7,000 patients and today over 20,000 patients.

From my experience, let me state it boldly: no one needs to die from COVID. No one should die from COVID. COVID is a treatable disease. If we treat COVID early, no one dies.

Let me repeat: If we treat COVID early, no one dies.

Yes, unfortunately, we experienced a few deaths in our practice. But it was with patients who presented at our clinics too late, or who did not adhere to the treatment protocol, or preferred to seek hospital care, where we have no influence on treatment.

All the patients we treated early, and who adhered to our treatments, lived. They were mostly adults with comorbidities. Sometimes, we treated elderly people, in their eighties or nineties. We treated only a few children, as they rarely develop a severe disease.

The vast majority of our patients presented early and adhered to our treatment. It's extremely fulfilling for me as a physician fulfilling my Hippocratic Oath, to tell you they all survived COVID, as they presented early and received treatment.

This is what I observed from the very beginning in March 2020. Yes, the disease has evolved with the variants, but our understanding of the disease, and the early, pre-hospital treatment protocols have also improved considerably.

It's why I can firmly state that no one needs to die from COVID. This should be our message. And we need to proclaim it, clearly and emphatically, to the world.

In early 2020, while the epidemic was already raging in Italy, we had just a few cases in California, so we had a bit of time to prepare.

We quickly learned and adapted from the work and studies of Professor Didier Raoult in France and Dr. Vladimir Zelenko in New York: two doctors I admire and who brought us, already in March 2020, what became the basis of an effective treatment for COVID.

In developing our treatment protocols, I had long discussions with my amazing colleague, Dr. Brian Tyson. We also consulted with the AAPS, the American Association of Physicians and Surgeons, and its leader, the amazing Dr. Peter McCullough, concerning the early treatment of COVID.

When COVID did strike in Southern California, we were ready, and we were able to confidently begin using a calculated treatment protocol. This treatment protocol, which evolved with time, has retrospectively proven to be effective—extraordinarily effective.

Partnerships with the general population, as well as with our patients, proved to be extremely important. In the beginning, there was skepticism in the community. But quickly, word of the successes of early treatment spread. The narrative became: "If you have COVID symptoms, and you get treatment with Dr. Tyson or Dr. Fareed, they will take care of you—and the chances are high you will not be admitted to the hospital."

The residents of our rural, predominantly low-income area quickly understood hospital treatment often led to a one-way street to death— and was to be avoided at all costs. They were right. Hospital mortality rates were high, and even now, in many hospitals, it remains high. Too high. Even if some hospitals have adopted much-improved treatment protocols.

Dr. Tyson's urgent care clinic is not a large operation. Due to the high volume and rapid spread of the virus, we quickly and literally invaded the parking lot in front of his clinic and installed a triage tent. Many people lined up for diagnosis and treatment while waiting in their cars. Soon, we were more efficient than a McDonald's drive-through as we diagnosed our patients and prescribed them the appropriate treatment!

Often, we saw 300 or more patients in a single day, all with a limited staff of two doctors, four nurse practitioners, five nurses, four lab and x-ray technicians, and office support staff. It was epic. And proved, a small operation can diagnose and treat considerable numbers of patients. We did follow-ups with our patients by phone. And in some cases, we also worked through telemedicine.

In the U.S., Canada, France, and many countries, a significant amount of COVID outbreaks, severe disease, and death occurred in nursing homes. As the medical director for the Imperial Heights nursing home in Brawley, CA, I witnessed a major outbreak of thirty-one patients presenting with and suffering COVID symptoms at the height of the pandemic in June 2020.

With this outbreak raging, I intervened with our protocol, with the consent of the patients and/or their families. Most residents survived, although unfortunately, two died. Perhaps I should have intervened earlier, but it was difficult, due to the negative publicity about hydroxychloroquine at the time.

We found that a combination of hydroxychloroquine, zinc, and antibiotics could serve as an extremely effective treatment, if they were administered as early as possible (within the first 5 to 7 days of illness). In fact, our results are nothing short of a *miracle*.

We know this is the way to treat COVID. There is no doubt about it. We know it's the way to avoid severe disease and its repercussions. We know it's the way to avoid hospital admissions. We know it's the way to avoid long-term COVID and extended recoveries. We know.

Our results: we saved 99.96 percent of 4,576 symptomatic patients we treated up to March 2021, according to the retrospective study conducted by Mathew Crawford about our work and published in early 2022 (Overcoming The Covid Darkness by Brian Tyson, M.D. and George Fareed, M.D., with Mathew Crawford)..

We know early treatment works. We know early treatment is safe.

It is a disgrace this is not the standard of care for COVID in the U.S. and globally.

It is more than a disgrace. It's a tragedy.

Despite the amazing success we achieved, all of the major medical organizations—from the WHO, to the NIH, to the CDC—did not welcome our information. Rather, they attempted to stop us from effectively treating patients, as well as suppress the information we knew the public needed to hear. We were even threatened with professional consequences if we were to continue providing this life-saving treatment to COVID-positive individuals.

Why? Why would anyone want to *stop* getting the word out, when a pandemic that rocked the globe could be effectively treated? Why would doctors on the front lines, saving lives each day, be threatened with punishment from their own colleagues?

Consider this: when the world was desperate to find a treatment or cure for a deadly disease, and when we provided that information . . . it was censored. Most people would say, WTF? But we wouldn't give up. In fact, we channeled our anger into collective action, by publishing a raw video of speeches that spoke the truth . . . and then posting and reposting again, as the videos were repeatedly taken down.

Despite making congressional statements, providing data to prove our success rates, and thousands of anecdotal stories of treatment and recovery, the CDC, NIH, or any other medical organization would not listen. They were too busy telling the public that there was no cure.

Despite the success of the HCQ treatment protocol, and despite the 100% success rate for our patients who were treated early, the unthinkable happened: the NIH, FDA, WHO, and CDC knowingly blocked effective early treatment for a virus.

The reason?

To sell a vaccine that turned out to be significantly ineffective in blocking new infections by variants and gain control of the populus.

If you're wondering why the development of a vaccine has anything to do with the HCQ treatment, then it's important to know a few important details about Emergency Use Authorizations (EUAs). The COVID vaccines were allowed to be administered because they were given an EUA. However, according to the FDA, an EUA may only be granted if there is "no adequate, approved, and available alternative to the candidate product for diagnosing, preventing, or treating the disease or condition." In other words, an EUA is possible only if there is *no* other safe, effective treatment.

Therefore, HCQ—and later ivermectin—had to be defeated. And the powers that be decided to take a two-pronged approach in their attack on a viable treatment:

1. Show that the protocol is dangerous. One study, published in *The Lancet* by Dr. Mandeep R. Mehra used faulty data to create the illusion that HCQ caused cardiotoxicity (damage to the heart) and lacked efficacy. . However, HCQ has been used for over fifty years to effectively treat malaria—providing more than ample evidence that this drug is safe and had previously been shown to have anti-COVID activity.

2. Show that the treatment is ineffective. The mainstream medical community waged this attack on the HCQ protocol in a study that not only used results from patients who were treated *late* (outside of the five-to-seven day window) but also did not use *all* of the cocktail's ingredients. Making matters worse, this particular study did not properly stratify (sort) the data, making the results and conclusions even more faulty and convoluted.[1]

As a result of this coordinated misinformation campaign, far too many physicians were severely tainted by the misinformation campaign being waged against HCQ. They were determined to follow the NIH/CDC's guidelines of the "no early treatment approach," without any appreciation for the ability to stem COVID-19 by stopping the multiplication early in the infectious process.

---

1   Ladapo, J. A., McKinnon, J. E., McCullough, P. A., & Risch, H. A. (2020, January 01). "Randomized Controlled Trials of Early Ambulatory Hydroxychloroquine in the Pre-vention of COVID-19 Infection, Hospitalization, and Death: Meta-Analysis." Retrieved from https://www.medrxiv.org/content/10.1101/2020.09.30.20204693v1

This assault against scientific facts continued for months. Even today, there is little to no support or encouragement for primary doctors, emergency room doctors, or frontline doctors in general.

With my fifty years of experience in medicine, I know, of course, about vaccines.

I support safe and effective vaccines. And I personally have administered hundreds of thousands of them. Regarding COVID, I have known since the beginning vaccines were not really necessary, were futile for highly mutable viruses if they didn't completely prevent reinfection and they would be difficult to develop. In addition, knowing that there was absolutely no good reason to suppress early treatment in order to open the way for mass vaccination, I was optimistic the vaccines would help us tackle this pandemic.

I was vaccinated early on. I had not previously had COVID. And it was a group decision within the medical team of the hospital where I work, in addition to my collaboration with Dr. Tyson (he didn't receive the vaccine since he recovered earlier in 2020 from the natural infection) at his urgent care, and also the nursing home.

However, my perspective today on COVID vaccination has changed. I personally witnessed too many vaccine injuries—some fatal. I have seen the VAERS voluntary reporting data. I have read estimates on the actual numbers of adverse events. The data are clear: these are the most unsafe vaccines in the history of medicine. Most importantly, these Spike gene vaccines place pressure on the virus to undergo mutations in the Spike gene, thereby modifying the Spike protein leading to new infectious variants and to the perpetuation of the pandemic.

We are living a new tragedy as we administer unsafe vaccines to healthy people, including children, who would most likely never develop severe disease or die from COVID if they receive early treatment. Far too many times, there are adverse events, serious adverse events, sometimes death, from these injections, and this is a tragedy.

In addition, I actually see fully vaccinated people in hospitals, because they had the false impression they were fully protected from COVID, when they were not. The authorities have called these cases "breakthrough" cases. They are actually cases of vaccine failure. And they are not rare. This is a new tragedy that was, again, avoidable if the authorities had done the right thing. In February 2021, there were clear signals these vaccines were not safe, but the campaign continues, despite the horrible safety signals stemming from reporting systems in the U.S., Europe, and the UK.

Today, the science is very clear. People are developing COVID-secure natural immunity. They develop robust, durable, natural immunity against COVID. This is better and more effective than the vaccine, because it is not limited to the spike protein.

So, in a sense, someone treated early for COVID, even with mild symptoms of the disease, will receive great natural immunities. In a sense, early treatment is a vaccine for COVID. This is much safer than the current vaccines.

I hope, one day, truly safe and effective vaccines against COVID will be developed. But today, such vaccines do not exist, and I am extremely concerned by the continued denial of this very fact by the authorities and their continued, unquestioned, mass vaccination policies, the various mandates, vaccination passes, and other measures implemented to essentially force vaccination on everyone.

I believe vaccines are intertwined with U.S. politics, and this is reprehensible. The former president, Donald Trump, pushed for the rapid development of the vaccines, in the belief he was doing the right thing: it would save lives. Our current President, Joe Biden, continues the same policy and is pushing for mass vaccination, including youth, who are at nearly zero risk from the disease, as well as advocating for booster shots, because of the waning effectiveness of vaccines.

This political push for mass vaccination has caused official agencies in the U.S. and elsewhere to cease acknowledgment of the considerable and real safety issues.

In addition, there is considerable disinformation being promoted about early treatment, causing most medical doctors not to prescribe them; many now believe viable early treatments do not even exist. In truth, they are by far the best way to handle this disease.

Medicine is in a very sad place today. Never in the history of medicine has it been advised that the best course is to not treat a disease in its early stages. Never has it been stated, in modern medicine, that someone should not be treated early and instead be left alone at home, fighting a deadly disease, without any form of treatment. Never. This is unconscionable.

Today, there is massive disinformation being disseminated. Our patients are told the vaccines are safe and effective, and they are being indoctrinated that there is no early home treatment for COVID. Nothing could be further from the truth.

What we are told contradicts the facts. The truth is, early treatment works exceptionally well, and vaccines, in their current versions, are NOT safe and are much less effective in preventing severe disease and death than the early treatments. That is the truth.

I am just a seventy-seven-year-old family doctor. Never would I think I would one day come to such prominence, testifying before the U.S. Senate, commenting on national television in front of millions of viewers.

This goes beyond medicine. It's about our freedom; it's about the world we are leaving to our children, and to our grandchildren. The future of humanity is at stake.

We must get our message across. We must tell the world early treatment is the way forward. We must encourage doctors everywhere to embrace early treatment. We must tell the people, we must tell everyone, whether they are vaccinated or not, that they absolutely must seek early treatment if they are infected with COVID.

We need to tell the truth about COVID. We need to dispel the fear. We must be relentless in our efforts to tell the truth. We must be united. And together, my friends, we will prevail.

CHAPTER 4

A Head Above the Parapet: Doing Right by Those Harmed by Covid-19 Vaccinations

Sir Christopher Chope

Conservative Member of the UK Parliament, Chair
of the UK Parliament's All-Party Parliamentary
Group on Covid-19 Vaccine Damage

Sir Christopher Chope OBE MP is a Conservative Member of the UK Parliament, and Chair of the UK Parliament's All-Party Parliamentary Group on Covid-19 Vaccine Damage. He was first elected to Parliament in June 1983. Sir Christopher was a Minister in the Governments of Margaret Thatcher and John Major. He has been the Member of Parliament for Christchurch since 1 May 1997.

It was in January 2021 that I first began trying to scrutinise the efficacy and potential adverse effects of Covid-19 vaccinations, with the goal of helping those suffering ill-effects. I was alone among MPs in doing this. My pressure on the Government included more than 100 Parliamentary Questions to the Department of Health and Social Care on the subject, two Adjournment Debates, three Private Members' Bills, multiple meetings with Ministers and other stakeholders, many press and related interviews and the establishment of the All-Party Parliamentary Group on Covid-19 Vaccine Damage, which I chair. At last, this effort seems to have been worthwhile with the Government now accepting what the general public already knew, that Covid-19 vaccinations were not absolutely safe.

Underpinning much of the UK Government's response to questions concerning harms from Covid-19 vaccinations has been a sense of denial. I challenged the Government on this in a speech in the House of Commons on 24 March 2023, after two years of asking the Government to provide help for those so harmed. My primary objective was to pressurise the Government into recognising that Covid-19 vaccinations have caused harm to a significant number of people, including, in a small number of cases, death. But it was not until June 2023 that the

Government was finally prepared to admit openly that people had died or suffered severe disablement as a result of Covid-19 vaccines. The Government's own Business Services Authority has now paid out over £12 million in recognition of the harm suffered by over 100 people (as recognised by the Government's own assessors).

The persistent denial by the Government of the adverse effects of Covid-19 vaccines for an unfortunate minority has caused immense distress to those affected, including some reports of suicide.

Other approaches

This is in stark contrast to members of other European Governments. Professor Dr Karl Lauterbach, Germany's Federal Minister for Health, for example, initially took a very hard line and publicly said on numerous occasions that Covid-19 vaccines were *"without side effects"*. In light of the increasing evidence to the contrary, he has publicly admitted that what he said was an exaggeration and accepts that, on his current understanding, one in 10,000 of those vaccinated against Covid-19 in Germany had experienced serious adverse effects. He has promised significant extra resources and said that he is in discussions with German Treasury Ministers to address issues around post-vaccine syndrome.

I am now trying to pressurise the UK Government to emulate Professor Lauterbach's approach by undertaking a wholesale review of the current UK Vaccine Damage Payment Scheme, which provides financial assistance to those harmed by Covid-19 vaccines. The legislation is wholly out of date.

During this exercise, I have uncovered the serious deficiencies with the UK's existing payment scheme for those suffering ill-effects from vaccines, and have received an overwhelming number of reports from members of the public regarding not only the poor care, but often the complete dismissal, of those who have suffered harm from a Covid-19 vaccination. Despite bringing these serious matters to the UK Government's attention, I am unable to report any substantial real progress. The only crumb of comfort is that the Vaccines Minister has now agreed to review the amount of the £120,000 compensation payment under the Vaccine Damage Payment Scheme, and the limitation period for legal claims following harm from a Covid-19 vaccination.

Secret monitoring

Disarmingly, my efforts and those of others to establish the truth, based on evidence, have been the subject of undercover monitoring by the UK Government, the full scale of which is not yet entirely known. Recent reports have shown, for example, that the UK's Cabinet Office, its Department of Digital, Culture, Media and Sport and even the British Army repurposed sub-departments to secretly monitor those purportedly spreading 'disinformation' concerning Covid-19 vaccinations and related matters. The 'disinformation' apparently stretches to any information which sought to scrutinise the UK Government's Covid-19 vaccination programme and response to the pandemic generally.

In answer to one of my Parliamentary Questions, the Cabinet Office clarified that its 'Rapid Response Unit' was tasked with understanding *"the spread of information and potential disinformation"*. The Minister stated that *"online disinformation is a serious threat to the UK, which is why we brought together expertise from across government to monitor disinformation, especially during the Covid-19 pandemic"*. Following Subject Access Requests I submitted to these departments, I discovered that my comments were being monitored by the Rapid Response Unit. In particular, it held records and commentary on my activity on the Covid-19 vaccine harm issue in a series of interview summaries, notes on Covid-19 communications and internal meetings and briefings for the

"Health Counter Disinformation Working Group". A similar picture came from the response to my Subject Access Requests to the Department of Health and Social Care's 'Counter Disinformation Unit'.

I have never campaigned against the UK Government's Covid-19 vaccination programme. My position has always been that those who have done the right thing by being vaccinated against Covid-19 but have been harmed or bereaved as a result should not be left behind, let alone actively ignored, treated with suspicion or even smeared. The issue does not end with me. A report by Big Brother Watch, a UK civil liberties campaign group, entitled *The Secretive Government Units Spying on your Speech*, summarised similar Subject Access Request responses from other Members of Parliament, and set out a full analysis of the monitoring, including a legal opinion from a senior barrister which gave an overview of the concerning legal implications of such monitoring.

Widespread harm

The extent of the issue indicates it deserves more attention than the Government and media have so far been willing to give to it. Since I started raising the issue publicly, I have received thousands of emails and letters from those harmed or bereaved from Covid-19 vaccinations. We now know that around 50 coroners' verdicts have confirmed that people have died as a direct result of Covid-19 vaccines (as at 23 March 2023), and the UK's reporting system (its 'Yellow Card' scheme) for Covid-19 vaccine harm received over 470,000 reports across Covid-19 vaccinations up to 23 November 2022 alone. Since then, the presentation of the information by the MHRA has been changed. What we do know, however, is that applications to the UK's Vaccine Damage Payment Scheme continue to increase and over 5,700 have been received as of 5 June 2023.

The Government has been aware of appreciable harm from Covid-19 vaccines on an international scale for some time. Following one of my representations, the then UK Health Minister, for example, willingly identified the *"growing international body of evidence supporting an association or link between the vaccines and certain adverse events"* (3 March 2023).

The reluctance of the Government to be open and transparent may well be now undermining public confidence in vaccines generally.

The Vaccine Damage Payment Scheme

The problem with the UK's current Vaccine Damage Payment Scheme ("**VDPS**") is that it offers no specific care arrangements for those with (often life-changing) illnesses following Covid-19 vaccinations. The existing framework for care relies upon the VDPS which grants a one-off payment of £120,000 if an applicant can show both causation and that they meet a 60% disablement threshold as a result of a Covid-19 vaccination.

This reveals a number of concerning deficiencies. Many applications are rejected on grounds of lack of causation, which is difficult or almost impossible to establish in circumstances where harms from Covid-19 vaccines are only recently becoming known and appreciated. Very few applications have been awarded where convincing evidence of causation has been provided, such as a coroner's report confirming death by Covid-19 vaccination, yet the Government has not provided commitments or even proper guidance as to when causation is taken to be established on any particular Covid-19 vaccine case, even with such compelling evidence. Instead, the Minister has confirmed that the Department of Health and Social Care has introduced extra unspecified 'quality assurance processes' when reviewing applications, the impact of which on outcomes is not known, but which may impact the alleged independence of the medical assessors. What is, however, known is that the processes cause considerable delays to the decisions and only 105 of 5,738 applications have been successful (as at 5 June 2023).

60% disablement threshold

Assessors are required to make a judgement, on the balance of probabilities, as to whether the applicant has met a 60% disablement threshold. But that threshold is linked to industrial injuries legislation which provides for an assessment against a list of physical injuries (such as loss of a limb). There are, for example, only two physical injuries listed in that industrial injuries legislation at the 60% disability threshold. These are loss of a leg below the knee and loss of a hand. Whereas the UK Courts have held that, in a VDPS context, the industrial injuries list is not to be deemed a "*straightjacket*", assessors are being asked to make unsuitable comparisons between largely autoimmune and related conditions resulting from Covid-19 vaccines and physical industrial injuries in circumstances where the 'quality assurance' monitoring to ensure consistency is conducted behind closed doors. It is not clear how such assessments are being made (and whether any accurate assessment could in fact be made), and how true consistency is ensured across assessments. Proper assessments with transparent and fair criteria are sorely needed, particularly for applicants who have lost the ability to work as a result of their disability, both now and in the future.

Quantum

Another key issue concerns quantum. The £120,000 available under the VDPS has not been revised since 2007, unlike that for similar schemes (such as industrial injuries, for example). Inflation has risen dramatically since then, and the UK Government will not commit to increasing it even by inflation or the Consumer Price Index. Those currently receiving state benefits have received little assurance that any

VDPS award will be carved out of their benefits entitlements. Part of the problem is that the VDPS was not designed to compensate for fatalities caused by a vaccination, but only for severe disabilities.

Civil claims

Many suffering lifelong conditions as a result of vaccination cannot support themselves on the VDPS payment, and are seeking recourse through other means, such as litigation. Only recently have some law firms publicly announced claims on behalf of those harmed, against Covid-19 vaccine manufacturers. But behind each claim faced is a confidential Government indemnity by which the manufacturers will likely be fully indemnified for any claims upheld against them.

The inequity is that those manufacturers have far greater resources than harmed individuals, and establishing even a *prima facie* case without professional legal support is very difficult indeed, and poses serious costs risks with no scope for legal aid. Philanthropic lawyers, whilst few and far between, have taken up the mantle for some individuals with the most obvious cases of manufacturer/Government liability, but they too do not have the resources needed to bring redress on a mass scale. A proper VDPS should, in any case, not require applicants to bring parallel Civil proceedings to achieve the level of award they so compellingly need.

One potentially positive development is that, responding to my questions on the issue, the Vaccines Minister agreed to review the limitation period for Civil claims in recognition of the danger that claims may be time-barred whilst VDPS applicants await a decision.

Appeals

Appeals against VDPS decisions can be both protracted and expensive, with almost no scope for recovery of legal costs unless recourse to the courts is needed. The process involves applying for a 'mandatory reversal', followed by an independent Tribunal decision, followed by, if needed, appeals to the appellate courts. Legal costs are a key barrier to such applications owing to the possibility of costs recovery attaching at only the latest, and most expensive, stages of the process.

Many of those who have written to me will shortly, however, have no option but to seek a 'mandatory reversal' in light of apparently failing the first application stage, whilst their long-term symptoms continue.

Proposed legislation

I have put forward bespoke legislation to address the shortcomings of the current system. This includes the following Private Members' Bills, the:

- Covid-19 Vaccine Damage Bill to establish an independent review of disablement caused by Covid-19 vaccinations and the adequacy of the compensation offered to persons so disabled;
- Covid-19 Vaccine Damage Payments Bill to place a duty on the Secretary of State to make provision about financial assistance to persons who have suffered disablement following vaccination against Covid-19 and to the next of kin of persons who have died shortly after vaccination against Covid-19. As part of this, the Bill requires the Secretary of State to report to Parliament on:
  o the merits of a no-fault compensation scheme to provide such financial assistance;
  o whether there should be any upper limit on the financial assistance available;
  o the criteria for eligibility; and
  o whether payment should be made in all cases where there is no other reasonable cause for the death or disablement suffered; and
- Covid-19 Vaccine Diagnosis and Treatment Bill to place a duty on the Secretary of State to improve the diagnosis and treatment

of persons who have suffered or continue to suffer ill effects from Covid-19 vaccines,

and, in each case, for connected purposes.

Without Government support, these Bills will not be passed. But the purpose is to draw attention to the relevant issues, provide solutions and widen support for this campaign.

Cross-party support

Building on this, I established the All-Party Parliamentary Group on Covid-19 Vaccine Damage (the "**APPG**"), which I formed to:

- ensure scrutiny of the safety profile of Covid-19 vaccinations;
- provide a forum for those harmed or bereaved from Covid-19 vaccinations and review financial arrangements available to them; and
- ensure that the health services respond and provide care to those who have continuing conditions caused by Covid-19 vaccinations.

So far, the APPG has held public meetings in Parliament, and has been instrumental in providing a forum for the various UK-based volunteer-led patient groups which have formed to support those suffering harm from Covid-19 vaccinations. The APPG has provided the means through which some of these groups may meet with relevant Ministers and other stakeholders. For example, on 5 June 2023, the Vaccines Minister met with the APPG and made commitments to review the level of VDPS compensation, the time limit on Civil claims and the treatment available for those who continue to suffer adverse effects.

An encouraging development has been the increased interest being shown by mainstream media which has helped raise the morale of Covid-19 vaccine victims by giving them hope that their plight is understood by a wider audience, including, ultimately, the Government.

Looking ahead

An alternative to the VDPS legislation or Civil claims could be to encourage manufacturers to pay into a redress fund for those harmed, in light of their recent exorbitant profits. There is increasing commentary on such a proposal, and it was referred to by Dr Lauterbach recently. Whilst we are a long way from securing such a commitment, it may well ultimately find favour as a way of resolving the current problems which continue to adversely impact so many individuals and families.

Whilst self-evidently it is incumbent on the Government and the health service to care for those harmed, it is distressing that it has proved so difficult to make progress. I am confident that in time the Government will be less defensive, the issue will be less politicised and those who are seeking to help victims will not be smeared as 'anti-vaxxers'. The increasing interest of the media in the Covid-19 vaccine saga could be decisive in encouraging Parliamentary colleagues and others to put their head above the parapet and do the right thing by those harmed.

CHAPTER 5

The Global Disinformation Campaign Against Ivermectin - The "Fix" at the WHO

Dr. Pierre Kory

Lung, pulmonary ICU specialist and co-founder of the FLCCC

Dr. Pierre Kory MD, MPA is a highly experienced lung/ pulmonary ICU specialist who has practiced medicine for 14 years. He has successfully treated more than 450 Covid patients during the pandemic. He is a co-founder and President of the Front Line COVID-19 Critical Care Alliance (FLCCC), together with Dr Paul Marik. He is also author of a new book titled *"The War On Ivermectin."*

This essay is published with the permission of Dr. PIerre Kory. It first appeared in his Substack. It has been edited for clarity and length and approved by Dr. Kory.

The biggest battle in the war on ivermectin was won by Pharma at the WHO and has since caused millions of preventable deaths. I had a front row seat to see how it all unfolded.

A researcher sponsored by the organizations Unitaid and the WHO by the name of Dr. Andrew Hill lectured on the 3rd day of an international conference put together by a French biotech company called MedinCell. Andrew Hill presented a systematic review of all the randomized trials on ivermectin in COVID. I was shocked. I thought our group was way ahead of everyone in our compilation of data (it turns out we were, more on that below). He had done an actual data synthesis of the 11 RCT's (Randomized Control Trial) which was mind-blowingly positive in terms of reduced time to viral clearance, time to clinical recovery, need for hospitalization, and death. At the time, those trials included over 1,000 total patients (note Paxlovid and Remdesivir got Emergency Use Authorizations based on less patients from just a single trial, using Pharma's well-established "one and done" fast track approval process built for Pharma at the PFDA (the P is not a typo).

I had an incredibly positive conversation with Andy, as any two researchers would when they think they may have stumbled upon data that potentially has global, historic implications. We started sharing our "origin stories" of how we had "discovered" the phenomenal data on the efficacy of ivermectin in COVID.

"Andy's" origin story of when he started to focus his research on ivermectin in COVID was that he had been hired in June 2020 by Unitaid, an international health care organization funded largely by the Bill and Melinda Gates Foundation (BMGF) and several other countries. BMGF is also the 2nd largest funder of the WHO after the United States. Unitaid was collaborating on the ACT (Access to Covid19 Tools) Accelerator program with the WHO (note that this program was completely run and staffed by BMGF). Andy was in charge of a *research team tasked with analyzing trials of repurposed drugs for use in COVID.* At the time, I thought this was phenomenal as it was exactly what I shouted about in my Senate testimony, i.e. that our governmental health agencies were not initiating a coordinated effort to identify effective, *readily available* drugs to "repurpose" them to fight COVID. And here he was, the head of a team doing just that at the global level!

Given this background, I asked Andy, "How and when did you come to choose to study ivermectin?" His answer, even then, was a little suspicious, "Well, we had been researching numerous repurposed medicines since June 2020, like favipiravir, hydroxychloroquine (I forget the others) and none of them showed efficacy" (*yeah right*). He then said, "I was told *by a Professor at my University* to look into ivermectin in early November." Note my ivermectin review paper was uploaded on a pre-print server on November 13th, 2020. Hmm. Do you think Big Pharma scientists were monitoring pre-print servers for emerging evidence on repurposed medicines?

The unknown Professor's identity will be revealed later in this essay, as I now know he was Big Pharma/BMGF's "point man" that distorted and suppressed the evidence of efficacy of ivermectin at the WHO. He was the one in charge of compiling the evidence on ivermectin to the WHO Treatment Guideline committee. Note the WHO's guidance is the most important in the world, influencing nearly every country on Earth (except the U.S. given Remdesivir is the standard of care here despite the fact the WHO says it doesn't work).

I have since become convinced that Andy's real mission was to find evidence of efficacy of repurposed drugs so that BMGF and Big Pharma could initiate their Disinformation campaign immediately upon identification of any effective *generic* drug which would threaten, well, everything really.

Andy was doing opposition research, but we, nor he, did not know it (yet). During the early period of our collaboration, it was clear to me that he thought his job was to identify a repurposed drug *for the WHO to actually recommend for use in the pandemic*.

When he finally found one (ivermectin), his paymasters quickly kicked off their historic and criminal disinformation campaign, first by getting Andy to no longer speak publicly about his findings. Andy told me that right after his last public lecture to a South African group on January 29th, 2021, his Unitaid sponsors told him he could no longer give public statements or interviews. Apparently Andy's last lecture was a bit too supportive and enthusiastic of ivermectin as he literally told the South Africans to "get ready, get supplies, etc." In later months, Andy would show up on Twitter and/or post preprints attacking the evidence base of ivermectin as fraudulent. He even retracted his later published review paper, which, just like the FLCCC's, found a massive reduction in mortality. His revised paper removed almost all of the evidence base and concluded that ivermectin had no impact on mortality. They eventually got to him, hard.

This mission of identifying effective generic drugs was critical to all the profits that Pharma was going to amass during COVID. Public awareness of any effective repurposed drug would have destroyed the global vaccine campaign as well as blown up the markets for all the pricey new patented COVID drugs that were currently in the pipeline of numerous pharmaceutical corporations. We in the FLCCC had no idea at the time that we were starting to mess with the big boys, the most powerful corporations on Earth and the FLCCC was poking that bear at a time when a hundred billion dollar marketplace for their wares was opening up. Gives me chills today thinking back on it. There are definitely moments when I wonder how we are still alive.

Anyway, here we were, discovering that a researcher from the WHO/Unitaid had found a strong signal of benefit amongst just the randomized controlled trials (the signal was blaring actually). Note that the FLCCC review paper I authored included all ivermectin data, not only the RCT's, but also many OCT's and the results of Health Ministry programs.

Soon after my senate testimony, a former Texas Health Commissioner named Reyn Archer reached out to me. Reyn was working as Chief of Staff for Nebraska Congressman Jeff Fortenberry who was on the committee that oversaw the budgets for the health agencies. Anyway, they convinced the NIH Treatment Guidelines committee to give me and Paul Marik an audience to present our findings.

The meeting was scheduled for January 6th, 2021. We decided to invite Andy Hill to present his more expansive RCT data along with us, plus he would bring more "credibility" because he was working for an international health care agency. Little did I know that meeting was going to be our first battle between the FLCCC and Fauci in what is now an ongoing 20+ month war. Actually it is not really an active war anymore because it has unfortunately reached a stalemate. All the countries and all the doctors who have used ivermectin successfully will continue to do so no matter how many high-impact journal trials and editorials claim it doesn't work. However, new adopters are likely near nil after the publication of history's most fraudulent trial in the New England Journal of Medicine put the final "nail in the coffin" (literally and metaphorically) of ivermectin.

So on January 6, 2021, Paul Marik, Andy, and myself teamed up to give a 20+ minute presentation to the NIH guidelines committee. Andy essentially gave the same presentation he gave at Medincell's conference 3 weeks earlier. I presented the epidemiological analysis paper by Juan Chamie, Jennifer Hibberd, and David Scheim which showed massive reductions in both cases and deaths in the wake of Peru's magnificent ivermectin distribution program called Operation Tayta. Paul presented newly released and as-yet-unpublished experimental data from Caly and Wagstaff of Monash University which found that indeed, standard doses of ivermectin do reach effective anti-viral concentrations in the blood.

The academics and health bureaucrats on the committee were full of questions, skepticism, and dismissiveness, especially in regards to the results of the Peru program that I had presented. I suppose this was to be expected, plus it is kind of their job. But not one showed enthusiasm or optimism. The most telling part of the meeting occurred at the very end, after the Committee discussion and questions, when first, Alice Pau, a Pharmacist in charge of coordinating the meeting, asked "Do you have any questions for us?" Paul Marik made a bold plea for the NIH to make a recommendation for ivermectin which I then emphasized and asked "Of all the medicines currently being used and/or studied for the treatment of COVID, all have had either weak recommendations for use or neutral ones in the form of 'there is insufficient evidence to recommend or not recommend' drug X. Yet since August of 2020, ivermectin **is the only medicine which had a negative recommendation to not use outside clinical trials**. Can I ask why that is?"

Second after second ticked by, then interrupted by Alice Pau trying to answer a question I really did not ask, so I cut her off and asked my question again. Another long pause ensued. There were over 20 "experts" on the zoom call, and not one answered. The silence got long enough and uncomfortable enough that I started saying, "OK, I guess no-one knows why," (I was pissed and, despite our plans of being collegial, decided to just be somewhat rude and dismissive of them). As soon as I said that, Chairman Cliff Lane talked over me and said to the group "Come on guys, we have to answer the question."

I will say that, whatever we presented and pleaded for did have an effect. Several weeks later, out of the blue, the NIH recommendation was changed. They no longer recommended "against use outside a clinical trial," and instead they changed it to a "neutral" recommendation, you know, the one where they write "there is insufficient evidence to recommend or not recommend" ivermectin.

A Win? Actually I thought not. Again, what these guys pull is so brazen to anyone knowledgeable, but no one's paying attention and very few are knowledgeable. But what you need to know is that there are many different strengths of recommendations, they can give a weak, moderate, or strong recommendation for a drug in the treatment of a disease. You can make a weak or moderate recommendation solely on observational trials data! Plus, the unparalleled safety profile of ivermectin combined with the existing highly positive data in over 1,000 patients and 12 randomized controlled trials should have led to at a minimum a weak recommendation in the midst of a humanitarian catastrophe (the winter of 2020-2021 was particularly brutal in U.S. hospitals). However, had they done that, the entire country's (and world's) doctors would have started treating all COVID patients with ivermectin. They knew they could not provide any recommendation stronger than "neutral." Plus Fauci would never let that happen (remember, as a public servant, it is well documented that he has worked in the service of the pharmaceutical industry his entire career). So that's what they did.

There was a lot of attention on ivermectin after my testimony so they had to do something. Knowing what I know now of the immense powers of Big Pharma, I suspect that even if they had delivered a "weak" recommendation for use, it may not have moved the needle much. I say this largely because the market competitors of ivermectin had many other tactics they could use (and did) to prevent widespread adoption i.e. their devastatingly effective "horse dewormer" public relations campaign deployed using synchronized messaging amongst all major TV, radio, and print outlets. Plus they probably knew that the WHO was going to update their recommendations based on Andy and his team's continued research over the next two months, so they punted. I would argue that they knew the fix was in at the WHO already. But this is when things get even crazier.

Although we knew the NIH was not going to recommend (actually we really didn't at the time as our collective naiveté and optimism was still profound), we became excited at another development. We were made aware of another renowned researcher and physician named Tess Lawrie from the United Kingdom (and a South African like Paul Marik). Apparently, she saw my testimony video and was highly intrigued by my presentation of the evidence supporting ivermectin. She asked herself, "What is this doctor talking about?

Tess has for decades been an expert reviewer of medical evidence. Her expertise is in conducting what are called "systematic reviews" and "meta-analyses" of the medical evidence for various therapeutics, just like Andrew Hill was doing for WHO/Unitaid. A systematic review and meta-analysis is considered the strongest form of medical evidence. She has published such reviews in the top medical journals, including many for the Cochrane Library, once considered the gold standard of such analyses (but no longer as they are now bought and paid for by Pharma/BMGF). Further, she has contributed to the development of treatment guidelines for the WHO, UK's NHS, and other national and international health agencies.

After watching my testimony, she immediately began to dig deep into the published and posted trials data on ivermectin in COVID. Note that experts generally rely on what is called "pattern recognition" and in her review of the evidence she recognized a remarkable pattern of results from the trials - consistent, often large magnitude benefits in time to clinical recovery, hospitalizations and death from varied countries and centers around the world.

So, not only the five of us highly published clinicians and researchers in the FLCCC, but here was a second independent, deeply expert researcher who was also impressed with the same data signal. Tess was so impressed with the strength of the data, she immediately sprang into action and recorded a video on January 7th pleading with Boris Johnson and the UK gov't and health authorities to look at and try to disseminate ivermectin to help her country. Her emotions were exactly matched with how I felt when I was uploading my paper to a preprint server two months prior on Nov 13, 2020.

Tess's video plea was quickly taken down by YouTube, one of the first distressing actions taken to suppress the evidence of efficacy of ivermectin. It was the first shot in what is now a 20+ month-long war.

We were so impressed with her decades of experience, thoughtfulness, and dedication - she knew we had identified an effective drug and that people were dying all over the world and that this information had to get to health authorities and treatment guideline developers.

I told her about Andy and his work so she reached out to him because she knew he had the most updated data from the randomized control trials that were being conducted. She invited him to work on a systematic review and meta-analysis for the Cochrane Library, a journal that had published many of her expert reviews in the past. She knew that time was of the essence because there were masses of people dying during the COVID surge in the winter of 2020. She knew that a review supporting ivermectin published in the Cochrane Library would immediately be noticed by doctors around the world.

He apparently agreed to collaborate on the review. Andy would be extremely important to such an effort because the scope of his work for Unitaid was to search the clinical trial registries from all over the world to find any registered RCT on ivermectin in COVID. He had already found 59 registered RCT's and had compiled a list of contacts of all the Principal Investigators for those trials and began having bi-weekly meetings with them. He was getting trial results way before any manuscript was being posted or published. And Andy was sharing the data with me and Paul. It was incredible hearing about positive results before anyone else in the world.

But suddenly everything went south, and fast. On January 16, 2021, Andy suddenly posted his review of the RCT's on a preprint server. Back then preprint servers were incredibly important in COVID, because researchers could post their data and have it publicly available without waiting for the many months of peer review and publication processing and proofing required prior to publication in an established medical journal.

Paul and I read his posted pre-print review and were shocked. ***The conclusions did not match the data.*** For the first time in my career, I found myself reading a scientific manuscript by a researcher presenting such profound and compelling data yet whose conclusions argued against the findings. If there is anything that scientists and researchers tend to do when publishing original work, it is that they tend to over-interpret the potential importance and impact of their data. But here there was such overwhelmingly positive data yet the paper and conclusions read as if the conclusions were very uncertain and too "heterogenous" to act on.

In addition, the paper was poorly written, with repeated expressions of the limitations of the data including false statements about how effective concentrations could not be reached with standard dosing (something we knew Andy knew was false). In addition the conclusion did not match the data presented. Paul and I immediately suspected scientific misconduct was occurring so we immediately wrote to Andy with our concerns and provided him with a complete peer-review of his paper containing our many comments and recommendations for changes. We demanded that he immediately take down his paper and implement the suggested revisions to be more consistent with the existing data. Among other demands, we asked that he remove the statements about how effective concentrations could not be reached in the blood with standard doses (we had as a group presented data disproving that to the NIH). Further we called out the numerous irregularities in his paper like the repetitive citation of the "limitations" of the data presented.

We knew something was off, like really off and so did Tess. But we didn't know exactly what was going on "behind the scenes." It was not until a year later when we found out who and what were behind these manipulations trying to distort and suppress the evidence of efficacy of ivermectin.

Those details were uncovered by a man named Phil Harper. I consider him a polymath with a diverse background of interests and accomplishments having worked in journalism and documentary filmmaking among other pursuits. He was a UK citizen and had been living in India during the early pandemic and was shocked when he returned to UK in mid-to-late 2021 and found a country without any early treatment strategy that was instead attacking, suppressing, and legislating against ivermectin which was in wide use at the time in India. So he dug into the topic. What he discovered about the events that occurred over those weeks is absolutely stunning.

In regards to Andy's preprint paper, again, the most stunning abnormality was the wording and content of the conclusion. It was markedly different from the version of his paper that Andy had sent Tess a week prior. I know this now because Phil performed a "document analysis" directly comparing all changes from the version that Andy had sent to Tess with the one that was posted on the preprint server. He found numerous changes inserted to the later preprint version. ***Every single change softened or reversed the importance of the findings and/or argued against the efficacy of ivermectin.*** A really weird statement about "what is sufficient for review by regulatory authorities" appeared. However, despite this paper and its muted conclusions and numerous limitations and suggestions, it went further and argued "more studies needed to be done." While people were dying at horrific rates around the world and all the available RCT evidence (plus OCT and Health Ministry data), were showing that one of the safest, least expensive, and widely available medicines in history could save lives in a global pandemic of a highly transmissible, viral illness.

Andy knew the importance of this finding too. In several public lectures he gave that month, he was as enthusiastic and supportive of ivermectin as Paul, Tess, and I were. He did an interview with a French publication called Bon Sens (they were one of my first interviews after my testimony in the Senate) and he even emphasized the "dose-dependent" effects of ivermectin. Note that a "dose dependent relationship" is one of the strongest pillars of support for efficacy of a therapeutic, defined as measuring greater benefits as the dose is increased). This is what he said at the time:

We are seeing very clear antiviral effects. We see smaller effects when the drug is given for one day, then in dose-ranging studies, we see more and more of an effect. And then if the drug is given at a high dose, for five days, we see the strongest effect. So, how could that be happening if the drug does not stop the virus from replicating? It simply does. It does. And we've got the evidence to prove it…. It's just a matter of time before it gets approved."

Tess knew even more than we did that something really rotten was going on. She knew that someone had altered his paper and his conclusions and his analysis. She asked him for a Zoom meeting to discuss, and he agreed! She recorded the meeting illegally and thus was reluctant to make it public for a time, but as the war went on with ever increasing devastation to the human race, she eventually decided to make the video public.

It is an astounding video. Andy actually admitted to Tess that his "sponsors" influenced the writing of the paper. Tess asked him for names but he refused. And we all know that whoever had altered that paper they were not listed as an author of the paper. This was clear scientific misconduct. Tess included the most relevant parts of this meeting in a devastatingly effective video called "A Letter to Andrew Hill" which essentially covers all of the most relevant and impactful events that I am detailing. It is a must watch and likely communicates more than I ever can with words.

So, who was the person making all the changes attacking ivermectin in Andy's paper? Not mentioned during the recorded meeting with Tess Lawrie and Andrew Hill, but Hill later referenced a person named Dominique Costagliola.

So what did Phil find out about Dominique Costagliola? She is a Pharma-conflicted individual just like all the other research and regulatory agency operatives working against ivermectin. She receives lecture fees from nearly every corporation with a competing product against ivermectin. Janssen, Gilead, Merck-Sharp & Dome (biopharmaceutical company), Viiv, Innavirvax and Merck Switzerland. She has taken money in the form of lecture fees, personal fees, and travel and meeting expenses.

What Phil discovered next, to me, is the "Scoop of the Century" given that I call what these people and others did to ivermectin, the "Crime of the Century." Phil discovered who was really in control of both Andy and the evidence supporting ivermectin. It was the Professor that Andy had mentioned to me in our first ever conversation.

Phil discovered the Professor's identity by simply looking at the "meta data" embedded in the PDF file of the preprint paper. It was finalized on the computer of Professor Andrew Owen of the University of Liverpool in the days leading up to the posting. Whoa. Thus, this was the same Professor that had suggested to Andy to "look into ivermectin" in November of 2020.

On what evidence do I make this claim? Not only the fact that Andy's paper was doctored on the computer of Professor Owen but also on his insane conflicts of interest against ivermectin. Again, I maintain he was getting Andy to do "opposition research" without Andy knowing he was working for the other side at the time.

Owen's Big Pharma conflicts with competing products to ivermectin are unparalleled. Costagliola's pales in comparison. To wit:

1. Owen studied molnupiravir for Merck, a direct competitor to ivermectin

2. Owen received research funding from ViiV Healthcare, Merck, Janssen, Boehringer Ingelheim, GlaxoSmithKline,

Abbott Laboratories, Pfizer, AstraZeneca, Tibotec, Roche Pharmaceuticals and Bristol-Myers Squibb.

3. Owen received consultancy fees from Gilead (another drug whose market ivermectin would decimate).

4. Owen is the Project Lead of the Center for Excellence in Long-Acting Therapeutics Program (CELT) at The University of Liverpool. CELT received *$40 million from UNITAID on January 12, 2021* (the importance of this financial influence simply cannot be overstated, so I won't. Just let it sink in for a moment).

Further:

a. CELT studies ways to use lipid nano-particles in pharmaceuticals, which is a foundational technology of the COVID mRNA vaccines.

b. The UNITAID grant was shared with a spinoff start-up company in which Andrew Owen was the top shareholder. Phil Harper finds it possible that the grant agreement may have granted Unitaid to "have a say" in the conclusions of any research it commissions. Andy basically told Tess that. A FOIA request by Phil for a copy of the grant agreement was denied, so I suppose we will never know. But we know.

Phil Harper also critiqued that on the very same day that the $40 million CELT deal was announced, the University of Liverpool *also* announced that it would be studying two new 'groundbreaking' therapies for COVID-19. They received "over £3m of investment from GlaxoSmithKline and Vir Biotechnology" to conduct this research. Notice that this was *an investment*, not a grant. The two therapeutics they were investigating were VIR-7831 and VIR-7832, novel therapies for COVID owned by the two companies. Andrew Owen was a part of that study. More than a year after the investment, no results have been published, with only an update on the recruiting progress for the planned trial.

Now, the importance of what I am about to reveal is inestimable in its impact on depriving the ***entire world*** of access and use of a life-saving drug to treat COVID.

Andrew Owen was also given the responsibility to prepare the evidence base upon which the World Health Organization would make their recommendation to not use ivermectin "outside of a clinical trial" on March 31, 2021:

Subgroup analysis

The MNA team performed subgroup analysis which could result in distinct recommendations by subgroups. From the available data, subgroup analysis were only possible by dose of ivermectin and considering the outcomes of mortality, mechanical ventilation, admission to hospital, and adverse events leading to drug discontinuation. The ivermectin subgroup dose subgroup analysis were performed from the direct comparison of ivermectin versus usual care. From these analyses, meta regression was used to evaluate the effect of cumulative dose as a continuous variable, and further adding a co-varlate for single vs. multiple dosing requirements. This approach was based on input from the pharmacology experts **(led by Professor Andrew Owen)** who performed pharmacokinetic simulations across trial doses, and found that cumulative ivermectin dose was expected to correlate with key pharmacokinetic parameters when single and multiple-dose studies were segregated. It should be noted that the included trials did not directly assess the pharmacokinetics of ivermectin and our approach was based upon simulations validated where possible against published pharmacokinetics in humans. The panel used a pre-specified framework incorporating the ICEMAN tool to assess the credibility of the subgroup findings (84).

A Professor swimming in financial conflicts of interests with pharmaceutical companies that had products directly competing with ivermectin in the now global "COVID marketplace" ***was put in charge of assessing the ivermectin evidence for the most powerful health care organization in the world.***

In Owen and his colleagues assessment of the evidence base for ivermectin, what they did to suppress the evidence of efficacy was so openly corrupt, I immediately wrote a white paper about their brazen manipulations of the existing evidence (which I spent many, many days on). The FLCCC sent out the paper via press release, trying to disseminate it as far and wide as we could. Good ole' FLCCC. The Bad News Bears trying to take down the Yankees with a white paper. We tried folks.

My paper extensively detailed how they whittled down the evidence base to as few trials as possible, using arbitrary exclusion criteria. Then they graded the few remaining trials that showed large, positive effects as "low quality" and a large Pharma conflicted trial that showed no benefit as "high quality." What is fascinating is that despite the fact that even amongst the paucity of remaining trials left, a massive reduction in mortality was found. They found a life-saving medicine in ivermectin. Yet they stated that this conclusion was of such "low certainty" it should not be acted on. Science baby. Disgusting.

Had the WHO recommended ivermectin, even using one of the conditional or "weak" recommendations available to them, it would have changed history and saved millions of lives across the world. Physicians would have adopted it globally at a time when there was no "official" early treatment option for COVID outside about a dozen low and middle income countries that had adopted ivermectin into their national or regional guidelines. A weak recommendation would have changed history by mitigating the disastrous scale and trajectory of the pandemic. And it would have prevented us from being subjected to the subsequent holocaust unleashed by lethal vaccines.

CHAPTER 6

COVID-19 and the Shadowy "Trusted News Initiative"

How it Systematically Censors the World's Top Public Health Experts

Elizabeth Woodworth

Retired Health Science Librarian,
BC Ministry of Health

Elizabeth Woodworth is a retired Head Health Sciences Librarian, Environmental Librarian (British Columbia Govt., 1971-2002) and author of "'What Can I Do?' Citizen Strategies for Nuclear Disarmament," carried by UN bookstores and discussed in Canada's House of Commons. Hon. BA, Phil. Hist. Eng.; Postgraduate BLS (Bach. Lib. Science)

Abstract: What do the inventor of mRNA technology; the lead author of the most downloaded paper on Covid-19 in the American Journal of Medicine; a former editor of the American Journal of Epidemiology; renowned epidemiologists at Harvard, Stanford, and Oxford; and France's leading microbiologist – have in common?

They have all been censored by a repressive media network that most people have never heard of. This network has monstrously conceived and conveyed a "monopoly of legitimate information."[1]

Exposing this censorship of eminent voices is especially vital to the fate of children and youth, who are being aggressively targeted for low-benefit, sometimes lethal, inoculations.

Since early in the COVID-19 pandemic, which according to the World Health Organization kills only 0.23% of those infected,[2] enormous fear and panic have been fuelled by the hourly drumbeat of a "one-voice" media.

An international process of editorial standardization has delivered unprecedented news coverage of the monopolized message:

1. The pandemic threatens the survival of all humanity
2. There is no therapy to cure the sick
3. It is necessary to confine the whole population, and
4. The delivery will come only from a vaccine.[3]

Many people have been dismayed by the singularity of this propaganda, and how it could possibly have been achieved. That is the subject of this essay.

Introduction: How the TNI Got Started

On June 24, 2021, a report from the Oxford-based Reuters Institute revealed that trust in the US media – ranking last among 46 countries – had descended to an all-time low of 29%. Meanwhile, Canadian trust in media has sunk to 45%.[4]

This downward spiral can only mean that people are going elsewhere for their news – a trend that has likely been accelerated by the emergence of a shadowy global censorship network called the Trusted News Initiative (TNI).

In July 2019, before the pandemic, the UK and Canadian governments hosted the FCO Global Conference on Media Freedom,[5] where then BBC Director-General Tony Hall announced:

"Last month I convened, behind closed doors, a Trusted News Summit at the BBC, which brought together global tech platforms and publishers. The goal was to arrive at a practical set of actions we can take together, right now, to tackle the rise of misinformation and bias....I'm determined that we use that [BBC] unique reach and trusted voice to lead the way – to create a global alliance for integrity in news. We're ready to do even more to help promote freedom and democracy worldwide."[6]

The initial Trusted News partners in attendance were the European Broadcasting Union (EBU), Facebook, Financial Times, First Draft, Google, The Hindu, and The Wall Street Journal.

This was the embryonic start of a soon-to-become global media-wide Early Warning System that would rapidly alert members to "disinformation which threatens human life or disrupts democracy during elections."[7]

Where did the idea come from?

The BBC had earlier responded[8] to a call for evidence from the House of Lords' Select Committee on Democracy and Digital Technology, citing in its first footnote a June 3, 2019 BBC blog entitled "Tackling Misinformation."[9]

The first point of that blog referred to a pre-pandemic March 3, 2019 BBC news report that anti-vaxxers were gaining traction on social media as part of a "fake news" movement spreading "misleading and dangerous information".[10]

The June 3 blog also claimed a "mammoth" online scale of deceitful business practices and hate speech as problems needing "algorithmic interventions". The online "information ecosystem" was "polluted"; the size of the problem "unprecedented." The BBC and other organizations would be looking at interventions "to address misinformation across the media landscape".

Looking back at this perception of pre-Covid problems, the motives of the TNI network appear to have been constructive and reasonable. However, there was no inkling at the time of how vast, repressive, and darkly persuasive these interventions were soon to become.

***

The action started. CBC/Radio-Canada publicly announced its participation in the TNI in September 2019, saying "this includes a commitment to collaborate on source authentication, civic information, media education, and other responses to disinformation."[11] The Hindu announced the Indian program simultaneously.[12]

Two weeks after WHO announced the Covid-19 pandemic on March 11, 2020, Canada's CBC reported that the Trusted News Initiative had announced plans "to tackle harmful coronavirus disinformation."

"Starting today, partners in the Trusted News Initiative will alert each other to disinformation about coronavirus, including 'imposter content' purporting to come from trusted sources. Such content will be reviewed promptly to ensure that disinformation is not republished." [13]

The media partners had now expanded to include Twitter, Microsoft, Associated Press, Agence France-Presse, Reuters, and the Reuters Institute for the Study of Journalism.

The TNI next agreed to engage with a new verification technology called Project Origin, led by a coalition of the BBC, CBC/Radio-Canada, Microsoft and The New York Times – with a mandate to identify non-authorized news stories for suppression.

In July, 2020, Eric Horvitz, Chief Scientific Officer for Microsoft, remarked about authorizing the news: "We've forged a close relationship with the BBC and other partners on Project Origin, aimed at methods and standards for end-to-end authentication of news and information."[14]

By December 2020, the BBC had reported that disinformation was "spreading online to millions of people," and included minimizing COVID-19 risks along with impugning the vaccine developers' motives.[15]

In a June 25, 2021 summary article by investigative staff, *TrialSiteNews* asked the question, "COVID-19 Censorship: Trusted News Initiative to Decide the Facts?" and began its reply with:

"Since time immemorial, those with power have used it to control those without. In the modern world, big government and big tech represent the seats of power when it comes to who is allowed to say what. Of course, many think that "private companies" can regulate speech in any way they see fit. But from either an ethical or legal point of view, this is false. The argument from the societal benefits of free speech works equally for posting YouTube videos and handing out flyers on a corner.

Legally, the [U.S.] Supreme Court has long held that when a private company creates something that functions as a public square (think of a company town), the First Amendment comes into play. Way back in April 2020, it was already clear that the then-existing online socio-political censorship was going to expand into the world of science, medicine, and academia in the new COVID-19 era."[16]

What is Disinformation?

This question has been sloppily handled by the mainstream media, which often confuses "misinformation" (unintentionally misleading information) with what they mean, "disinformation," which is *deliberate.*

Several dictionary definitions agree on that point:

American Heritage: "Deliberately misleading information announced publicly or leaked by a government or especially by an intelligence agency in order to influence public opinion or the government in another nation."[17]

Merriam-Webster: "False information deliberately and often covertly spread (as by the planting of rumors) in order to influence public opinion or obscure the truth."[18]

The OED (Oxford English Dictionary): "The dissemination of deliberately false information, esp. when supplied by a government or its agent to a foreign power or to the media, with the intention of influencing the policies or opinions of those who receive it."[19]

Given that these definitions specify deliberate government action, it seems odd that the TNI has identified a scattered online public as the source of intentional false information and propaganda – especially concerning elections and health policy.

What are the TNI's Public Health Sources? Are They Trustworthy?

The TNI reports Covid-19 health policy from the world's major public health agencies, including the World Health Organization (WHO), the US Centers for Disease Control (CDC), the US Food and Drug Administration (FDA), and the US National Institutes of Health (NIH).

This policy is passed down through national and state governments, who convey it to the public via their media and websites, along with local case reports (based on the questionable PCR test) and deaths.

Unfortunately, this top-down leadership has at best been illogical and inconsistent, and at worst corrupted by the vast profits of the vaccine industry.

Examples of either incompetent or corrupt public health leadership include NIAID director Dr. Anthony Fauci's extraordinary contradictions concerning the protection offered by masks.[20]

The PCR test had a checkered history: Its recommendation had been very suddenly approved by WHO after being hurriedly rushed to publication in Eurosurveillance,[21] one day after its submission date of

January 22, 2020. Incredibly, it lacked peer review – an irregularity that was formally challenged by 22 scientists seeking its retraction.[22]

Worse yet, this global PCR test, which amplifies fragments of live or dead virus found in nose swabs, shows many false positives (which are officially deemed "cases," regardless of symptoms). A study conducted last year by the Infectious Diseases Society of America found that at 25 cycles of amplification, "up to 70% of patients remain positive in culture" tests. Fine, but at 30 cycles culture verification dropped to 20%, and by 35 cycles, less than 3% of cultures remained positive.[23]

Misleadingly, most European and US labs have been basing their frightening "case" numbers – published 24/7 through the TNI – on 35 cycles or higher.[24]

The most shocking – if not criminal – Covid leadership failure of all is that the WHO, NIH, CDC, and FDA have consistently denied the existence of the 85%-effective, cheap, safe and abundant early treatments for Covid-19.

Their only recommended option until November 2020 – a month before the vaccines arrived – was to sicken at home until you couldn't breathe; then go to the hospital. (In November the FDA and the NIH allowed anti-SARS-2 monoclonal antibody products for mild outpatient disease in high-risk patients – but nothing else.[25])

There was to be no government-sanctioned cure until a vaccine arrived.

The obedient TNI – not into investigative journalism – followed suit. In spite of extensive evidence supporting early treatment efficacy,[26] and although 56 countries have adopted early treatments,[27] there have been no TNI-approved media statements that any early treatments, including hydroxychloroquine (HCQ), ivermectin (IVM), quercetin, zinc, budesonide, or Vitamins C and D, are effective in treating Covid-19 outpatients during the first 5-7 days of flu-like symptoms.

The denial has been so strong that in early 2020 many US state pharmacy boards – in unprecedented disrespect for the authority of physicians – banned pharmacies from filling HCQ prescriptions to treat outpatient Covid-19.[28]

In August 2020, it came to light that pre-licensure Emergency Use Authorizations (EUAs) for the mRNA vaccines could not be legally approved if there was an available alternative – that is, if the FDA had already issued an EUA for outpatient use of HCQ, as shown in the final item of this in-house FDA slide.[29]

Apart from early op-ed exposés by eminent Yale epidemiologist Dr. Harvey Risch,[30] where was the investigative journalism?

Who and What Have Been Most Censored by TNI's Early Warning System?

To support individual acts of censorship, the social media giants refer to the WHO, CDC, FDA, and NIH policies as their justification. Discussions such as the source of the virus, early treatments, and vaccine adverse effects – if they originate outside of these agencies – are quickly suppressed by the coordinated TNI network.

We will look at seven of these suppressions, in order of their first occurrence:

Suppression #1: The Source of SARS-2

The Trusted News Initiative very quickly got to work silencing "disinformation" about a SARS-2 connection to the inadequate Wuhan levels 2 and 3 biosafety labs. However, since former NYT writer Nicholas Wade's thorough investigation in May 2021,[31] and the FOIA dump of Dr. Fauci's emails[32] in June, the TNI partners, including Facebook and Twitter, gave up censoring free speech about a Wuhan lab escape.

Suppression #2: Denial of Early Treatments for Covid:

As we have seen, the medical literature is full of peer-reviewed published studies showing both the prophylactic and early treatment efficacy of a range of safe, inexpensive, readily available drugs and substances.

During the March-December 2020 period, these were claimed to be ineffective by government and the media in order to pave the way for FDA Emergency Use Authorizations for remdesivir (whose efficacy is now under question[33]) and the mRNA vaccines.

Scandalously, hundreds of thousands of people died while waiting for the vaccines to arrive in December 2020. Why did they die? Because their doctors were blocked from prescribing the repurposed drugs HCQ and IVM that have long been on the WHO list of essential medicines.

The TNI, by censoring the truth that the public so desperately needed, has been a primary enabler of this catastrophic, vaccine-friendly policy.

During July 2021, instead of acknowledging the early treatment evidence they had housed[34] all along (thus being directly complicit in these deaths), the government-media complex doubled down on its intense campaign to vaccinate every one of us.

Incredibly, on August 3, 2021, 16 months and 612,386 deaths too late, Anthony Fauci, in an excerpt supplied by TNI partner Reuters, "floats [a] pill to 'knock out' COVID early," given once daily for seven to ten days.[35]

Suppression #3: The Voices of Dissenting Health Professionals

While major health policy-makers such as WHO, CDC, FDA, and Anthony Fauci have careened from one unprecedented society-killing edict to the next, many eminent public health professionals at the tops of their fields have stepped forward to offer sane, traditional, contagion-control measures.

However, they have not been welcome in the media or on social media. TNI Director Jessica Cecil explained why, at the *Trust In News Conference,'* in April, 2021:

"First, those pushing disinformation...are using apparently trustworthy sources. Anti-vax content often uses interviews with people who have medical degrees for instance.

And there is frequently a grain of truth to what is claimed. That makes untangling the true from the false harder..."[36]

In "untangling the true from the false," untrained media personnel have censored the following prominent professors and researchers with outstanding publication histories[37] and conflict-of-interest-free credentials. Further information can be found at his or her Google Scholar publication record:

Dr. Jay Bhattacharya, epidemiologist, Stanford University

Dr. Sunetra Gupta, infectious disease epidemiologist, Oxford Univ.

Dr. Martin Kulldorff, epidemiologist, Harvard

Dr. Robert W. Malone, inventor of mRNA technology platform

Dr. Peter A. McCullough, former Vice-Chair Int. Med., Baylor Univ.

Dr. Didier Raoult, microbiologist and director, IHU Méditerranée Infection; Professor at Aix Marseille Université

Dr. Harvey A. Risch, Prof. Epid., Yale School of Public Health

Dr. Knut M. Wittkowski, biometrician, 20-year head, biostatistics/ epid., Rockefeller University

Dr. Michael Yeadon, former VP of respiratory research, Pfizer.

The TNI has also vigorously censored frontline physicians who have saved thousands of lives with early Covid-19 treatments: Dr. Zev Zelenko in New York,[38] Drs. George Fareed and Brian Tyson in California;[39] America's Frontline Doctors,[40] founded by Dr. Simone Gold; and the Frontline COVID-19 Critical Care Alliance (FLCCC),[41] led by ICU/critical-care physician Dr. Pierre Kory.

A member of FLCCC, Dr. Joseph Varon, who is chief of staff at United Memorial Medical Center in Houston, has had more than 1,600 media interviews, yet he told local Fox reporter Ivory Hecker that reporters will never discuss his highly successful MATH+ hospital treatment protocol – "because the news producers will not allow it."[42]

Why not? Because his hospital-based protocol using cheap, safe, plentiful drugs such as methylprednisolone, fluvoxamine, thiamine, heparin, and ivermectin, combined with zinc, ascorbic acid, and vitamin D,[43] has yielded about half the inpatient death rate reported by the CDC.[44]

And that is not allowed by those who direct the media – those whose inferable mission is a vaccine policy based on millions of questionable PCR tests, followed by a vaccine passport that by all appearances is the endgame.

Suppression #4: The Record Number of Serious Post-Vaccine Side Effects and Deaths

Record post-vaccine side effects and deaths have been reported online by the US CDC VAERs (Vaccine Adverse Effects Reporting system), by the UK Yellow Card System, by the EU Vaccine Injury Reporting System, and by Israel.

In the United States, VAERS reported 491,218 adverse effects and 11,405 deaths from February 10 until July 24, 2021.[45]

However, connecting these deaths directly to the vaccines is not straightforward.

In England, Dr. Tess Lawrie of the Evidence-based Medicine Consultancy (EbMC), stated in June 2021 that there were "at least 3 urgent questions that need to be answered by the English equivalent to CDC, the MHRA:

"How many people have died within 28 days of vaccination?

How many people have been hospitalised within 28 days of vaccination?

How many people have been disabled by the vaccination?"[46]

Also in June, Dr. Lawrie wrote a highly-referenced 11-page letter to the MHRA Chief Executive showing that "the MHRA now has more than enough evidence on the Yellow Card System to declare the COVID-19 vaccine unsafe for use in humans."[47]

Suppression #5: Natural Immunity Stronger than Vaccinated Immunity

Very simply put, the mRNA vaccines only generate antibodies against the single synthetic spike protein that they instruct the body first to make, and then to provide immunity against. But if the original wild SARS-2 spike mutates, the altered virus is less easily recognized by the immune system and often escapes its antibodies.

Meanwhile, natural immunity, which has fought off the whole virus and remembers it through both antibody and T-cell immunity, is much more robust and effective – in spite of minor spike mutations.[48]

Given this fact, the world's governments and media should have allowed proof of immunity through tests such as T-Detect, which is authorized "for detecting and identifying the presence of an adaptive T-cell immune response to SARS-CoV-2"[49] – in lieu of being vaccinated, for those who preferred them.

Instead, the confusing, superficially informed TNI has pushed only the highly profitable but increasingly failed experimental vaccines, which now, although they reduce risk in high-risk people, have "almost no value as a way of protecting others, so there is no benefit in vaccinating children, introducing vaccine passports domestically or internationally, or coercing young people to get a vaccine which to them is almost all risk and no benefit."[50]

Suppression #6: Worrying Evidence of Pathogenic Priming/ADE

During early mRNA clinical trials, cats, ferrets, monkeys, and rabbits have experienced Antibody Dependent Enhancement (ADE), also known as pathogenic priming or a cytokine storm. This occurs when the immune system creates an overwhelming, uncontrolled inflammatory response upon being confronted with the virus in the real world, and then dies.

The director of the Pathological Institute of the University of Heidelberg, Peter Schirmacher, has carried out over 40 autopsies on people who had died within two weeks of vaccination. Schirmacher was alarmed to cite on August 3, 2021, "rare, severe side effects of the vaccination – such as cerebral vein thrombosis or autoimmune diseases."[51]

On August 5, 2021, Israeli Dr. Kobi Haviv, at the Herzog Hospital in Jerusalem, reported that "95% of the severe patients are vaccinated...85-90% of the hospitalizations are in fully vaccinated people...We are opening more and more COVID wards...The effectiveness of the vaccine is waning/fading out."[52]

Dr. Robert Malone, inventor of mRNA technology, has explained that the susceptibility to ADE is greatest precisely during the long phase in which the vaccine tapers off: "The vaccine in its waning phase is causing the virus to replicate more efficiently than it would otherwise, which is called Antibody Dependent Enhancement," adding that all previous coronavirus vaccine development programs led to ADE.[53]

It is essential that informed consent for Covid-19 vaccines include notification of the possibility of ADE, *especially with regard to parents*, whose children should be protected at all costs:

"The specific and significant COVID-19 risk of ADE should have been and should be prominently and independently disclosed to research subjects currently in vaccine trials, as well as those being recruited for the trials and future patients after vaccine approval, in order to meet the medical ethics standard of patient comprehension for informed consent."[54]

How many people receiving mRNA vaccines have been told this? Certainly their *Trusted* News Initiative has not told them.

Suppression #7: The Central Role of Co-Morbidities in Serious Covid Disease

Only 4% of Covid deaths in England died without pre-existing conditions.[55] In the US, 94.9% had pre-existing conditions.[56]

How often has the pharma-backed media hinted that 78% of US Covid hospitalizations are overweight or obese? Or suggested that "hey folks, you might save your life by dieting?"[57]

How often have we been warned that 59% of hospital admissions are deficient in Vitamin D?[58] [59]

Has the government-media complex ever mandated Vitamin D intake standards to take pressure off Intensive Care Units?

Has Tony Fauci ever told people to take enough Vitamin D when – according to his FOIA'd emails – he takes 6,000 IUs a day himself?[60]

Or would it have created insufficient fear to drive people to unguaranteed experimental vaccines for the TNI to let us know?

Conclusion: The Media and Democracy

A primary motive behind the formation of the TNI may have been to eradicate the so-called "disinformation" that an insulted, indignant public prefers to the creatively irrelevant corporate-led media, aka "the presstitute".

It's not as if the media has a track record of being right about pandemics. For example, it trusted worst-case scenario modeler Neil Ferguson and the pharma-controlled World Health Organization over the 2009 swine flu "pandemic"– which fizzled out leaving governments to incinerate millions of dollars in vaccines.[61]

Such industry achievements use "influencers" – falsely independent "experts" including specialist journalists, think tank facilitators, and academics whose research is funded by industry or government.

Regarding Covid-19, Dr. Piers Robinson, co-director of the Organisation for Propaganda Studies, has judged, "It wouldn't be an underestimation to say that this is probably one of the biggest propaganda operations that we have seen in history," concluding "what happens is down to how people resist and how much force and coercion the authorities use."[62]

Indeed, the very foundation of democracy is that public wisdom should be consulted and given its head in self-rule. The public has the constitutional right to full information to form and express its own conclusions and does not need a coordinated TNI to corral and contain it.

It is utterly outrageous that the voices the public needs, from its top public health figures, at its best universities, are being denied a hearing.

A far superior job of investigative reporting is being done by the hard-working alternative media researchers without Big Pharma's blood-stained advertising dollars.

Perhaps the *TrialSiteNews* staff has said it best:

"We think that disallowing good-faith medical information because the public can't be presumed to properly weigh claims is infantilizing said public, along with dismantling the free speech culture that perhaps peaked in the 20th Century. The efforts now underway to completely suppress positive data associated with early-onset treatment prospects such as ivermectin or the squelching of any discussion of vaccine safety issues is completely unacceptable in a civilized, democratic market-based society. Those perpetuating such offenses are in fact on the wrong side of history."[63]

Endnotes

[1] Pierre Bourdieu, *Sur la télévision*, Paris, Seuil, 1996, 82.

[2] Ioannidis J. "The infection fatality rate of COVID-19 inferred from seroprevalence data," *Bull World Health Organ.*, Epub Oct. 14, 2020 (https://pubmed.ncbi.nlm.nih.gov/33716331/).

   The *British Medical Journal*, citing this article, reported: "Clearly, mortality is age-stratified from covid-19. The corrected median estimates of IFP [Infection Fatality Rate] for people aged lower than 70 years is currently 0.05%, [2] which, for the population less vulnerable to deaths, is similar to influenza. However overall estimates for covid-19 are higher [i.e., 0.23%], due to the higher fatality rate in elderly people." *BMJ* October 6, 2020 (https://www.bmj.com/content/371/bmj.m3883/rr).

[3] Laurent Mucchielli, "How is built the 'legitimate information' on the Covid crisis," UMR 7305, CNRS and Aix-Marseille University, April 2020 (https://www.mediterranee-infection.com/wp-content/uploads/2020/04/MS-Mucchielli.pdf). *Translation from French.*

[4] Rick Edmonds, June 24, 2021, by Rick Edmonds, "US ranks last among 46 countries in trust in media, Reuters Institute report finds," June 24, 2021 (https://www.poynter.org/ethics-trust/2021/us-ranks-last-among-46-countries-in-trust-in-media-reuters-institute-report-finds/).

[5] Global Conference for Media Freedom: London 2019 (https://www.gov.uk/government/topical-events/global-conference-for-media-freedom-london-2019). The Conference website states that "It is supported by Luminate," (https://luminategroup.com/) which in turn was founded by the Omidyar Group (omidyargroup.com).

[6] Tony Hall, "Media Freedom: What is it and why does it matter?" BBC, 11 July 2019 (https://www.bbc.co.uk/mediacentre/speeches/2019/tony-hall-fco).

[7] Leila About, "News groups and tech companies team up to fight disinformation; BBC-led project aims to build an 'early warning system,'" *Financial Times*, September 6, 2019 (https://www.ft.com/content/6857149a-d0b2-11e9-99a4-b5ded7a7fe3f).

[8] BBC – written evidence (DAD0062), undated (https://committees.parliament.uk/writtenevidence/429/html).

[9] Ahmed Razek, "Tackling Misinformation," June 3, 2019 (https://medium.com/bbc-design-engineering/tackling-misinformation-30d39f6d02e9).

[10] "Vaccination deniers gaining traction, NHS boss warns," *BBC News*, 1 March 2019 (https://www.bbc.com/news/health-47417966).

[11] "CBC/Radio-Canada joins global charter to fight disinformation," 9 September 2019 (https://cbc.radio-canada.ca/en/media-centre/trusted-news-charter-fight-disinformation).

[12] "News majors to fight disinformation," 07 September 2019 (https://www.thehindu.com/news/national/news-majors-to-fight-disinformation/article29356124.ece).

[13] "Trusted News Initiative announces plans to tackle harmful coronavirus disinformation," 27 March 2020 (https://cbc.radio-canada.ca/en/media-centre/trusted-news-initiative-plan-disinformation-coronavirus).

[14] EBU: Operating Eurovision and Euroradio, "Trusted News Initiative steps up global fight against disinformation and targets US presidential election," 13 July 2020 (https://www.ebu.ch/news/2020/07/trusted-news-initiative-steps-up-global-fight-against-disinformation-and-targets-us-presidential-election).

[15] BBC, "Trusted News Initiative (TNI) to combat spread of harmful vaccine disinformation and announces major research project," 10 December 2020 (https://www.bbc.com/mediacentre/2020/trusted-news-initiative-vaccine-disinformation).

[16] *TrialSiteNews* Staff, "COVID-19 Censorship: Trusted News Initiative to Decide the Facts?" 25 June 2021 (https://trialsitenews.com/covid-19-censorship-trusted-news-initiative-to-decide-the-facts/).

[17] (https://ahdictionary.com/word/search.html?q=disinformation)

[18] (https://www.merriam-webster.com/dictionary/disinformation)

[19] (https://www.europarl.europa.eu/RegData/etudes/ATAG/2015/571332/EPRS_ATA(2015)571332_EN.pdf)

[20] A video compilation from Justin Hart, @justin_hart, San Diego, embedded in his tweet, 26 July 2021 (https://twitter.com/justin_hart/status/1419833290421272580?s=12).

[21] Victor M. Corman, et al., "Detection of 2019 novel coronavirus (2019-nCoV) by real-time RT-PCR," *Eurosurveillance*, Vol. 25, Issue 3, 23 January 2020 (https://www.eurosurveillance.org/content/10.2807/1560-7917.ES.2020.25.3.2000045).

[22] CORMAN-DROSTEN REVIEW REPORT. CURATED BY AN INTERNATIONAL CONSORTIUM OF SCIENTISTS IN LIFE SCIENCES (ICSLS). "Retraction request letter to Eurosurveillance editorial board," 8 November 2020 (https://cormandrostenreview.com/retraction-request-letter-to-eurosurveillance-editorial-board/)

[23] Rita Jaafar et al, "Correlation Between 3790 Quantitative Polymerase Chain Reaction–Positives Samples and Positive Cell Cultures, Including 1941 Severe Acute Respiratory Syndrome Coronavirus 2 Isolates," *Clinical Infectious Diseases*, Vol. 72, Issue 11, 1 June 2021, page e921 (https://academic.oup.com/cid/article/72/11/e921/5912603). 28 September 2020 at https://doi.org/10.1093/cid/ciaa1491

[24] Swiss Policy Research, "The Trouble With PCR Tests," updated June 2021 (https://swprs.org/the-trouble-with-pcr-tests). The authors note: "From a lab perspective, it is safer to produce a 'false positive' result that puts a healthy non-infectious person into quarantine, than to produce a 'false negative' result and be responsible if someone infects their grandmother."

[25] NIH. "Therapeutic Management of Nonhospitalized Adults with COVID-19, last updated July 8, 2021" (https://www.covid19treatmentguidelines.nih.gov/management/clinical-management/nonhospitalized-adults--therapeutic-management/).

[26] 14 Peter A. McCullough, et al., "Pathophysiological Basis and Rationale for Early Outpatient Treatment of SARS-CoV-2 (COVID-19) Infection," *Am J Med*. 2021 Jan; 134(1): 16–22 (https://www.ncbi.nlm.nih.gov/pmc/articles/PMC7410805/).; Published online 2020 Aug 7. doi: 10.1016/j.amjmed.2020.07.003. See also the very extensive website, c19study.com; see https://swprs.org/on-the-treatment-of-covid-19; and see PubMed for further outpatient Covid early treatment, (https://pubmed.ncbi.nlm.nih.gov/?term=%28%22early+outpatient+treatment%3A%29+AND+%28covid-19+OR+sars-2%29&sort=).

[27] "Global adoption of Covid-19 early treatments" (as of July 30, 2021), (https://c19adoption.com/).

[28] "State Rules and Recommendations Regarding Chloroquine, Hydroxychloroquine and Other Drugs Related to COVID-19," posted March, 2020 (https://www.nashp.org/wp-content/uploads/2020/03/State-covid-drug-chart-3-27-2020.pdf).

[29] FDA. "Considerations for FDA Licensure vs. Emergency Use Authorization of COVID-19 Vaccines," July 29, 2020; see 10:20 min. (https://youtu.be/UkXQ09T6f94).

[30] Harvey A. Risch, "The Key to Defeating Covid-19 Already Exists. We Need to Start Using It," *Newsweek*, 23 July 2020 (https://www.newsweek.com/key-defeating-covid-19-already-exists-we-need-start-using-it-opinion-1519535); "FDA obstruction: Patients die, while Trump gets the blame," *Washington Examiner*, 19 October 2020 (https://www.washingtonexaminer.com/author/harvey-risch).

[31] Nicholas Wade, "Origin of Covid – Following the Clues: Did people or nature open Pandora's box at Wuhan?" May 2, 2021 (https:/nicholaswade.medium.com/origin-of-covid-following-the-clues-6f03564c038).

[32] See Dr. Chris Martenson's Fauci takedown videos, episodes 7, 8, and 9 (https://www.youtube.com/user/ChrisMartensondotcom).

[33] Owen Dyer, "Covid-19: Remdesivir has little or no impact on survival, WHO trial shows," *BMJ* 2020; 371 doi: https://doi.org/10.1136/bmj.m4057 (Published 19 October 2020) (https://www.bmj.com/content/371/bmj.m4057).

[34] For example, it was reported in 2005 that "Chloroquine is a potent inhibitor of SARS coronavirus infection and spread," Martin J. Vincent et al, *Virology Journal*, vol. 2, no. 69, 2005 (https://virologyj.biomedcentral.com/articles/10.1186/1743-422X-2-69). *Virology Journal* is well known to the NIH, and is available on its website: https://www.ncbi.nlm.nih.gov/pmc/journals/273/

[35] Interview with J. Stephen Morrison, Senior Vice President, Center for Strategic & International Studies, Reuters excerpt, 3 August 2021 (https://www.reuters.com/video/watch/idOVEOQEL7J).

[36] Trust In News Conference. BBC, April 8, 2021 (https://www.bbc.co.uk/mediacentre/articles/2021/trust-in-news-conference).

[37] A scientist's credibility can be estimated by how often his/her published articles are cited in the indexed, peer-reviewed literature. This is quantified as the h-index number, and can be found by searching an author's name on Google Scholar, e.g., Harvard Medical School bio-

statistician and epidemiologist, Dr. Martin Kulldorff, has been cited 26,087 times and has an h-index of 77. (https://scholar.google.com/citations?user=WNEj34MAAAAJ&hl=en).

[38] Board Certified Family Physician Vladimir Zev Zelenko, M.D. (https://vladimirzelenkomd. com/about/).

[39] Brian Tyson and George Fareed, "Doctors story of Light and Life: the Covid-19 Darkness Overcome," *The Desert Review*, 2 August 2021 (https://www.thedesertreview.com/news/ local/doctors-story-of-light-and-life-the-covid-19-darkness-overcome/article_97b53ca6-f3b7-11eb-8773-c7ecbb9070e7.html).

[40] (https://americasfrontlinedoctors.org/).

[41] (https://covid19criticalcare.com/).

[42] "Ivory Hecker Exposes Fox News Managers Censoring Her for Reporting on Hydryoxychloroquine," 16 July 2021; see 1-2 min. (https://www.bitchute.com/ video/8y5VHbdFfkji/).

[43] (htpps://covid19criticalcare.com/covid-19-protocols/math-plus-protocol/).

[44] Holmquist, Annie, "The Media May Be Responsible for Countless COVID Deaths," *Chronicle: A Magazine of American Culture*, 29 June 2021 (https://www. chroniclesmagazine.org/blog/the-media-may-be-responsible-for-countless-covid-deaths/). Dr. Varon's bio and awards are shown on Dr. Been, July 2021(https://www. youtube.com/watch?v=YGKD8c51UmU).

[45] United States. CDC. VAERS (https://wonder.cdc.gov/vaers.html), via Karen Selick, 25 July 2021 (https://www.bitchute.com/video/3bmfKOGpkuGD/).

[46] Kathy Gyngell, "Expert's damning vaccine evidence," *The Conservative Woman*, 14 June 2021 (https://www.conservativewoman.co.uk/doctors-damning-evidence/),

[47] Lien Davies, "Open Letter from Dr Tess Lawrie to Chief Exec MHRA Dr Raine – URGENT Report – COVID-19 vaccines unsafe for use in humans," 10 June 2021 (https://freedomalliance.co.uk/2021/06/10/open-letter-from-dr-tess-lawrie-to-chief-exec-mhra-dr-raine-urgent-report-covid-19-vaccines-unsafe-for-use-in-humans/).

[48] Sharyl Attkisson, "Covid-19 natural immunity compared to vaccine-induced immunity: The definitive summary," 6 August 2021 (https://sharylattkisson.com/2021/08/covid-19-natural-immunity-compared-to-vaccine-induced-immunity-the-definitive-summary/).

[49] (https://www.t-detect.com/).

[50] Will Jones, "Devastating New Data From PHE Shows Vaccine Effectiveness Down to 17% and No Reduction in Infectiousness – But Mortality Cut by 77%," *The Daily Sceptic*, 6 August 2021 (https://dailysceptic.org/2021/08/06/devastating-new-data-from-phe-shows-vaccine-effectiveness-down-to-17-and-no-reduction-in-infectiousness-but-mortality-cut-by-77/).

[51] Free West Media, "German chief pathologist sounds alarm on fatal vaccine injuries," 3 August 2021 (https://freewestmedia.com/2021/08/03/german-chief-pathologist-sounds-alarm-on-fatal-vaccine-injuries/).

[52] "Israel: "85-90% of the hospitalizations are in fully vaccinated people," 5 August 2021 (https://www.coronaheadsup.com/coronavirus/israel-85-90-of-the-hospitalizations-are-in-fully-vaccinated-people/).

[53] Robert Malone, "The Vaccine Causes The Virus To Be More Dangerous," 29 July 2021 (https://www.eastonspectator.com/2021/07/29/the-vaccine-causes-the-virus-to-be-more-dangerous/).

[54] Timothy Cardozo and Ronald Veazey, "Informed consent disclosure to vaccine trial subjects of risk of COVID-19 vaccines worsening clinical disease," *Int J Clin Pract*. 2021 Mar;75(3):e13795. doi: 10.1111/ijcp.13795. Epub 2020 Dec 4. (https://pubmed.ncbi.nlm.nih.gov/33113270/).

[55] Table: "COVID-19 deaths by age group and pre-existing conditions", 4 February 2021 (England.covid19dailydeaths@nhs.net).

[56] United States. CDC. "Underlying Medical Conditions and Severe Illness Among 540,667 Adults Hospitalized With COVID-19, March 2020–March 2021," 1 July 2021 (https://www.cdc.gov/pcd/issues/2021/21_0123.htm).

[57] Berkeley Lovelace Jr., "CDC: 78% of people hospitalized for Covid were overweight or obese," *The Journal of Nursing*, 1 March 2021 (https://www.asrn.org/journal-nursing/2517-cdc-78-of-people-hospitalized-for-covid-were-overweight-or-obese.html).

[58] Dieter De Smet, et al., "Serum 25(OH)D Level on Hospital Admission Associated With COVID-19 Stage and Mortality," *Am J Clin Pathol*., 2021 Feb 11;155(3):381-388. doi: 10.1093/ajcp/aqaa252 (https://pubmed.ncbi.nlm.nih.gov/33236114/).

[59] Mustafa Demir, et al., "Vitamin D deficiency is associated with COVID-19 positivity and severity of the disease," *J Med Virol*. 2021 May;93(5):2992-2999. doi: 10.1002/jmv.26832. Epub 2021 Feb 9 (https://pubmed.ncbi.nlm.nih.gov/33512007/).
Vitamin D deficiency is associated with COVID-19 positivity and severity of the disease
Mustafa Demir 1 , Fadime Demir 2 , Hatice Aygun 3

[60] (https://vitamindwiki.com/Dr.+Fauci+takes+6%2C000+IU+of+Vitamin+D+daily+%E2%80%93+Sept+2020).

[61] CBS News, "$260M of Swine Flu Vaccine to be Incinerated," 1 July 2010 (https://www.cbsnews.com/news/260m-of-swine-flu-vaccine-to-be-incinerated/).

[62] Piers Robinson, "Covid is a Global Propaganda Operation," *Asia Pacific Today*, 4 August 2021 (https://rumble.com/vkppo0-covid-is-a-global-propaganda-operation.html).

[63] *TrialSiteNews* Staff, "COVID-19 Censorship: Trusted News Initiative to Decide the Facts?" 25 June 2021 (https://trialsitenews.com/covid-19-censorship-trusted-news-initiative-to-decide-the-facts/).

CHAPTER 7

Fact-checking the 'fact-checkers': Standing up for the Truth in the Age of COVID Censorship

Dr. Michael Nevradakis

Journalist and senior reporter for The Defender and CHD TV host

Michael Nevradakis, Ph.D., based in Athens, Greece, is a senior reporter for The Defender, published by Children's Health Defense (CHD), and part of the rotation of hosts for CHD.TV's "Good Morning CHD." For 10 years, he produced and hosted the "Dialogos" radio program and podcast, and he has previously been published by The Guardian, the Huffington Post, the Daily Kos, Truthout, Mint Press News and other outlets. He completed his Ph.D. in media studies at the University of Texas in 2018 and holds a masters degree in public policy from Stony Brook University. He is an instructor in communications and journalism and has taught at various institutions of higher education in Greece and the U.S.

Long before I had the privilege of joining Children's Health Defense (CHD) as a reporter for its daily publication, *The Defender*, I had already become highly acquainted with censorship in its modern-day form. Living in Greece during the decade of its crippling financial crisis, producing and hosting an independent radio program and podcast known as *Dialogos Radio*, I presented narratives which ran contrary to the establishment orthodoxy that 'there is no alternative' to severe economic austerity. In sharing such narratives, I placed myself in the firing line on social media. Anonymous trolls were one issue, but it was those operating eponymously that really crossed the line, including 'foreign correspondents' for 'reputable' media outlets—who, acting with the impunity that comes with the knowledge that you're protected— brazenly harassed and slandered me.

'Covidian' censorship, therefore, did not surprise me. Writing for *The Defender*, I have seen countless articles of ours, including some of mine, receive fact-free 'fact-checks,' and I have seen CHD gradually deplatformed from many social media sites. In an increasingly polarized world where the balance of power is highly uneven, those who hold that power have the disproportionate ability not just to control the narrative, but to manipulate it—and to stigmatize, ridicule, marginalize, censor, and eliminate any opposing voice.

If indeed you've felt, at any time over the past three-plus years, that the mainstream media seem to be operating in 'lock step,' you are not far off the mark. A lawsuit filed by CHD and other entities that have also been at the receiving end of COVID-era censorship, alleges precisely this. On May 31, 2023, CHD, Creative Destruction Media, *Trial Site News*, Ty and Charlene Bollinger (founders of *The Truth About Cancer* and *The Truth About Vaccines*), independent journalist Ben Swann, Erin Elizabeth Finn (publisher of *Health Nut News*), Jim Hoft (founder and editor-in-chief of *The Gateway Pundit*), Dr. Joseph Mercola, and chiropractor Ben Tapper filed a groundbreaking novel lawsuit against the Trusted News Initiative (TNI), making antitrust and constitutional free speech claims.[1]

This represents a refiling of a lawsuit first filed by the above parties, plus Robert F. Kennedy, Jr., in January 2023. The initial lawsuit was filed in U.S. District Court, Northern District of Texas, Amarillo Division[2], but was voluntarily withdrawn by the plaintiffs after the presiding judge mistakenly transferred the case, following a motion by the defendants for a change of venue. The new lawsuit is essentially identical, sans the participation of Kennedy, who is now chairman on leave of CHD after declaring his candidacy for the 2024 U.S. presidential election. Kennedy, however, remains involved in the case as volunteer counsel for CHD. The new lawsuit was also filed in a different court: the U.S. District Court for the Western District of Louisiana, Monroe Division. This is significant, as the same court is currently hearing three other censorship cases, including another CHD case: *Kennedy v. Biden,* a class action lawsuit filed March 24, 2023 against President Biden, Dr. Anthony Fauci, and other top U.S. government officials and federal agencies, alleging the defendants "waged a systematic, concerted campaign" to compel the three largest social media platforms to censor constitutionally protected speech.[3] I covered the TNI lawsuit for *The Defender* when it was first filed in January 2023, closely reviewing the legal documents and interviewing several of the plaintiffs.[4]

TNI is a self-described "industry partnership" launched in March 2020 by several of the world's largest news organizations, including the BBC, The Associated Press (AP), Reuters, and *The Washington Post*— all of whom are named as defendants. The lawsuit alleges they partnered with Big Tech firms to "collectively censor online news," including stories about COVID-19 not aligned with official narratives. Aside from the named defendants, "core partners" of the TNI include Agence France Press (AFP), CBC/Radio-Canada, the European Broadcasting Union (EBU), the *Financial Times*, *First Draft*, Google/YouTube, *The Hindu*, *The Nation* Media Group, Meta, Microsoft, the Reuters Institute for the Study of Journalism, and Twitter.

All of the plaintiffs allege that they were censored, banned, deplatformed, 'shadow banned,' or otherwise penalized by the Big Tech firms partnering with the TNI, as their content was deemed 'misinformation' or 'disinformation.' The lawsuit further alleges that TNI's legacy media and Big Tech firms would act in concert to remove such voices from their platforms. As the plaintiffs argued, such censorship resulted in a major loss of visibility and revenue for their content and limited the wider dissemination of COVID-related counternarratives. As described by Mary Holland, president on leave of CHD, TNI operates "a global media monopoly in the English language." Jed Rubenfeld, lead attorney for the plaintiffs, said "When social media companies collude with government to censor critics of government policy, that violates the First Amendment. When they collude with major mainstream news organizations to censor rival online news publishers, that violates antitrust law."

The plaintiffs allege violations of the Sherman Antitrust Act based on evidence of horizontal agreement and economic collusion among the defendants and Big Tech firms. While only the TNI and its founding members are named as defendants, Big Tech firms prominently figure in the case. As the lawsuit alleges a conspiracy between the TNI and its media outlets on the one hand, and the Big Tech firms on the other, any successful finding of a conspiracy between these entities would likely hold them all liable. This strategy also bypasses legally binding arbitration provisions Big Tech platforms impose in their terms of service.

The lawsuit states that "The TNI exists to, in its own words, 'choke off' and 'stamp out' online news reporting that the TNI or any of its members peremptorily deems 'misinformation.'" According to the lawsuit:

> TNI members have targeted and suppressed completely accurate online reporting by non-mainstream news publishers [and] have deemed the following to be 'misinformation' that could not be published on the world's dominant Internet platforms: (A) reporting that COVID may have originated in a laboratory in Wuhan, China; (B) reporting that the COVID vaccines do not prevent infection; (C) reporting that vaccinated persons can transmit COVID to others; and (D) reporting that compromising emails and videos were found on a laptop belonging to Hunter Biden"—[stories that were] true or, at a minimum, well within the ambit of legitimate reporting.

"Moreover," states the lawsuit, TNI members "publicly declared—categorically, as if it were established fact—that the lab-leak hypothesis of COVID's origins was 'false.'" Lending credence to the plaintiffs' claims, soon after the lawsuit against TNI was filed, the FBI, the Department of Energy, and the State Department all began publicly supporting the "Wuhan lab leak" theory. The lawsuit goes on to claim that "The TNI did not only prevent Internet users from making these claims; it shut down online news publishers who simply reported that such claims were being made by potentially credible sources, such as scientists and physicians." As a result, "TNI members not only suppressed competition in the online news market but deprived the public of important information on matters of the highest public concern."

The lawsuit further alleges collusion—a "group boycott" in legal terms—stating that "TNI members confer and coordinate in making their censorship decisions," noting that "TNI members' parallel treatment of prohibited claims further evidences concerted action" by "engaging in strikingly similar viewpoint-based censorship of plausible, legitimate news reporting relating to COVID-19." As an example of this, the lawsuit references a March 2022 statement by Jamie Angus, then-senior news controller for BBC News, who explained TNI's "strategy to beat disinformation":[5]

Of course, the members of the Trusted News Initiative are ... rivals ... But in a crisis situation like this, absolutely, organizations have to focus on the things they have in common, rather than ... their commercial ... rivalries. ... [I]t's important that trusted news providers club together. Because actually, the real rivalry now is not between, for example, the BBC and CNN globally, it's actually between all trusted news providers and a tidal wave of unchecked [reporting] that's being piped out mainly through digital platforms. ... That's the real competition now in the digital media world.

Perhaps unsurprisingly, Angus has since left the BBC to take a position with Saudi Arabia's state-owned television broadcaster.[6] Saudi Arabia ranked 166th out of 180 countries in Reporters Without Borders' Press Freedom Index for 2022.[7]

The lawsuit refers to Supreme Court precedent—specifically, a 1945 ruling in *Associated Press v. United States*,[8] where a news industry partnership of that era, led by the AP, "prevented non-members from publishing certain stories." Non-members sued under the Sherman Act, and despite AP's claim that *its* arguments were the ones protected by the First Amendment, the court sided with the plaintiffs. In the majority opinion, Justice Felix Frankfurter wrote that the First Amendment:

> ... rests on the assumption that the widest possible dissemination of information from diverse and antagonistic sources is essential to the welfare of the public, that a free press is a condition of a free society.

> Surely a command that the government itself shall not impede the free flow of ideas does not afford non-governmental combinations a refuge if they impose restraints upon that constitutionally guaranteed freedom.

> Freedom to publish means freedom for all, and not for some. Freedom to publish is guaranteed by the Constitution, but freedom to combine to keep others from publishing is not. Freedom of the press from governmental interference under the First Amendment does not sanction repression of that freedom by private interests.

Returning to Big Tech, the lawsuit describes the TNI's Big Tech members as "platform gatekeepers," with the power to cripple or destroy publishers by excluding them from their platforms." It was noted by the plaintiffs, for instance, that "TNI members agreed in early 2020 that their 'ground-breaking collaboration' would target online news relating to COVID-19 and that TNI members would 'work together to ... ensure [that] harmful disinformation myths are stopped in their tracks'"[9] and "jointly [combat] fraud and misinformation about the virus."[10] These efforts included the development of a "shared early warning system of rapid alerts" to quickly identify and remove 'disinformation.'[11] The nature of this "shared early warning system of rapid alerts" was described as "the only place in the world where disinformation is discussed in real time" by Jessica Cecil, founder and then-head of TNI and former chief of staff for the BBC who, in a clear indication of the 'revolving door' among such entities, now works for the Reuters Institute for the Study of Journalism.

The lawsuit noted Cecil's admission that TNI's members, at "closed-door" meetings and through inter-firm communications, "signed up to a clear set of expectations on how to act" upon such "misinformation" and "disinformation." Moreover, the lawsuit also alleges TNI's Big Tech partners often knowingly removed or otherwise blocked content they knew was true. For instance, at a TNI presentation titled "Big Tech's Part in the Fight," Nathaniel Gleicher, a senior Meta information moderation officer, said "it was a mistake to think of 'misinformation' as consisting solely of 'false claims,' because a great deal of it is 'not provably false.'"[12]

The lawsuit alleges that the collusion was so all-encompassing that it expanded beyond just the confines of TNI and its Big Tech partners. One example involves payment processors such as PayPal and Stripe—known for their sanctimonious stance vis-à-vis several categories of perfectly legal transactions—who banned several of the lawsuit's plaintiffs, including CHD and Creative Destruction Media, soon after social media suspensions or bans were levied against these organizations. The lawsuit refers to the "temporal proximity" of such actions, suggesting they were coordinated.

More examples of censorship are referenced in the lawsuit. One involves Dr. Joseph Mercola, who was deplatformed by YouTube on September 29, 2021. Mercola learned of this via a *Washington Post* article published that morning[13]—*before* he was notified by YouTube. As part of my own research, I discovered that the *Washington Post* later changed the timestamp of the article to a time later that day. However, the *Internet Archive* has preserved the original article with the original timestamp,[14] which itself has been memorialized for posterity on *archive.ph*.[15]

The discovery process in a lawsuit filed by the attorneys general of Missouri and Louisiana against the Biden administration,[16] also revealed a memo from Meta detailing efforts to reduce the visibility of CHD content, while a White House email to Twitter revealed a demand for one of Kennedy's tweets to be "removed ASAP." Kennedy's January 22, 2021 tweet concerned the death of baseball great Hank Aaron, 18 days after he received the Moderna vaccine, describing Aaron's death as "suspicious."[17] This tweet was 'fact-checked' by *The New York Times* based on the claim that the medical examiner who examined Aaron confirmed his death was unrelated to the COVID-19 vaccination. Kennedy subsequently spoke with the medical examiner and discovered that he had not examined Aaron's body. In March 2023, these revelations were further confirmed via a 'Twitter files' release focusing on the activities of the 'Virality Project,' an initiative of the Stanford Internet Observatory which collaborated with the Biden administration and social media platforms.[18] The Virality Project categorized true stories of vaccine-injured individuals as "actionable content," developed a "Rumor Control" proposal (subsequently adopted by the U.S. Food and Drug Administration, or FDA) to combat 'misinformation,'[19] and called for the creation of a government 'disinformation' body—one day before the Biden administration did so.

This is far from the only instance where the federal government censored content. The FDA, for instance, argued that it needed 75 years to fulfill a Freedom of Information Act (FOIA) request to release 400,000-plus pages of documents pertaining to the Emergency Use Authorization (EUA) issued to the Pfizer-BioNTech COVID-19 vaccine.[20] When a federal court ruled that the FDA would have eight months instead of 75 years to release these files,[21] Pfizer (unsuccessfully) asked to "intervene" in the files' release—with the FDA's support.[22] These files became known as the "Pfizer Documents," revealing multiple irregularities—and deaths—during the vaccine trials.[23] Similarly, the U.S. Centers for Disease Control and Prevention (CDC) attempted to stonewall a FOIA request for the release of data regarding adverse events following COVID-19 vaccination collected via the V-safe app.[24] Several lawsuits and a court order later, the data was released, revealing over 3.35 million adverse events that were reported out of approximately 10 million people who submitted reports to the app.[25] The federal government also refused to intervene in a lawsuit filed by whistleblower Brook Jackson, who worked at one of the Pfizer-BioNTech COVID-19 vaccine trial sites, claiming that under the False Claims Act, such lawsuits could be dismissed even if fraud was proven, as long as the federal government continued paying for the product in question.[26] This argument was successful, as the suit was dismissed.[27] And the *Kennedy v. Biden* lawsuit lists several allegations of government censorship, including "substantial evidence of coordinated efforts by Fauci and others to suppress the lab-leak theory,"[28] "threats by congressional representatives, senators and Biden to break up Big Tech if they did not improve censorship practices,"[29][30][31] and 'Twitter files' documents, news reports, and documents received through Freedom of Information Act requests that have shown evidence of numerous and ongoing White House communications with Facebook, Twitter, and Google about how to take action against 'misinformation' related to COVID-19. It would therefore not be inaccurate to say that, as taxpayers, we are paying for our own censorship.

However, as the 'Twitter files' and the TNI lawsuit have shown, such broad censorship would not have been possible without the collusion of private actors, including the media—and academia. The case of New York University (NYU) media studies professor Mark Crispin Miller (a member of my dissertation committee who was, by far, the most supportive of my research—some other members no longer even respond to me) is indicative, as he was ostracized by NYU's administration and his peers simply for asking students in his propaganda course to examine peer-reviewed literature from both sides of the 'mask debate.'[32] A November 2022 study, "Censorship and Suppression of COVID-19 Heterodoxy: Tactics and Counter-Tactics," found that scientists and academics who countered establishment COVID-19 narratives were habitually censored, defunded, or fired.[33] My own experience as an academic has confirmed this, as at one institution where I was previously affiliated, my request regarding a legally recognized medical exemption resulted in hostility towards me and, ultimately, the non-renewal of my contract.

Under such conditions, it is no surprise that society has, in recent years, become more polarized and divided. This is so because such polarization and division have been imposed from the top. While many are (rightly) disenchanted with the legal system, in a society where not all sides are heard on an equal playing field, exercising our legal and constitutional rights via the legal system—and pressuring it to enforce the law and the constitution—becomes imperative.

Endnotes

[1] https://childrenshealthdefense.org/wp-content/uploads/Trusted-News-Initiative-Louisiana-Complaint-Dkt-1-05-31-2023.pdf

[2] https://childrenshealthdefense.org/defender/lawsuit-trusted-news-initiative-antitrust-first-amendment-censoring-covid-content/

[3] This lawsuit has now been consolidated with Missouri v. Biden. See https://childrenshealthdefense.org/defender/chd-lawsuit-consolidate-censorship-big-tech/ and https://childrenshealthdefense.org/defender/lawsuit-rfk-jr-chd-biden-free-speech/

[4] https://childrenshealthdefense.org/defender/lawsuit-trusted-news-initiative-antitrust-first-amendment-censoring-covid-content/

[5] https://www.bbc.co.uk/beyondfakenews/trusted-news-initiative/role-of-the-news-leader

[6] https://www.dailymail.co.uk/news/article-10964951/BBC-chief-Jamie-Angus-leaves-corporation-job-Saudi-state-TV-channel-Al-Arabiya-News.html

[7] https://rsf.org/en/country/saudi-arabia

[8] https://supreme.justia.com/cases/federal/us/326/1/

[9] https://www.bbc.com/mediacentre/2020/trusted-news-initiative-vaccine-disinformation

[10] https://www.usatoday.com/%E2%80%8Cstory/tech/%E2%80%8C2020/03/16/coronavirus-tech-google-microsoft-facebook-misinformation/5064880002

[11] https://www.ebu.ch/%E2%80%8Cnews/2020/07/trusted-news-initiative-steps-up-global-fight-against-disinformation-and-targets-us-presidential-election

[12] https://www.bbc.co.uk/beyondfakenews/trusted-news-initiative/big-tech/

[13] https://www.washingtonpost.com/technology/2021/09/29/youtube-ban-joseph-mercola/

[14] https://web.archive.org/web/20210929133304/https://www.washingtonpost.com/technology/2021/09/29/youtube-ban-joseph-mercola/

[15] https://archive.ph/rZT86

[16] https://nclalegal.org/state-of-missouri-ex-rel-schmitt-et-al-v-biden-et-al/

[17] https://twitter.com/robertkennedyjr/status/1352748139665645569

[18] https://childrenshealthdefense.org/defender/twitter-files-virality-project-covid-misinformation/

[19] https://childrenshealthdefense.org/defender/fda-robert-califf-combat-misinformation/

[20] https://childrenshealthdefense.org/defender/fda-75-years-release-pfizer-vaccine-documents/

[21] https://childrenshealthdefense.org/defender/fda-eight-months-produce-pfizer-safety-data/

[22] https://childrenshealthdefense.org/defender/pfizer-fda-delay-release-covid-vaccine-safety-data/

[23] https://phmpt.org/pfizers-documents/

[24] https://childrenshealthdefense.org/defender/cdc-data-covid-vaccine-injuries-vsafe-app/

[25] https://childrenshealthdefense.org/defender/women-covid-vaccine-injuries-v-safe-data/

[26] https://childrenshealthdefense.org/defender/pfizer-whistleblower-lawsuit-fraud/

[27] https://childrenshealthdefense.org/defender/pfizer-whistleblower-brook-jackson-lawsuit-dismissal-fraud/

[28] https://childrenshealthdefense.org/defender/emails-nih-virologists-covid-lab-leak-theory-rtk/

[29] https://www.wsj.com/articles/save-the-constitution-from-big-tech-11610387105

[30] http://www.warner.senate.gov/public/index.cfm/%E2%80%8C2020/10/statement-of-sen-mark-r-warner-on-facebook-s-decision-to-finally-ban-qanon-from-its-platform

[31] https://www.whitehouse.gov/briefing-room/press-briefings/2021/05/05/press-briefing-by-press-secretary-jen-psaki-and-secretary-of-agriculture-tom-vilsack-may-5-2021/

[32] https://childrenshealthdefense.org/defender/covid-mask-vaccine-mandates-cities/

[33] https://link.springer.com/article/10.1007/s11024-022-09479-4

Did these chapters help you in some way? If so, we would love to hear your honest opinion. Please rate and review "Canary In a Covid World" on Amazon.

CHAPTER 8

I Believe Fraud Has Occurred at Pfizer

Edward Dowd

Former Wall Street analyst and Blackrock portfolio manager & author of "Cause Unknown: The Epidemic of Sudden Deaths in 2021 & 2022."

Edward Dowd is currently a Founding Partner of Phinance Technologies, a global macro alternative investment firm. He is also author of the new book, *"Cause Unknown: The Epidemic of Sudden Deaths in 2021 & 2022."* (Release Date: Dec 13, 2022, Skyhorse Publishing). Edward has worked on Wall Street most of his career, spanning both credit markets and equity markets. Some of the firms he worked for include HSBC, Donaldson Lufkin & Jenrette and Independence Investments. Most notably, he was promoted to Managing Director at Blackrock, where he managed a growth equity portfolio, increasing it from $2 billion over a ten year span to $14 billion.

This essay is based on an interview between Ed Dowd and Robert F Kennedy Jr. It has been edited for length and clarity and turned into an essay format. It has been included in this book with the generous permission of Ed Dowd.

I believe fraud has occurred at Pfizer. What tipped me off to the fraud was primarily the FDA's decision to hide the data for 75 years. In my world, when I see that, I don't need The Wall Street Journal or The New York Times to tell me fraud has occurred. Throughout my whole career, I've seen fraud, over and over again. I make bets with capital. And my bet was that's fraud. The FDA is in on the cover up.

A friend of mine from the biotech industry discovered that Pfizer had failed their all-cause mortality endpoint and that information was not available to us. When we learned that - it came out in a FOIA request (Freedom of Information Request) - I was aware that if you miss the all-cause mortality endpoint, the drug doesn't get approved. It's the gold standard of the FDA. Well, they missed that endpoint, the vaccine got approved and that's a big deal. I started to really believe that fraud had occurred. And then I started to think, if the FDA is in on it, this reminds me of the great financial crisis of 2008-2009 where the rating agencies became corrupted and allowed that fraud to happen. It's called the institutional imperative where over time an institution acts in the interests of itself rather than its shareholders or in the case of the FDA, the stakeholders. We also know that the FDA has 50% of its budget from the pharmaceutical industry. So I believe over time it's been corrupted.

Then, with this Operation Warp Speed, which I thought was a disaster from the get go; corners cut, things rushed, safety protocols ignored. I knew that anything rushed is writ large with errors. It takes seven to 10 years for a normal vaccine to be tested for safety before it's put into the arms of people. The clinical trial only lasted 28 days, and I knew something was fishy there. I came to the conclusion that the FDA didn't really look at this clinical trial data. They rushed it through due to political pressure. Maybe, straight up bribes; we don't know. But what we do know is that this should never have been approved.

I was able to speak to Brook Jackson, the Ventavis whistleblower who went public in November 2021. Everybody ignored her. The mainstream media ignored her. She called me. What she saw was so much fraud. It was mind boggling.

Jackson oversaw 1,000 patients of the 44,000 patients in the original clinical trials study done by Pfizer. All of them were unblinded, all 1000. When that happens, that data is supposed to be thrown out per Pfizer protocol. But it was not. It was rolled up. When she became aware of this, she alerted more senior people in her company. That's when the tone changed with her. Then, when they wanted her to get involved in a cover up, she went to the FDA, and made an anonymous whistleblower complaint. This happened at nine in the morning. By three in the afternoon, she was fired. Five days later, a Pfizer lawyer reached out to her. She ignored him.

I think there's enough proof for people to investigate fraud in the clinical data and the FDA's complicity in this. I think, unfortunately, we have had to wait for real world evidence. And the real world evidence is so awful that there's going to be a public outcry. Tragically, it's showing up in real world data insurance companies and funeral homes. And this is a disaster. The CDC data, their own data shows what's going on. This is a disaster of epic proportions.

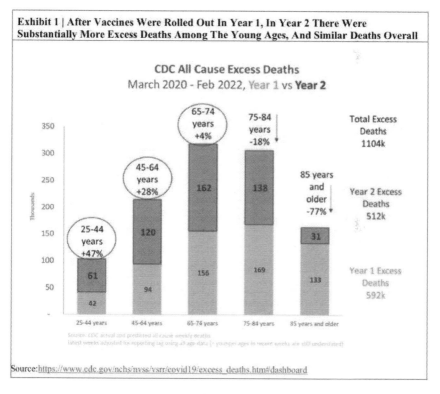

Exhibit 1 | After Vaccines Were Rolled Out In Year 1, In Year 2 There Were Substantially More Excess Deaths Among The Young Ages, And Similar Deaths Overall

Source: https://www.cdc.gov/nchs/nvss/vsrr/covid19/excess_deaths.htm#dashboard

The millennial age group saw 61,000 deaths, excess deaths in a one year time frame, correlated with an acceleration in the mandates and the boosters in the fall of 2021. They just experienced a Vietnam War in a year. I don't know how this is going to be hidden for much longer. Eventually the reckoning will come. I have faith that this is going to come to light and there will be consequences.

This is an excerpt from my book, *Cause Unknown The Epidemic of Sudden Death in 2021 and 2022 (Skyhorse Publishing)*. "By 2017, around 2.8 million Americans died. 2018 was the same again, 2019, about the same again. Not surprisingly, 2020 saw a spike in deaths smaller than you might imagine, some of which could be attributed to COVID and to initial treatment strategies that were not effective. But then in 2021, the stats people expected went off the rails. The CEO of the One American Insurance Company publicly disclosed that during the third and fourth quarters of 2021, death in people of working age, that is 18 to 64 was 40% higher than it was before the pandemic. Significantly, the majority of the deaths were not attributed to COVID."

EXCESS MORTALITY BY DETAILED AGE BAND

Age	Q3 2020	Q4 2020	Q1 2021	Q2 2021	Q3 2021	Q4 2021	Q1 2022	Q2 2022	4/20-6/22	% COVID	Non-COVID %	% Count
0–24	124%	104%	101%	119%	128%	112%	95%	100%	111%	3.1%	7.8%	2%
25–34	132%	121%	118%	132%	179%	136%	122%	123%	132%	11.9%	20.1%	2%
35–44	133%	127%	129%	133%	200%	158%	131%	124%	140%	20.7%	19.1%	4%
45–54	126%	129%	133%	119%	180%	152%	129%	120%	134%	24.3%	10.2%	9%
55–64	123%	129%	129%	114%	153%	140%	125%	112%	127%	21.2%	5.7%	18%
65–74	115%	133%	130%	108%	130%	125%	117%	100%	119%	16.8%	2.6%	17%
75–84	113%	133%	123%	105%	119%	123%	121%	99%	117%	13.0%	3.6%	20%
85+	103%	124%	111%	92%	105%	107%	104%	86%	105%	9.7%	-4.7%	27%
All[11]	115%	128%	123%	107%	134%	127%	117%	102%	119%	15.5%	3.3%	100%

SOA Research- Group Life Covid-19 Mortality Survey Report
https://www.soa.org/4a368a/globalassets/assets/files/resources/research-report/2022/group-life-COVID-19-mortality-03-2022-report.pdf

For the insurance industry, that's equivalent to a one in a 200-year flood. A 10% increase would be a three standard deviation, an unheard of event in the insurance industry. It's such a catastrophic number. And the injuries are going to continue to be created for years. They just poisoned 220 million Americans. This is too far and it's too fast, too much death and injury. Unlike regular life insurance which has had pretty slow, steady rates of death over extended periods of time, the insurance industry did not price this. They make their money off pretty steady death rates and injury rates. The key to their profit is predicting it. Predicting it and then charging a premium that covers the losses that happen.

I got an insurance expert from Wall Street to help me analyze the insurance results. Two PhD physicists are helping me analyze the excess mortality. We have a website called the Humanity Project that has all the excess deaths that have occurred in Europe, UK, Germany, Australia and the U.S. We have the data. We have the evidence and there's a large global murder scene that just occurred. The facts are that excess mortality has risen in 2021, 2022 and continues into 2023.

In 2020 / 2021 I think there were two pandemics. There was the pandemic from COVID and then the vaccine pandemic. Whereas the virus started killing people in 2020, it was primarily older Americans that died. And we're starting to hear that early treatment was suppressed to make way for the vaccine.

So I think about 500,000 Americans died excessively in 2020, mostly old with comorbidities. Had early treatment been allowed, I think we could have avoided a lot of those deaths. So there was a crime in year one, in my humble opinion. In year two, 2021, there was a shift from mostly old people who died in 2020 to 500,000 excess deaths in 2021. The mix shift was from old to young. That's when the young folks started dying. You can see it globally across the Western nations. Below, I show country example after country example of younger age groups suddenly experiencing excess death once mass vaccination was introduced into the country.

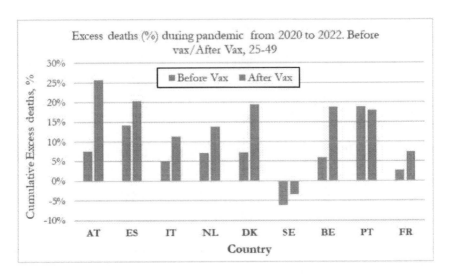

Excess deaths (%) during pandemic from 2020 to 2022. Before vax/After Vax, 25-49

In the U.S. the FDA is critical to this fraud, not least for the doctors who trust the FDA. That's why it's just like the financial crisis with the rating agencies. The rating agencies vetted the bonds, gave them triple-A ratings, and people trusted the rating agency so they didn't look too hard. The doctors who don't read clinical data, trial studies, who don't have backgrounds in statistical analysis, trust the FDA. So the key to this fraud was the FDA regulatory capture. The pharmaceutical industries have done a fabulous job of doing that. That's what occurred with this vaccine. That's why so many of these doctors, when you try to talk to them, and I've tried to talk to some, think I'm crazy. But I've been a cynic my whole life. I know how fraud works and I know how psychopaths work. You corrupt the third party trusted institution.

Some doctors were early to call this because of what they were seeing. I applaud all the frontline doctors who came forward early when they started seeing strange things, but especially in the first year with early treatment and now with vaccines. Doctor Ryan Cole saw in his practice biopsy cancer shooting up in 2022. He's what I call a stock-picker of doctors. He saw a trend. That's what I do for a living; notice trend changes and pattern recognition. Dr. Cole didn't need someone from the CDC or FDA to tell him something was wrong. He figured it out early and said this is a signal.

That's why he's been such a critical voice in all this. Dr. Robert Malone also, these are people that can think by themselves. I would say all the people that have been vilified are critical thinkers. If you don't take the marching orders and you question the orthodoxy you're vilified and pushed aside. This is literally a crisis of critical thinking across all industries.

I've labeled this "total fraud" we've seen with Pfizer. It's a multi-siloed fraud, a conspiracy of interests. It started with Pfizer and Moderna, with the help of the government and the regulators. And then the tech titans and the media titans are complicit, accessories to murder in my mind. That's how I'm seeing it, through their censorship. I believe that they were incentivized by large amounts of ad spend from Pfizer, and we learned that it looks like the government's been giving the media companies money to propagandize the nation into getting the vaccine. They got money to censor.

Let's also not underestimate the influence of intelligence agencies here, because we do know that a lot of these tech titans have contracts with intelligence agencies that they can't disclose. They've had these for years. They'll never talk about these contracts, but we know they're there. Once you sign these secrecy agreements, you essentially become a vassal of the military intelligence agencies or the CIA. I think there's over three million Americans who have signed those. But we know that In-Q-Tel and the CIA focus their investments in Silicon Valley. I suspect undue influence and strong-arming from the intelligence agencies for these guys to censor, because what they said initially about what they wanted to do with their companies is not what they're doing now. They pulled a 180-degree from their original promises to democratize the Internet. Now they've become the primary instrument of control, of authoritarian and totalitarian control.

I have total commitment to this. No fear. I literally don't care what anybody thinks of me, because I know I'm right. And I know that what has happened to our country has been the most awful thing that could ever be imaginable. I have decided I'm not going to live in a world where I'm going to be mandated to take poison.

CHAPTER 9

Interpreting Vaccine Adverse Events Reporting System Data (VAERS) to Show the Harms Caused by COVID-19 Vaccinations

Dr. Jessica Rose

Researcher

Jessica Rose is a Canadian researcher with a Bachelor's Degree in Applied Mathematics and a Master's degree in Immunology from Memorial University of Newfoundland. She also holds a PhD in Computational Biology from Bar Ilan University and 2 Post-Doctoral degrees in Molecular Biology from the Hebrew University of Jerusalem, and in Biochemistry from the Technion Institute of Technology. Her more recent research efforts are aimed at descriptive analyses of the Vaccine Adverse Event Reporting System (VAERS) data in efforts to make this data accessible to the public.

Data analysis has always been a critical component in my academic life. As part of presenting final analyses or experimental results to colleagues, or for publication purposes, data analyses and clear presentation is vital. My role since 2020 has been to clearly and accurately present data in the context of the COVID-19 pandemic, and specifically, in the context of the potential harms of the COVID-19 injectable products.

The COVID-19 mRNA injectable products were rushed through clinical trials. A conventional vaccine typically takes about 10 years to get to market. This timeframe was reduced to less than a year in the context of the COVID-19 injectable products. The rushed trials have been used as the springboard upon which all safety evaluations have been subsequently made and they quite simply and clearly are not sufficient to prove safety or efficacy, as time has revealed.

The exclusion criteria lists for the Phase III clinical trials for the Pfizer and Moderna products was very long. Basically, only people who were healthy and of a certain age requirement were allowed to participate. It has been very difficult for me to understand how anybody could make claims of safety with regard to these products, when there simply wasn't enough time to make this assessment. **Genuine safety testing was not possible.** That is a fact. Furthermore, rather than a two-year follow up of the patients in the trial, in the case of the Pfizer phase III clinical trial, the placebo participants were unblinded and injected with the product, so the placebo group was intentionally lost. This means that any ongoing trial or experimental data being collected would be null and void - it's lost without a placebo group because you have no comparison. At that point, and perhaps many points prior, the trial should have been halted.

In her presentation to the FDA, Rachel Zhang, Team Leader Clinical Review Staff, confirmed that the placebo group was lost and that therefore we can't say anything about efficacy. But what she didn't say is that we can't say anything about safety either. To do this – to inject the placebo group during the Phase III trial was ghastly and is absolutely unprecedented. Furthermore, the (immunological) effects of rushing these trials in the first place and performing them improperly in the context of novel transfection technologies is absolutely unknown.

This is a fact. We do not know the effects – short term or long term. Although, we are beginning to learn the short-term effects through pharmacovigilance. We should have done studies for years, perhaps even decades, to see if this was going to become a problem from a genomic point of view. A quick word on transfection for people who do not know that transfection is not the same thing as exposure to foreign proteins which is the basis of conventional vaccines. We either kill/attenuate a virus or we send in proteins in a carrier package like an innocuous virus. The idea is to get the immune system to mount a response against these proteins such that an immune army is established ready to fight upon challenge with the 'real' virus. But that's very different from the mechanism of action of these COVID-19 injectable products.

As an aside, I really would like to know how many people of the billions who have been injected with these products knew that they were being injected with something that wasn't a traditional vaccine? I can pretty much guarantee that most people didn't know this. I don't even think people know today. Even a lot of medical professionals don't know this because they're turning a blind ear to it when it is merely suggested to them. Because it's been made out to be a conspiracy theory.

According to the United States pharmacovigilance database VAERS, there was enough of a safety signal emitted with respect to death reports to stop the roll-out of these products in January 2021. Yes, just one month after the roll-out began on December 17th, 2020. We had almost 90,000 reports in VAERS spread across many age groups, and almost 700 deaths in the context of just 3 products: the COVID Moderna, Pfizer and Janssen products.

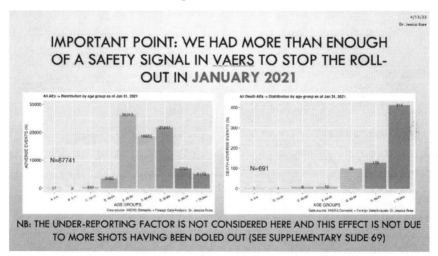

The last time a product went onto the market and killed more than 50 people, that product was pulled. VAERS *functions* as a pharmacovigilance tool, in that when a safety signal is detected, such as was the case in 1999 when a handful of intussusception cases was detected in VAERS, a causality assessment was done, and the rotavirus vaccine was subsequently pulled based on a verdict of 'very likely' causal relationship. This isn't intussusception, this is death. What's the cut off for the number of people who are considered allowed to die, become disabled or have neurological conditions manifest before these products are pulled? Why aren't the CDC and the FDA asking these questions? The owners of this data are **not** asking these questions. Why aren't they doing the assessments that they always have done in the past, such as causality assessments or Bayesian analysis or PRR assessments?

VAERS was introduced 30 years ago essentially as a trade-off for immunity from liability for pharmaceutical companies. We got VAERS, and they got immunity from liability. So if they're not going to be using VAERS as a pharmacovigilance tool now, then I propose that the immunity from liability should also be waived. It only seems fair, does it not?

One of the main problems with VAERS, contrary to what you might have heard, is underreporting. There have been studies done that actually claim that only 1% of reports are ever filed to VAERS. That means for every 100 people who are suffering, only one of them might make a report. I don't know if that's accurate in the COVID-19 context, but there is only a percentage of people who ever file an adverse event report to VAERS.

VAERS is a database that is very easy to access. Anyone can simply download the CSV files for analysis. For the past ten years, the number of adverse event reports has increased slightly. That makes sense because there are more products on the market and there are more shots being administered indicating that there is a proportional increase in the number of reports. What we see in 2021 is not typical and certainly an exceedingly anomalous up-turn in the number of reports. Something is strange there. Something is different. Something is atypical. And there is certainly no way to misinterpret this. This is just what it is – it is raw data. This is a safety signal that you simply cannot ignore.

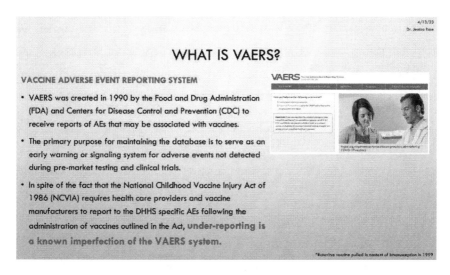

There is a 1,400% increase in file size and 1,300% increase in the number of reports in the domestic set between 2020 and 2021. Again, there is no interpretation required here. These are people who have submitted reports of injury and/or suffering in the context of a biological product that was meant to be prophylactic, for a virus that has a near zero infection fatality rate. There is no age group that is immune from damages or reporting.

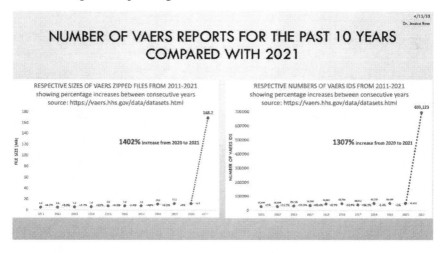

Why are we seeing these adverse events in association with these particular shots? What is in them? The Pfizer and the Moderna products both have specifically modified mRNA. Basically, as we understand the technology today, the mRNA is useless without lipid nanoparticle envelopes (LNPs). This is a very important secondary technology that is also novel in this context. Moderna and Pfizer both have their own recipes for the LNPs. They comprise four lipids each, two of which include polyethylene glycol (PEG) molecules which coat the surface, and cationic lipids, which are notoriously toxic. It has been the bane of the existence of this industry to design cationic lipids for use in humans that are not hyper-toxic. Just at about the same time when we needed them, both of these companies developed ionizable cationic lipids that are allegedly safe for use in humans. In all of my research, I couldn't find safety data sheets that explicitly state that either of these have a version that is safe for use in humans. The safety data sheets, in fact, both explicitly state that these two products are not safe for use in humans or for veterinary use. This remains a big question mark for me.

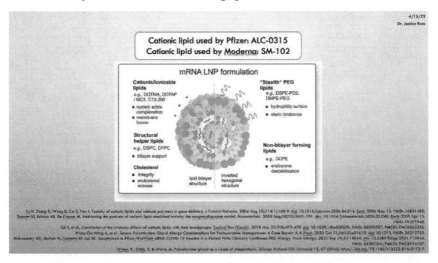

PEG does have a well-documented allergenic profile in humans. It induces anaphylaxis. Cationic lipids have a well-documented toxicity profile. There are many papers that have been published to date that show that both the modified mRNAs and the spike protein are very durable and long lasting in the human body. There are a number of different characteristics of this spike protein that remain questionable from a safety perspective according to published studies. The ubiquitous adverse event reporting and case study reports raise serious and fundamentally vital questions about *the way* in which the spike protein is doing damage, and where the lipid nanoparticles traffic. They have been shown to traffic to the ovaries and accumulate there, and also in the liver which is one of the organs where the LNPs are found at the highest concentrations - second only to the injection site itself. This is problematic for two reasons: complications with both the Renin Angiotensin Aldosterone System (RAAS) and the clotting pathway. The RAAS regulates blood pressure and electrolyte levels.

There might be a common etiology with regard to many of the adverse events that we are seeing submitted to pharmacovigilance databases that revolve around these potential dysfunctions associated with the liver - thrombotic events, clotting and micro-clotting. The reason why I am starting to think that this is absolutely the case is because the liver, our big detox organ, is the place where the LNPs traffic to and accumulate at the highest levels.

The numbers that I report *never* include an underreporting factor. The range of reported adverse event *types* is far greater than has ever been reported in the past for any and all of the vaccines combined. This is also compelling evidence that there is something very different about these shots and that it might be liver-related.

The number of thrombotic adverse event reports in VAERS as of mid-May, 2023 is well into the hundreds of thousands without the underreporting factor, distributed across all ages. No one is immune, not even the babies. All you have to do is talk to clinicians or anyone on the ground. It's ubiquitous right now.

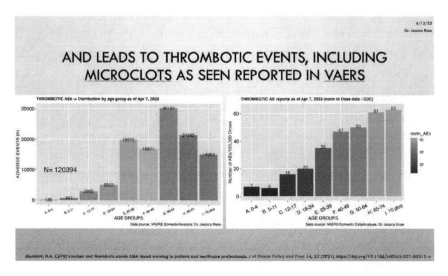

When I began investigating the VAERS data in January 2021, I noticed that there was a systemic nature to the adverse events being reported. It was and is not exclusive to the cardiovascular system or to the neurological system or to the immunological system. The adverse events were involving every system.

Myocarditis is one of the adverse events that has come to the attention of even the lay-person. The VAERS myocarditis reports have a very interesting dose response pattern. There is an approximate four times higher reporting rate of myocarditis in young people – as in, 15 years old – following dose 2. This is most prevalently reported in males. This is a very compelling finding in terms of causality because if there was no causal effect, if there was no impact of subsequent shots, then we would not see this difference. Or at the very least, what else could explain this difference if not a causal effect? This is not seen in any other type of adverse event and this finding is very unique to myocarditis in young children. This is not a secret. Even the CDC has admitted that this is a problem and has amended their website to include warnings about myocarditis as a potential 'side effect.'

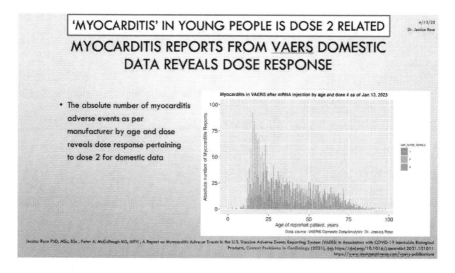

I was lead author on a paper with Dr. Peter McCullough, who is a renowned cardiologist. That paper, entitled *"A Report on Myocarditis adverse events in the U.S. Vaccine Adverse Events Reporting System,"* was accepted in a peer-reviewed journal to be published, but five days before a Vaccines and Related Biological Products Advisory Committee (VRBPAC) meeting to determine whether or not these COVID-19 injectable products should be approved for use in children aged 5 to 11, the journal withdrew our paper. I do not believe in coincidences. I think this was done intentionally to hide the findings.

The thing that breaks my heart the most is that people did not have an opportunity to freely read this paper and to make their own minds up having done so. It is criminally tragic because many children have been injected with the COVID-19 shots unnecessarily (infection fatality rate of next to 0 in children) because their parents thought they were safe and effective because they were told they were. It is a tragedy. There is no other word for it.

We have 1.5 million reports in VAERS, which is a nice sized data set, but it is still just a tip of the iceberg in one dataset.

CHAPTER 10

The Dangers of Self Censorship During The COVID Pandemic

Dr. Joseph Fraiman

Emergency medicine physician and researcher

Dr. Joseph Fraiman is an Emergency Medicine physician currently working in New Orleans, Louisiana, and the surrounding rural region. Dr. Fraiman served as the medical manager of Louisiana's Urban Search and Rescue Disaster Task Force 1. As an independent clinical scientist he researches harm benefit analysis of clinical interventions, and has published analyses linking the COVID-19 mRNA vaccines with serious harm.

At first, I hesitated to contribute a chapter to this book due to the fear of being associated with some of the other authors. It wasn't personal dislike of the other writers, but given that so many of us have had our reputations destroyed these past years, I feared further damage to my own.

It dawned on me that my hesitation was itself a form of self-censorship, and I saw the irony in refusing to write a chapter in a book on censorship. So instead I decided to offer my exploration of self-censorship during the COVID-19 pandemic.

Self-censorship is a common aspect of our daily lives as it is a basic skill we begin to learn in childhood. Toddlers learn that curse words are fun to say, then quickly learn to censor themselves to avoid punishment. As children, most of us read the Emperor's New Clothes, a fable teaching us that too much self-censorship can become dysfunctional. I believe this fable provides a timeless lesson that fits our current moment.

Self-censorship during the COVID pandemic has taken many forms. As a medical professional and scientist, one might assume that I'm immune to such pitfalls, but the opposite is true. Facing fear of professional repercussions, I have downplayed and withheld discussing valid scientific concerns publicly. Other medical professionals have done the same, thus stifling productive debate, preventing critical variables from being evaluated, and creating the illusion of scientific consensus where one may have never existed. The media, taking its cue from the experts, disseminated information that fit a specific narrative, ignoring or ridiculing everything questioning it. Journalists who attempted to challenge the narrative came up against the resistance of their superiors and, more often than not, decided to play it safe. To compound this any expert or publication that dared raise a challenge would be investigated by fact checkers and predictably labeled as misinformation and subsequently censored. Everyday citizens, on the receiving end of this distorted information machine, were left without any previously respected outlet for any well-founded skepticism. A few spoke out and were virtually ostracized from mainstream society. Many others saw the writing on the wall and, wishing to maintain their relationships and avoid uncomfortable situations, kept their opinions to themselves.

In this way, medical professionals, mainstream media, and everyday citizens, combined with the power of fact checkers to label misinformation, created a feedback loop resulting in an overly self-censored society. In the remainder of this chapter, I'll explain these aspects of self-censorship in greater detail through my own experience as a physician and scientist.

***

While today I am an outspoken critic of COVID-19 orthodoxy, I have not always been so. Early in the pandemic, I trusted "the experts." I publicly advocated support for their policies and sometimes an even more aggressive approach. As an Emergency Room Physician, I witnessed first-hand a massive amount of death and devastation caused by COVID-19. The ER doc in me was thinking only about saving lives

– anything to stop the death around me. I became publicly outspoken on the topic, doing interviews with journalists, writing op-eds and publishing in medical journals.

I believed more aggressive measures would save lives. It's interesting to note that every time I offered an opinion criticizing federal policy recommendations as not aggressive enough, I found medical journals and news media more than willing to publish my views, even in cases where the evidence supporting my positions was questionable at best.

Despite publicly calling for more aggressive measures without quality supporting evidence, fact-checkers never censored me, labeled my views as misinformation, nor publicly smeared me. During this time I was easily able to publish in medical journals and in the news media. Many journalists began contacting me for my opinions, and I became friendly with several of them. It wouldn't have occurred to me to hold back or hesitate before sharing my ideas and opinions. However, those advocating for less restrictive measures were fact checked, labeled misinformation spreaders, censored, and publicly smeared as COVID-deniers, anti-maskers, and anti-vaxxers.

Soon, however, it was my turn. I remember the first time I felt the impulse to censor myself on COVID-19 policy. A friend of mine, a teacher, asked me to speak against school reopening at a Louisiana public hearing in the summer of 2020. Initially I had supported school closures, but by this time I was worried that the data demonstrated that school closures were likely more harmful than beneficial for children and society-at-large. But I didn't speak my views at the hearing, or anywhere. I self-censored. I was worried that I did not have enough data to back up my opinions on this topic, even though previously I had felt comfortable advocating for more aggressive policies with considerably less evidence.

***

A few months later, I undertook a study to investigate the mysterious global pattern of COVID-19. Some countries appeared to be suffering far less than others. With two other scientists, we hypothesized that demographics and geography likely explained these unusual patterns. To test our hypothesis, we performed a worldwide analysis. The results of our study[1] explained 82 percent of the national differences in COVID-19 burden, with the major finding suggesting that island nations with aggressive border closures were successfully able to reduce their COVID-19 infection rates. Our results implied restrictive policies could reduce the burden of COVID-19 in island nations. However, for non-island countries, population age and obesity rate were the major determining factors. We realized that if these demographics explained the majority of differences in COVID-19 burden among non-island nations, this strongly suggested policy decisions didn't have much influence on the rate of spread in these countries.

At this point, I was forced to conclude that I was likely wrong to have advocated for more aggressive policies for the U.S., a non-island nation in the months prior. However, had I truly been operating according to my scientific principles and without concern for public perception, I would have spoken out publicly regarding the implications of my own research. Instead, I self-censored.

I told myself I needed more data to support such a radical position. Why did I feel comfortable advocating for more aggressive policies on flimsy evidence, but uncomfortable advocating against these policies with more solid evidence? I did not realize it at the time, but I was experiencing a clear double standard on the evidence; somehow mine wasn't quite good enough, while the limited evidence supporting

---

1   https://www.medrxiv.org/content/medrxiv/early/2021/06/22/2021.06.14.21258886.full.
     pdf

more aggressive measures rolled out across the nation by the "experts" *was* more than adequate.

***

There is a political science term called the Overton Window, which gives us a way to understand that there is a range of viewpoints believed to be "acceptable" to mainstream society. Current policy is considered to be at the center of this window. Views on both sides of this window are "popular," while views a little farther from the center and existing policy are "sensible" and those still farther, "acceptable." However, views just outside the Overton Window are termed "radical;" and views even farther are termed "unthinkable." In most contexts, people who hold views outside the window censor themselves in public to avoid backlash.

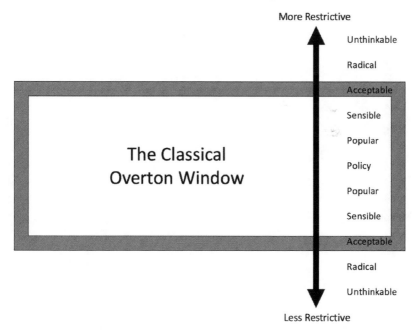

Looking back on the evolution of my opinions regarding COVID-19 policy, the Overton Window provides a useful model that shows how social pressures came to bear on many of my viewpoints. Furthermore, the COVID pandemic was a unique socio-political event in that it distorted the shape of the Overton Window itself. While the normal window of acceptable attitudes and policies occurs in both directions with the 'radical' and 'unacceptable' extremes at both sides, the Overton Window during the pandemic was unidirectional, in that any policy or attitude that was less restrictive than current policy was immediately deemed 'radical' or 'unthinkable' and would often garner epithets like "COVID-denier" or "grandma-killer." Meanwhile, it was infinite, in that on the other side, policies and attitudes remained in the window of acceptability no matter how restrictive the policy or attitude was. In other words, as long as it was seen as a tool to reduce transmission of the virus, it remained in the Window. Thus, when the COVID-19 vaccine was developed and initially sold as the ultimate tool to stop transmission, it fit squarely into this unidirectional Overton Window, while anyone raising questions or concerns regarding its efficacy or potential harm fell outside the Window.

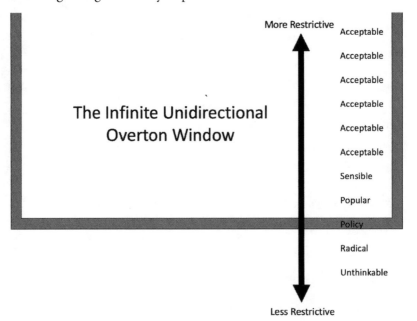

Here's an example that will make this idea more concrete. When the Pfizer vaccine was authorized by the FDA in December 2020, I read the FDA briefing in full and put together a summary for a physician-run site called TheNNT.com. In my review of the Pfizer FDA briefing, I noticed a strangely worded portion in which they discussed, "suspected but unconfirmed," COVID-19 cases, of which there were thousands, raising serious questions on the efficacy of the vaccine. Initially, I was reluctant to speak out, as I was concerned that raising the issue prematurely could unnecessarily cause vaccine hesitancy. I felt that I needed to confirm if this was a problem worth discussing. Expressing this concern with various scientists, we understood the potential seriousness of the issue and I was put in touch with Biden's COVID vaccine Chief Officer David Kessler through email. Kessler assured me this was not an issue, but would not offer the data. I was not reassured. After being denied this data directly from the President's Chief Officer, I decided I had done my due diligence and was ready to pursue this inquiry on its scientific merits.

My concern was that overestimating efficacy could result in more reckless COVID behavior, subsequently increasing transmission. However, I was unable to get anything published on the topic in medical journals or news op-eds. This surprised me for two reasons: First, up to that point, any report that raised concerns of increased transmission of the virus would have received immediate media attention; and second, other prominent scientists had already felt the issue was important enough to bring it to the attention of the country's highest authority on the topic.

Despite these setbacks, I continued writing papers highlighting the lack of evidence the vaccines reduced transmission, and raising concerns about the longevity of protection that they offered. I continued to get rejected from publication after publication. Next, I contacted the same journalists who had been calling me earlier in the pandemic and a predictable pattern emerged. At first they would show immediate interest, but soon after, their enthusiasm would evaporate. I began to lose hope that I would successfully publish on any of these topics in a medical journal or newspaper.

This was my first run-in with the "publishing firewall", which is what I call the barrier that prevents the dissemination of ideas that fall outside the distorted unidirectional Overton Window. It seems that the Window had shifted so that it had become unacceptable to even raise questions regarding the safety and efficacy of COVID vaccines, presumably because the COVID vaccines were touted to reduce transmission of the virus.

Around this time, I didn't see any articles in any major medical journal or major newspapers that raised these concerns. One exception worth noting was Dr. Peter Doshi. He was able to publish articles on these controversial topics in The BMJ, a top medical journal where he also served as an editor. However, it was his role as editor at BMJ that allowed him to bypass the firewall; thus, he was an exception that proved the rule.

But given that I was not an editor at a medical journal, the media firewall crushed my spirit and drove me to an entirely different form of self-censorship. I no longer censored myself due to fear of repercussions or a false sense of not having enough evidence, but simply to stop wasting time.

***

My experience as a doctor has taught me that novel medications often fail to deliver on their optimistic promises and it is not until later that we learn they are more harmful or less beneficial than initially believed. That said, other than this general concern regarding all novel medications, when the vaccines were first authorized, I didn't harbor any specific safety concerns.

My concerns for COVID-19 vaccine safety became much more specific in April 2021 when it was discovered that the spike protein was a toxic component of COVID-19, which explained why the virus caused such diverse harmful effects such as heart attacks, blood clots, diarrhea, strokes, and bleeding disorders. This discovery prompted me to design a study that re-analyzed the original trials and took a magnifying glass to the data regarding reported serious harm. Lo and behold, the preliminary results suggested that in the original trials there was evidence the vaccines were causing serious harm at a level higher than previously recognized. Given my past experiences, I was not optimistic at this point that I'd be able to publish, so I tried to hand off the study to Peter Doshi, the very editor at The BMJ who had shown success publishing on these controversial topics previously. In the end, he convinced me to stay on and work with him.

We put together a team of seven internationally renowned scientists. Along with myself and Peter Doshi were Juan Erviti, Mark Jones, Sander Greenland, Patrick Whelan, and Robert M Kaplan. Our findings were highly concerning. We soon found that the mRNA COVID-19 vaccines in the original trial could be causing serious harm at a rate of 1 in 800.

Prior to publication, we sent the paper to the FDA to alert them of our concerning findings. Several top FDA officials met with us to discuss the study, indicating that they recognized its significance. Despite that interest from the policy-makers, we still came up against the publishing firewall as our paper was rejected by journal after journal. It was only after much persistence that we were able to publish the paper in the peer-reviewed journal, *Vaccine*[2].

---

2   https://www.medrxiv.org/content/medrxiv/early/2021/06/22/2021.06.14.21258886.full. pdf

Now with a carefully performed study published in a preeminent journal, I learned about some of the other drivers that encourage experts to censor themselves : public smearing, misinformation labels, and reputation destruction. As I will show, these forces were being driven in part by a dysfunctional system of media fact checking that ironically suppressed scientific debate in favor of accepted narratives.

It's easy to forget that before 2020, fact checking played a very different role in our media and journalism. Traditionally, a fact check article might appear as a corollary to the original article for readers who doubted or wanted to verify its credibility. This meant that the reader would read the original article and then, if they were curious, read the fact check, coming to their own opinion on the balance of two or more sources. According to a 2016 national survey[3], less than one third of Americans trusted fact checkers, so it wasn't even a given that a critical fact checking piece would spell doom for the original article. Furthermore, fact checks rarely, if ever, weighed in definitively on controversial medical science claims.

This model had already started to change with the dominance of social media, but the pandemic, and with it the 'infodemic,' accelerated this transformation. In response to growing concerns of misinformation on social media, fact checkers and social media companies stepped up their efforts to control it. They began displaying misinformation labels on article links and outright preventing people from seeing and/or spreading articles deemed 'misinformation.' With this newly granted power, fact checkers became our society's arbiters of scientific truth, tasked with separating fact from fiction.

Science is not a collection of facts. It is a process that allows us to better understand the world around us. This might come as a surprise

3   https://www.rasmussenreports.com/public_content/politics/general_politics/september_2016/voters_don_t_trust_media_fact_checking

to those of us who were taught scientific 'truths' in the classroom that we had to memorize for tests, but in reality, medical science is premised on uncertainty. Generations of medical school students have been told: "Half of what we taught you is wrong; the only problem is we don't know which half." The point is that no one, not even the world's top medical scientists, can determine absolute truth. Yet, fact-checkers were tasked with just this, and in their effort to do so they confused confident expert opinion for facts, when expert opinions are not facts. Indeed, even a consensus of medical experts is not a fact.

For these reasons, fact checking is a flawed system even in the most ideal circumstances. Once political context and unavoidable bias are taken into consideration though, the situation becomes even more concerning. At the outset of the pandemic, the pattern that emerged was that only certain types of statements and articles were getting fact-checked. Specifically, articles that contradicted or challenged official policy tended to face relentless scrutiny from fact-checkers, while the original government statements themselves somehow evaded fact-checking altogether. For example, in March 2021, CDC director Rochelle Walensky stated that vaccinated people, "don't carry the virus," and "don't get sick." Fact checkers did not write articles investigating the validity of Walensky's statement. Yet, months later when this quote was mocked on social media videos and posts, fact checkers saw it as necessary to publish articles[4] describing these social media posts (which were mocking a false statement from a federal official) as misleading. The fact-checkers argued that Walensky's statement was taken out of context and reminded us that CDC data showed that the vaccine reduced hospitalizations and death. However, neither of these defenses spoke to the effect of the vaccine on transmission rates and so neither one refuted the fact that Walensky's original statement was false and should

---

4   https://www.reuters.com/article/factcheck-walensky-clips-idUSL1N2PX1IZ

have been subjected to at least the same level of scrutiny as social media posts made months later. Nonetheless, the social media[5] posts mocking Walensky's statement were subsequently either censored or subjected to a 'false information' warning label while her original statement never received[6] such treatment.

Interestingly, the only examples I have found where people challenged government policies and statements and did not garner aggressive fact checks were those that advocated *more* restrictive policies. In this way, fact-checking decisions mirrored the distorted unidirectional Overton Window that I had come across previously.

As one would expect, these dynamics have helped to create the illusion of 'scientific consensus' which is actually just a case of circular logic. Here's how it works. A federal agency makes a statement, which is then criticized or challenged by a scientist, journalist, or viral social media post. Fact checkers then ask the federal agency about the veracity of their original statement. The agency predictably claims that their statement is accurate and those challenging it are incorrect. The fact checker then goes to the experts to verify the agency's claim. The experts, who by now instinctively understand which answers are safe and which ones risk reputational harm, confirm the agency's claim. The result is that fact-checking agencies consistently label articles and statements outside the unidirectional Overton Window as 'misinformation'. In this manner, government 'expert opinions' morph into 'facts' and dissenting opinions are stifled.

This is how our paper, with its carefully worded conclusion that "these results raise concerns that mRNA vaccines are associated with more harm than initially estimated at the time of emergency authorization," written by a team of internationally renowned scientists,

---

5   https://www.instagram.com/p/CS8yaqvBG1s/?img_index=1

6   https://www.instagram.com/p/CNIbj2upfWz/

peer-reviewed by experts in the field, and published in a preeminent journal of vaccinology, got slapped with a 'misinformation' label and censored on social media.

***

At this point, it's important to consider how the unidirectional Overton Window, the publishing firewall, and the fact checking feedback loop all work together to create an ecosystem that engulfs medical professionals, media figures, and everyday citizens.

For healthcare professionals and scientists, a 'misinformation' label given by a fact checker can serve as a scarlet letter, destroying reputations and threatening careers. As a response to these negative incentives, healthcare experts with critical views of existing policy often do the most natural and reasonable thing: they censor themselves. The result of this is that the exact experts on whom we rely to provide us with unbiased, science-based information are themselves compromised.

Now consider the journalist who gets their COVID information from the experts. Even if we presume that they are operating according to the most thorough methodologies and reporting with an open mind and the best intentions, they are most likely only going to be able to find experts promulgating opinions within the distorted Overton Window. In addition to eliminating valid scientific ideas that fall outside the Window, this has the effect of manufacturing a consensus even if one doesn't exist. Furthermore, even for the intrepid journalist who *is* able to find an expert opinion outside the Window, they will most likely find that their boss is unwilling to publish something that will probably get labeled as misinformation and hurt their organization's bottom line.

Finally, consider the effect on the everyday citizen who is listening to these experts and consuming the products of these media companies.

Given all the filters that have distorted the information to this point, it's no wonder that the range of acceptable opinions on the pandemic is so narrow that it creates the illusion of a scientific consensus. Furthermore, we now have a clearer picture of why everyday citizens might feel the need to self-censor, even if they have a well-founded, thoroughly examined, scientifically-based opinion. After all, if the "expert consensus" that is being communicated by the media is able to say confidently, for example, that the COVID vaccines prevent transmission of the virus, that means that any conflicting opinion on the matter must be 'misinformation.'

***

All of us self-censor every day. Sometimes we withhold statements that might hurt the feelings of a loved one; other times we refrain from offering an unpopular opinion when around friends; often we express our views in a way we think others will find more palatable. All of this is understandable and, to a certain extent, unavoidable. When a global pandemic upended the way of life for virtually every person on the planet, these patterns were bound to play out on a larger scale. That, too, to a certain extent, is understandable. However, hundreds of years ago our ancestors devised an ingenious method to help us reduce uncertainty in a highly complex world. This method differed from prior belief systems in that, instead of deferring to authorities who claimed a monopoly on absolute knowledge, it acknowledged, and even celebrated uncertainty.

The method was not a blanket defense for something we *want* to be true, nor a reframed version of what we previously believed. This was science, an evolving method of questioning and still the most effective tool we've devised to gain information about the world around us. When experts fail to live up to their scientific duties because they are stuck in their own self-perpetuating cycles of self-censorship, it is detrimental to the cause of science. I am one of those experts who failed to live up to my scientific duties and I value science above all else, yet *still* I failed to live up to my own standards of truth-seeking. Consider what that means on a mass scale when even the most staunch proponents of science can be made hesitant in the face of societal pressures. Now consider what kind of society we want to live in and ask yourself: what duty does each of us have to make that a reality?

I propose it is time we all yell out loud "The Emperor has no clothes!"

CHAPTER 11

Cruel Seasons

Trish Wood

Producer, director and investigative journalist formerly
of CBC's The Fifth Estate, she now hosts Trish Wood
is Critical, a popular podcast on critical thinking

Trish Wood is an award-winning former science journalist, producer and director, who started her podcast Trish Wood is Critical, in May of 2020 to counter Covid 19 propaganda. She has hosted CBC's flagship investigative broadcast The Fifth Estate for ten years, wrote an acclaimed book about the Iraq War and produced investigative true crime documentaries, including Ted Bundy: Falling for a Killer for Amazon Studios. She lives in Toronto, Canada.

In March of 2020, just as the gates surrounding the free world were slamming shut, I sent an email to an American journalist I didn't know but who had a reputation for critical thinking. Desperate to prick a hole in the ballooning lockdown narrative, I supplied him with strong evidence it was a dangerous mistake.

It was an attempt to, perhaps tamp down the COVID-19 hysteria that was setting up house in virtually all of our institutions, especially legacy media. Aside from a few outlying grumps, like me, my former industry went *all-in* on the government's obscene gambit of jacked-up fear messaging designed to scare us into obedience.

Even the mighty Joe Rogan faltered briefly. Early in the pandemic he interviewed Dr. Michael Osterholm – who downplayed risk stratification, suggesting all of us were vulnerable. It was an unfortunate misstep for Rogan but he has since redeemed himself many times over and he is one of the few who changed course based on clear-headed analysis.

My email note, time-stamped March 18th, 2020, warned of Dr. Anthony Fauci's history: dissembling and playing politics with pathogens and the humans they affect. It was based on my experience reporting on Fauci during the AIDS crisis. I had come away from that story traumatized by the death count and the callousness, ego and incompetence of the man running the response. Here is part of what I wrote:

Doctors and scientists are as vulnerable to groupthink, hubris and greed as any other profession. Treating them as Gods, not to be questioned, and handing them the reins to public health policy and the world's economy without accountability is absolute folly. I watch as every news program takes without question or accountability, pronouncements that have no underpinnings in actual data.

I had hoped that reaching out might prompt a phone call and a chance to discuss what I knew, but I never heard back.

In fact, the journalist to whom I'd reached out kept his head down for three years, not questioning the official line and even publicly supporting vaccines. He was a dutiful narrative stitcher, like the rest of legacy media who collected their paychecks by reporting uncritically whatever the government was saying.

Media played along with CDC, NIH and any of the seemingly hypnotized scientists developing a side hustle in television as *talking heads* – fawned over by facile anchors while working to buttress the official narrative. I suspect few of the media's go-to experts are worried about future funding which flows from the very officials they avoided critiquing.

The architects of the pandemic game plan needed the public to believe there was a consensus – that they were following something they called, *The Science*. Social media companies and legacy newsrooms were a critical component of this propaganda campaign. They also indulged in the dangerous censorship/silencing of esteemed voices bringing evidence that *lockdowns were not working* and were desperately harmful to humans and society more generally.

That list is long and includes Jay Bhattacharya and Scott Atlas, both of Stanford University, an august school with big science credentials that continues to embarrass itself. Indy reporter Matt Taibbi called an email he discovered during the Twitter Files investigation *devastating*.

Here is Stanford's Virality project — which partners with multiple state agencies — recommending against "stories of true vaccine side effects" and "true posts that could fuel hesitancy." A conscious decision to emphasize narrative over truth.

Both Bhattacharya and Atlas are good people who have been professionally and personally shunned on the Stanford campus, despite being correct about the lockdown's tragic effects and a better plan for dealing with Covid-19.

If I had children attending Stanford, I would pull them out. A gentle, but brave scientist from Harvard and another from Oxford, were also smeared and made virtual outcasts – for supporting focussed protection, which is now becoming policy. We should protect the vulnerable, not lock down those at zero risk, which was the vast majority of the world's population.

Vaccine efficacy failure and adverse reactions from the shot plus panic-driven lockdown policies killed people. That's a fact. The soaring mental health crisis born of loneliness and the long-term psychic damage of crushing government oppression and betrayal are played out every day now in news reports of violence and social depravity.

The homogeneous blob that has taken over newsrooms enabled it all by acting like the menacing, central mind-hub in a science fiction movie, ruthlessly parroting in unison the same policy talking points no matter how cruel or absurd. *Anti-vaxxer. Stay home, stay safe. Safe and effective. All in this together. Follow the science.* Media supported and promoted the biggest public policy failure of our lifetime by attacking anyone who called it out, no matter how credentialed.

The utter and total abandonment of critical thought by our media and the managerial class leaves us in a post-covid dystopia of crime, captured medicine and social debauchery they caused but refuse to acknowledge. *It's time to move on*, they say.

The media blob won't make the connection between its own complicity and the rampant random stabbings, shootings and beatings, soaring addiction rates and education's lost children. With dire consequences, a large cohort of children will never recover their learning losses. A few, sad victims of the legacy-media-public-health *partnership,* will remain isolated, lonely, and psychologically barricaded in plastic-draped rooms – only venturing out wrapped in cling film for necessities while breathing through snorkel gear tightly affixed to their heads. They remind me of Hiroo Onoda, the Japanese intelligence officer who never understood the war had ended so he stayed hidden in the jungles of a small Philippine Island for nearly thirty years. Alone for all that time, Onoda refused to surrender to an enemy that had long ago stopped fighting.

Like the devoted Japanese officer, those most indoctrinated by Covid-19 propaganda are waiting for a signal that it's safe to come out. They peer uneasily at us from behind their triple-layered masks, give us a wide berth on the sidewalk and avoid all social invitations. They are waiting for the *all clear* that will never come from public health because it impugns the entire effort. Better to let them stay crouched behind those protective jungle ferns in case we need to scare them again. *The war will never be over; it's just a temporary ceasefire.*

Recently my email target emerged as a mild Covid-19 policy critic in a new high profile television job, with what I suspect is a big salary bump. There were no payday interruptions for journalists who took this route and played along.

No one will call them conspiracy theorists, anti-vaxxers or the silliest epithet of them all – Trump supporters – an accusation hurled about by pandemic *experts* when confronted with uncomfortable truths. They recoil from critical thinking as if it is the torture of the damned – like Holy Water sprinkled on the demon-possessed twelve-year-old in *The Exorcist. It burns! It burns!*

When I wrote that journo in 2020, I'd been thinking about a night in New York City about thirty-five years ago. I was filming a documentary interview in the penthouse of the Royalton, a swank Manhattan hotel. Dramatic, full-height windows framed twinkling lights embedded across the darkness below in a city I had loved my whole life. My interview subject was soon to die of AIDS after surviving for 11 years. Michael Callen, whom I'd known since the 80s had become an historic figure in the *people with aids* movement and knew his time was up. Facing the end, his big questions weren't about the meaning of life and death but rather about the moral landscape inhabited by Tony Fauci.

He recalled a desperate meeting at the NIH a few years before. Michael and his doctor begged Fauci to smooth the way for Bactrim – a simple sulpha drug being used off-label successfully to stave off a catastrophic pneumonia that often meant the end. That night, Michael's fighting spirit was gone and in its place was a deep sadness that Fauci refused to send a life-saving alert. In the halls of the NIH, the ultimate bureaucracy, things had to be done the correct way – even if that meant people dying – which they did for two more years.

I was a high profile TV reporter back then and booked an interview with Fauci to ask him myself – why wouldn't he tell AIDS clinicians about the success with Bactrim? I was aggressive and Fauci was, well, Fauci – a man accomplished at spinning while taking offense at even being asked. I persisted and it was quite a showdown. Even though it is said that thousands of AIDS patients died as a result of the two-year delay, Fauci wouldn't acknowledge his mistake. But he did reveal something about his nature that's been on full display during the pandemic; a loose relationship with the truth and an expectation he won't be held to account – by anyone.

The documentary itself was never finished and given the historical importance of Michael Callen's final words and the grilling of Tony Fauci by an unexpectedly tough Canadian reporter (me), it is heartbreaking that the tapes were never archived. They simply disappeared somewhere inside the CBC. That conversation would be absolute gold today --- but alas it has most likely been erased.

Like with AIDS, legacy media dropped the ball on Covid-19 early and never picked it up. Their reporting on Covid was a new low.

Fear porn, out of context test results erroneously called *cases* and worst of all, the annihilation by edict of what it means to be human were protected ideas. How quickly we snitched on each other, bowed to the power of unelected bureaucrats and threatened fellow citizens who refused to be vaccinated. It took no time at all for our civic bonds to be broken, perhaps permanently. Once you see children being used as human shields by the teachers' unions and hysterical parents, you begin to view your community differently. Naomi Wolf calls it *The War Against the Human* and I think she is correct.

For the three years I've been producing my show and attending events with Covid-19 policy critics and I've heard a lot about the other big story that was mostly censored by social and legacy media; mental illness caused by lockdowns and public health's brutal and insensitive approach. It is reported mostly as statistical but many people have reached out to me with their sorrows. Our pain was depersonalized, perhaps the worst kind of censorship because it meant *we were dehumanized*. We had no value once they reduced us to nothing more than the results of our C-19 tests. I received this from a young man whose identity I'm protecting.

I am staying alive and trying to keep my head above water. I want to believe the truth cannot be stopped but I'm not sure. The only thing keeping me alive is the hope that the truth does come out one day. I will dance like I never danced before when I see those who are accountable being taken to account. If the people understand what I see they will freak out. They will know they've all been under a spell and the things you spoke about regarding why good people do bad things will come to be known. They will turn on the powers that be and I will feel sorry for those I hate at this moment because my heart does not like to hate; anyone. I just love freedom. I love love.

We (or maybe just I - the only person I can speak for) need you to keep talking in order to make everyone care about human rights again, please please please don't stop. It's freedom itself, we are about to lose the world... you must understand this.

A few more months of this and a once healthy vibrant person is going to give up. They won. I can't believe it but my soul doesn't want to be here anymore. I'm tired of being non-essential. Not needed. I'm tired of arguing with people I know share my values but are somehow sleepwalking. I'm tired of feeling like a freak. Please don't stop, it may keep someone like me from killing myself. Hearing just a little truth gives me hope, the only nourishment I have left.

The story of Covid-19 censorship told truthfully is a condemnation of every single institution we rely on. Our foundations have been breached. We can no longer trust that government, and the media that keeps them in power, have our best interests at heart. It's all here in the ugly tale of disaster, steeped in fake consensus and nurtured by a multitude of mistaken groupthink pronouncements. The powerful sacrificed some of us to appease the safety obsession of others – an obsession ignited by their own foolish plan. Then those injected with the poison of irrational terror made escalating and prolonged demands for rescue – from the very people too corrupt and self-interested to stop making them afraid.

CHAPTER 12

Observation as Misinformation

Dr. Ryan Cole

Pathologist

Dr. Ryan Cole, MD is a pathologist and physician based in Boise, Idaho. He received his medical degree from the Medical College of Virginia at Virginia Commonwealth University, and further specialty at the Mayo Clinic in Rochester, Minnesota, also at the Ackerman Academy of Dermatopathology, in conjunction with the Columbia School of Medicine, in New York City. He is a board certified Anatomic and Clinical pathologist with a subspecialty training and 20 years experience in dermatopathology and particular interest in molecular diagnostics. Dr. Cole is licensed in states from coast to coast.

When COVID hit, I noticed that the guidelines coming out of the CDC and NIH did not seem consistent with my knowledge of viruses, on many levels. Social distancing and recommendations to stay indoors did not make sense. School closures did not make sense. Masking requirements and plexiglass dividers did not make sense. The types of businesses allowed to remain open and those required to close did not make sense. The lack of basic public health guidelines for overall healthy living and disease prevention did not make sense. Most of all, the treatment of patients in the hospitals did not make sense. At no time in the history of medicine has the general rule been to tell patients, "Go home until your lips turn blue, and then we will see what we can do," or that "we don't have any treatment, just wait for the vaccine."

My journey to involvement in the medical freedom movement began long before we knew anything about COVID. As a board-certified pathologist, I have spent my career making observations about patterns and reporting my findings. My job is to tell the truth about what I see and I have practiced medicine by the maxim that "the cells don't lie." I never could have anticipated the ways that sharing these observations would be twisted and construed as "mis-, dis-, and mal- information" by scientific "authorities," government agencies, and numerous media outlets.

Pattern observation seems to be a natural gift for me, which I developed through many facets of life - playing the trumpet in orchestra and band during high school and college, learning to speak Spanish fluently, studying aeronautical engineering at the U.S. Air Force Academy, recognizing bird songs and flight patterns as an amateur ornithologist, and classifying tree species for woodworking. When I was in medical school, this gift was especially evident in our required histology courses. My professors and fellow students quickly perceived that I had a knack for cell pattern recognition through the microscope. In my fourth year of medical school, I completed rotations in family medicine, dermatopathology (skin pathology) and forensic pathology, as I was trying to decide what kind of doctor I wanted to be when I grew up. I was drawn to the personal interaction and continuity of care of rural family medicine, and at the same time knew I had a gift for pathology that was not common amongst my colleagues. Both specialties utilized my observational skills, though in different ways.

A rotation with the pathology department at the Mayo Clinic in Rochester, Minnesota, helped finalize my decision, and I applied to several pathology residency programs, ultimately matching with the Mayo program. There I spent 4 years in general pathology training, and one additional year as the chief fellow of the surgical pathology fellowship. The Mayo Clinic is unique in both the volume and complexity of cases that come through the pathology department, and my experience there honed my pattern recognition skills for all different types of cancers and disease conditions. In addition to my required residency and fellowship hours, I took on 30+ hours per week moonlighting at a family practice clinic and several local emergency departments to deepen my clinical skills. Treating patients in these environments requires thorough observation, rapid assessment and definitive diagnosis and treatment. Frequently, patients would ask if I could be their regular doctor, and the nursing staff was always reassured to see my name on the schedule, knowing they could trust me to provide excellent care to every patient that walked through the door.

Upon completion of my fellowship at Mayo, I was selected as a fellow at the prestigious Ackerman Academy of Dermatopathology in New York City. The Academy was directed by the late Dr. A. Bernard Ackerman, then considered the eminent expert in the field of dermatopathology. I served as Dr. Ackerman's chief fellow for the year, where my skills of observation and pattern recognition were applied to the diagnosis of skin disease. Dr. Ackerman was an excellent teacher, and during my time at his microscope, I was steeped in the philosophy of diagnostic medicine, in addition to learning how to differentiate skin conditions. Part of our required training was also in the dermatology clinics, allowing me to correlate clinical diagnoses and treatment with microscopic diagnoses. One of the main tenants that Dr. Ackerman reinforced was the importance of providing the clinician with a clear and concise diagnosis. A description of findings was not enough – I needed to classify those findings as a specific diagnosis to give the clinician the best information for treating the patient.

After a year in New York, I took a staff pathologist position at a hospital in Idaho. It was a change of pace to be in a community-based practice, instead of the high volume setting of a large reference institution. I developed good relationships with many of the referring clinicians and my pathology colleagues, and they quickly came to trust my diagnostic skills. However, I was not content working within a multi-layered, bureaucratic hospital system, with little autonomy over my workload, my schedule, and my reporting style. I thought pathology could be better, and I wanted the opportunity to explore my own ideals about the practice of medicine. At the end of my first year, I started my own solo practice, Cole Diagnostics. Building on the lessons I learned from Mayo and Dr. Ackerman, I based my practice on accurate, concise, and actionable diagnoses with a rapid turn-around time, including photos on every report, and being available to my clients for questions and concerns at any time. We started the lab in our garage and living room, with the initial support of a few busy dermatologist friends who sent biopsies to me, growing the practice to 10,000 cases per year within 3 years, continuing to steadily grow our case numbers every year, until we eventually moved to our own laboratory building and added additional staff.

In 2015, we decided to expand the lab from primarily outpatient dermatology diagnostics to a full-service clinical laboratory. With a heavy investment in lab equipment, and hiring of key clinical technologists, we opened the blood testing side of Cole Diagnostics. This allowed us to develop deeper relationships with clinicians in our community – primarily family medicine and women's health groups. As more and more clinics of all specialties were gobbled up by large hospital systems, we focused on serving independent practices. These groups shared our values that medical care should be primarily about the relationship between the patient and their clinician, and there should not be multiple levels of bureaucracy dictating the type of care a patient should receive.

Having a full-service laboratory poised us to quickly become involved when the COVID pandemic arrived in the U.S. in 2020. As we began to hear about the virus spreading in China, I started reading scientific articles and watching YouTube medical lectures, learning as much as possible as I consumed information on SARS-COV-2 as quickly as it was available on the internet. I had done one year of PhD research in virology and immunology, in addition to having had training in those areas during medical school and residency, so I had an excellent background for understanding viral mechanisms and pathophysiology. Almost immediately, I had questions and concerns about the approach toward the illness, as directed by the medical "authorities" and communicated to the public through the mainstream media. The approach they were taking did not seem to line up with my observations and understanding of this type of virus.

One of the first areas I started studying was COVID testing, since this was particularly applicable to my specialty as a pathologist. There was a great deal of demand in the early days for testing for SARS-COV-2, however, it took several weeks for laboratories to ramp up their ability to test for the virus at the scale of the demand. For the first several months, patients were waiting 7-10 days for results of a PCR test, considered the gold standard in diagnosis. With this delay, the results were basically worthless. By the time patients received their results, they were either better or critically ill. We looked at antibody testing as an alternative. Supplies for antibody testing were more readily available, and results from a rapid antibody test could be available within hours instead of days. We began to offer this testing on a large scale in our community, particularly to those in the nursing homes. While not an ideal test, an early IgM antibody result was more informative than the delayed PCR test. The medical director of a local nursing home spoke with us extensively about this plan. With some trial runs, he found that our antibody testing was very helpful to him and his staff in making important decisions about the care of his nursing home patients and was instrumental in preventing a wider spread of infection in his facility.

Simultaneously, our laboratory molecular team and I were working on validating a PCR test for our lab. We began offering our PCR platform in July 2020, and within days were testing hundreds of samples per day. I personally learned the testing procedure and actually lived at the lab for 3 months, to get patient tests processed within a short time frame. One of the hospital systems asked for help with testing for their pre-surgical patients. Nursing homes continued to use our lab for their routine resident screening, and individual patients came to us for their pre-travel testing because they knew they could get results quickly. I was featured on the evening news for my role in helping our community. Our staff was exhausted and yet we continued to test at our maximum capacity in service to our patients. My motto from the day our lab opened has been "The patient always comes first," and we pushed through many obstacles to provide our patients with the best possible diagnostic results.

At the same time we were performing high volumes of testing, I continued to observe and study the patterns of spread, diagnosis, and treatment of COVID. I noticed that the guidelines coming out of the CDC and NIH did not seem consistent with my knowledge of viruses, on many levels. It was at about this time that my younger brother, with Type-1 diabetes and moderate obesity, tested positive for COVID. He called me one evening as he was headed to the emergency room, telling me he felt like an elephant was sitting on his chest. I had been studying extensively the repurposed drugs being used for COVID treatment and was aware that some areas of the world were experiencing success by treating with Ivermectin and/or hydroxychloroquine. The mechanisms of action for these medications made perfect sense to me from a pathophysiologic point of view, and I asked my brother to instead go to the pharmacy, where he would find a prescription ordered for him for Ivermectin and a couple of other routinely used medications. He trusted me, picked up the medications and went home to take his first doses. Twenty-four hours later, he called me again, incredulous at how quickly his symptoms disappeared.

Among the independent providers in my local area, I became the go-to expert on COVID, and through those connections, I was invited to speak at a lunch seminar in the state Capitol building, sponsored by our Lieutenant Governor, on the topic of prevention of disease and possible early treatment options. I focused primarily on general public health messages including the role of Vitamin D in overall immune health and the importance of good lifestyle choices in preventing illness.

Unbeknownst to me, the talk was filmed and was posted online a few days later. Within a matter of days, it had several thousand views, snowballing quickly to tens of thousands and eventually millions of views, and I started getting calls and messages from people around the world who wanted to talk to me about this message. I received invitations for other speaking engagements, podcast interviews, and public appearances with like-minded groups. Since then, I have spoken around the world and around the country, including before members of the E.U. Parliament, and with members of the U.S. Senate. I have testified before state legislators in an effort to influence policies protecting freedom, medical autonomy and scientific truth. I have listened to countless patients and families share their stories of illness, treatment, vaccine side-effects, and in many heart-breaking cases, death of loved ones.

My goal in speaking up about COVID has been to share observations and patterns and to tell the truth about what I see and what I understand about pathophysiologic mechanisms. For example, I was concerned from the first discussions about vaccine development. I understood that these vaccines would be ineffective and potentially harmful because of the rapidly mutating nature of coronaviruses. Soon after the vaccine roll-out I began to see disturbing trends in the types of cancers and infections I was seeing under the microscope in my lab. This is the very nature of scientific discovery – to make truthful observations and study this through rigorous and repeatable application of the scientific method. I have learned through this process that the truth is not always appreciated.

As with many of my colleagues, my talks and interviews have been censored, blocked, removed from internet searches, and labeled "mis-, dis-, or mal-information." I have been "fact-checked" and discredited in many mainstream media sources, including my local news stations that praised my early efforts to bring testing to my community. My comments have been taken out of context and misconstrued. I have been blamed for the spread of COVID, labeled an "anti-vaxxer," reported to multiple state medical boards for unprofessional conduct and as a threat to patient safety, and had my fellowship in the College of American Pathologists revoked without a hearing. Insurance companies pulled their contracts from my practice, resulting in the loss of clients who could no longer send patients to me because their insurance didn't cover our routine pathology tests, and ultimately causing me to fire-sell my practice. I am still in a legal battle in one state over my licensure, having to spend excessive legal fees to defend my license to practice, without any patient complaint of harm.

For me, this journey has become about more than a pandemic and more than a virus. The COVID pandemic has exposed the deep-seated flaws in our medical system, our public health institutions, and in our democracy as a whole. It has exposed the private special interests that dictate government policy, and the ties to media that reinforce that message from the government. As I observe the larger patterns, we are now in a fight for our very freedoms – our freedom from the influence of state-controlled media, our freedom of bodily autonomy and self-expression, our freedom of speech, and our freedom to find truth. I will continue to stand for freedom and truth despite the personal and professional costs. Those with me in this fight were born for this time and will continue to stand strong in the belief that truth will ultimately prevail.

CHAPTER 13

How Pharmaceutical Overreach, Corruption and Health System Failures Birthed COVID

Dr. Aseem Malhotra

British Cardiologist

Dr Aseem Malhotra is an NHS-trained Consultant Cardiologist, and visiting Professor of Evidence Based Medicine, Bahiana School of Medicine and Public Health, Salvador, Brazil. He is a world renowned expert in the prevention, diagnosis and management of heart disease. He is honorary council member to the Metabolic Psychiatry Clinic at Stanford University School of Medicine California, and is Cardiology MSc examiner at the University of Hertfordshire, UK. He is a founding member of Action on Sugar and was the lead campaigner highlighting the harm caused by excess sugar consumption in the United Kingdom, particularly its role in type 2 diabetes and obesity.

For societies to progress in a cohesive manner, people need access to the truth and to be able to trust each other. What are the barriers that are inhibiting our ability to access the truth and therefore leading to more divisions in society today?

I think the current situation we've been in the last few years with the pandemic has probably taught us quite a lot about how important truth is. So I'm going to start by addressing the issue of psychological barriers, because I believe that science alone isn't enough. Opposition from powerful vested interests needs to be overcome.

The first psychological barrier I want to share with you is one of willful blindness. This is when human beings - we're all capable of this - turn a blind eye to the truth in order to feel safe, reduce anxiety, avoid conflict, to protect prestige, egos and reputations.

Another barrier to us getting to the truth is one of fear. If we are gripped by fear, many of us, most of us to some degree, were gripped by varying levels of fear with the COVID pandemic. That inhibits our ability to engage in critical thinking.

What's worse than ignorance? The late, great Stephen Hawking teaches us, the illusion of knowledge. I'm a practicing cardiologist. More than anything, I'm interested in health, in trying to improve my patient outcomes. This is a really nice definition of health. It was coined by the World Health Organization. They're not in my good books at the moment, but actually, their definition of health is a wonderful one. It is a state of complete physical, mental and social well-being and not merely the absence of disease or infirmity.

Why are we not achieving this? Why in the UK has life expectancy stalled in the last ten years? Why are more and more people living with chronic disease? We are regressing mentally and physically, worldwide. The question is why?

As doctors practicing and teaching medicine, the analytical framework that we use is the evidence-based medicine triad. In order to improve patient outcomes, manage risks, treat illness, relieve suffering, we need to incorporate these three components. Our individual clinical expertise as doctors - our knowledge, our experience, our clinical intuition - the best available evidence and last but not least, the most important thing is incorporating patient values and preferences. In other words, informed consent. To have informed consent, people need to have all the information given to them. Consent that isn't fully informed is not consent at all. The problem is that over the last few decades, evidence based medicine has become an illusion. Evidence based medicine has been hijacked by powerful vested interests. The best available clinical evidence has been corrupted. And if doctors are making clinical decisions on biased and commercially corrupted information, it doesn't take a rocket scientist to figure out, at best, it's going to lead to suboptimal outcomes for patients. At worst, it's going to do harm. Now, we have complete health care system failure, and a pandemic of misinformed doctors and misinformed and unwittingly harmed patients, based upon a number of factors.

These factors are: biased funding of research that is funded because it's likely to be profitable, not beneficial for patients; biased reporting in medical journals; biased patient pamphlets, and biased reporting in the media. This is a big, big issue. Combine this status quo with commercial conflicts of interest, defensive medicine and last but not least, medical curricula that fail to teach doctors how to comprehend and communicate basic health statistics.

John Ioannidis is the most cited medical researcher in the world. I call him the Stephen Hawking of Medicine. He wrote a paper in 2017 *"How to Survive the Medical Misinformation Mess."* He makes some very clear, important points I think people need to fully acknowledge and understand. Much, if not most published research is not reliable, offers no benefit to patients and is not useful to decision makers. Most health care professionals are not aware of this problem. One of the barriers to overcoming these system failures is awareness. Most doctors are not aware, they then lack the necessary skills to evaluate the reliability and usefulness of medical science. Patients and families frequently lack relevant, accurate medical evidence and skill guidance at the time of medical decision making.

If we just take a step back and also think about what these entities are disseminating - so-called medical information - that we take as gospel truth. We need to understand what their primary interests are; we're talking about the pharmaceutical industry here.

In 2018, with almost two decades as a practicing doctor, I tried on a number of occasions to call for public inquiries on this issue. I took this to the European Parliament in 2018 and I gave a talk entitled, "Big Food and Big Pharma, Killing for Profit?" I made some key points there that people need to appreciate. First, the pharmaceutical industry has a fiduciary obligation to make profit for their shareholders. They do not have a legal requirement to give you the best treatment, although most of us would like this and would hope this to be the case. The real scandals are that medical regulators fail to prevent misconduct by industry. Those with responsibilities to scientific integrity and patients, namely doctors, academic institutions and medical journals, collude with industry for financial gain.

The situation has become so dire; doctors can no longer practice honest medicine. Why is this a public health issue? Well, one estimate suggests that prescribed medications (Peter Gaucher, co-founder of the Cochrane Collaboration) are the third most common cause of death after heart disease and cancer globally, because of side effects that are mostly preventable. Why? Because doctors are making decisions on information where the drug industry exaggerates the benefits and the safety of their drugs.

What most people don't know, in fact, most doctors probably don't know is that if you look at the increase in life expectancy in the Western world from 1850 to now, there's about a 40-year increase in life expectancy. Of those 40 years, modern medicine has added about three and a half to five years maximum. A lot of the low-hanging fruit of great achievements we made in medicine happened decades ago. Most new drugs now, unfortunately, according to one analysis in America, are just copies of old ones. Only 11% are truly innovative. And one of the reasons for that is the drug companies spend 20 times more on marketing than they do on basic science research.

These are problems with the system. We have an innovation crisis because of system failures. What's worse, it is no longer possible to trust much of the clinical research that's published or to rely on the judgment of trusted physicians or authoritative medical guidelines. "I take no pleasure in this conclusion, which I reached slowly and reluctantly over my two decades as an editor of the New England Journal of Medicine," said Marcia Angell. The New England Journal of Medicine is considered the highest impact medical journal in the world. Is she alone? No, she's not.

Richard Horton, editor of The Lancet, wrote an editorial in 2015 in which he said that possibly half the published literature may simply be untrue. He concluded that science has taken a turn towards darkness. Who's going to take the first step to cleaning up the system? Nothing has changed to this point.

Richard Smith, former editor of the BMJ attended a meeting a few years ago in London with academics from some of Britain's most prestigious institutions. He asked the audience how many of them were aware of a colleague or someone in their department fabricating data? A third of the audience put their hand up. He asked them, how many of you reported it? All of them put their hands down. This is a cultural problem.

I'm going to get to the roots of this cultural problem shortly and the downstream effects. Misleading health statistics are important because without understanding the numbers involved, doctors, patients, and members of the public are vulnerable to exploitation of their hopes and anxieties by political and commercial interests. Sound familiar during the COVID pandemic? Yes, it was devastating. There's no doubt a lot of people died and a lot of vulnerable people suffered at the beginning. But there was a hugely exaggerated fear of COVID amongst the population. One survey in America suggested that 50% of adult Americans thought their risk of being hospitalized if they got COVID was 50%. In other words, one- in-two, when the figure was closer to 1 in 1000.

Medical professionals use something called relative risk or absolute risk, also known as the numbers needed to treat. And if you communicate relative risk as opposed to the absolute risk, then it leads doctors and laypeople to overestimate the benefit of interventions.

For example, if you look at the data on the use of statin drugs in people with type 2 diabetes based upon randomized controlled trials, it will tell you the relative risk reduction is 48% in having a stroke over four years. In other words, I could say to the patient, "listen, if you take this drug religiously for the next four years, you're 48% less likely to have a stroke." That sounds very impressive. What does it actually mean when you look at the data and follow up with the 1,000 people with type 2 diabetes over four years? In the placebo group - those taking a dummy pill - 28 of them had a stroke. Of those taking statins, only 15 in 1000 had a stroke over the four year period. So you've reduced the number to 13 out of 1000. The relative risk reduction would say 13 divided by 28, times 100 offers a 48% relative risk reduction. But in reality, in the absolute risk terms, it's only 1.3%. 13 out of 1000 people have been saved from having a stroke because they took the statins.

Framing in medical journals has made the issue worse. A third of articles published in The Lancet, the BMJ and JAMA between 2004 and 2006 use mis-match framing. This is a method of manipulating statistics to amplify the risk reduction and minimize harms, when in reality the data may be the same. This is not ethical. This is not scientific. This is marketing in a medical journal, leading doctors - in their heads - to exaggerate the benefits of a drug and underplay the harms.

In September 2022, I published an article called "Curing the Pandemic of Misinformation on the COVID 19 Vaccines through the Principles of Real Evidence-Based Medicine." I wanted to look at the best available evidence that we have, to come to a conclusion about the absolute benefits of the COVID vaccines, versus the harms. Only recently, the UK was able to look at the benefits of the mRNA vaccine.

Data, supplied by the UK Government, allowed data experts to compare one million vaccinated versus one million unvaccinated people. There are confounding factors here, so the figures may change up or down with more data, but it gives you a rough idea. After taking two doses of the Pfizer jab, for those over the age of 70, you have to vaccinate 2500 people to prevent one person being hospitalized with severe COVID. For those aged 50 to 69, then 18,700 people need to be vaccinated to prevent one person being hospitalized. Younger than that and we are getting into the hundreds of tens, to hundreds of thousands of people. That's the absolute benefit of the vaccine to prevent severe hospitalization. Not what people were led to believe about the benefits.

What about the harm? As a proponent of evidence-based medicine, the highest quality level of evidence is what we call the double blinded, randomized controlled trial. This is what led to the approval of the vaccines in the first place from Pfizer and Moderna. Just those single trials. And we were sold on a 95% effectiveness figure, which in the end, actually meant a less than 1% (.84) in absolute risk reduction in infection prevention. How many would have taken the vaccine had they known it had less than 1% benefit?

Near the end of 2022, some eminent scientists published a reanalysis of the original trials in the peer reviewed journal Vaccine. They concluded that you were more likely to suffer a serious adverse event from the COVID mRNA vaccines; disability, life changing event, hospitalization, than you were to be hospitalized with COVID, from the very beginning. If you take just that data on its own, that means that these vaccines should never have been approved for anybody in the first place. What was the rate of serious adverse events that they found in two months? At least 1 in 800 suffered a serious adverse event.

Historically, other vaccines have been suspended for much less harm. The 1976 swine flu vaccine was suspended because it was found to cause a debilitating neurological condition called Guillain-Barre syndrome in 1 in 100,000 people. Rotavirus vaccine was suspended 1999 because it was found to cause a form of bowel obstruction in kids in 1 in 10,000. But here we're talking at least 1 in 800.

I'm a clinician that took two doses of the Pfizer vaccine and went on Good Morning Britain and told people it was safe because I believe in traditional vaccines. Traditional vaccines have an adverse event rate thought to be about one per million. This is almost a thousand-fold higher.

When the vaccines were being approved, the World Health Organization endorsed a list of potential serious side effects, which doctors were not aware of. Anything and everything that can go wrong with the heart is on this list. I'm now managing vaccine injuries. Everything is happening; heart attacks, cardiac arrests, rhythm disturbances, heart failure, etc. This is unbelievable. It is shocking. I don't even think those words do it justice. And in terms of the serious adverse events, we know it's at least 1 in 800, but it may well be much higher.

In medicine, 80% of your diagnosis comes from patient history. If you're a good doctor and you know your stuff, you will get your answer from the patient, from the conversation in most cases. However, a U.S. survey published in BMC Infectious Diseases, a high impact journal, looked at people who felt they had suffered a vaccine injury or they knew of somebody that had died or suffered an injury. The study concluded that the COVID vaccination may have killed as many as 278,000 people in America in 2021. And the serious adverse event rates were about a million. So we're talking about serious adverse events, about maybe as high as 1 in 300. From my own clinical experience, I think that's probably closer to the truth than 1 in 800.

What about the regulators? The problem is the regulators have been captured. Most of the regulators around the world and in developed nations get most of their funding from pharma. Most doctors, even senior doctors I've spoken to, didn't know this. The FDA gets 65% of its funding from pharma. The MHRA in the UK gets 86% of its funding from pharma. Donald Light in the BMJ, in an investigation that exposed all these conflicts of interest in terms of funding, said, "It's the opposite of having a trustworthy organization independently and rigorously assessing medicines. They're not rigorous, they're not independent, they are selective, and they withhold data. Doctors and patients must appreciate how deeply and extensively drug regulators can't be trusted so long as they are captured by industry funding."

So how do big corporations exert their power, their influences over health policy that ultimately influences us patients? They have power over decision making and control over the political agenda. They influence politicians through lobbying. They have the power to define issues and potential issues; they shape preferences, they can capture the media. They have influence over philanthropic organizations. Think about the Bill and Melinda Gates Foundation which is the second largest funder to the W.H.O. BIll Gates is heavily invested in stocks in McDonald's, Coca-Cola and the pharmaceutical industry. Bill Gates himself has made hundreds of millions from investments in these drug companies that have been producing vaccines. This is a gross conflict of interest. He shouldn't be anywhere near the decision making process, but he is the second biggest funder to the W.H.O.

Margaret Chan, the former director of the W.H.O. recently said 70% of the W.H.O.'s funding comes with strings attached; control over the knowledge environment, funding medical research. Most medical research now is funded by pharma. They have control over the legal environment, limited liability for Pfizer for example. They have immunity from liability from most governments around the world. If there were vaccine injuries, they weren't liable. Why did we allow this to happen? Because we didn't know about it. The general population doesn't know what's happening and they don't even know that they don't know.

Next, these people engage in opposition fragmentation. When an issue is raised and it makes it to the public discourse through the mainstream media - which is also being captured - they will smear and attack those people who are calling them out.

In 2011, Merck was fined $950 million for fraud in relation to their drug Vioxx. It was thought to be better than Ibuprofen as an anti-inflammatory because it didn't give people stomach issues. Ultimately, that was found to be false, but also it was determined that it doubled the risk of heart attacks and it was estimated that it probably killed about 60,000 Americans. John Abramson was involved in the litigation process that led to the ultimate criminal investigation against Merck. He was privy to internal emails that were circulated amongst the company. One email from the chief scientist of Merck said this when the drug was being rolled out: "It's a shame that the cardiovascular effect is there, but the drug will do well and we will do well." What do you call that kind of behavior? Psychopathic. Reckless disregard for the safety of others, deceitfulness, repeated lying and conning others for profit.

I've lost both my parents, both doctors, both general practitioners, prematurely in the last few years. My mother suffered unnecessarily in hospital. My father suffered a sudden cardiac death, which I attributed ultimately, to the Pfizer vaccine. The ambulance to take him to hospital was delayed by 30 minutes and he probably would have been saved if the ambulance had come on time. I subsequently learned that the Department of Health knew there were ambulance delays across the country for months before my father died. So, I published a piece on this subject, but was warned not to do so by another senior cardiologist who advised that I'd only make enemies.

What about our duty to patients and the public? This is a cultural problem. People are scared of speaking out. Why have we created a society and a system where it becomes not safe to speak the truth?

Keep speaking the truth. I look at it rationally. It is even less safe to not speak the truth. Because a problem only gets bigger.

There are some clear solutions here when it comes to pharma. Although the drug industry plays an important role in developing new drugs, they should play no role in testing them. All results of all trials that involve humans must be made publicly available, and the regulators should not be taking money from industry. Medical education should no longer be funded or sponsored by the pharmaceutical industry.

These big corporations now are essentially oppressing society. It's corporate tyranny and I think we need to understand that freedom from these external systems of oppression is directly linked to liberation from our own internal mechanisms of suffering. Ancient wisdom tells us that to lead a good and happy life, for societies to function cohesively, for us to be able to trust each other, to speak the truth, we have to come from a position of virtue. Of all the virtues, courage is the most important. Without courage, you can't practice any other virtue consistently.

Let's all go back to thinking about how important it is to speak the truth, even though it may be difficult, because ultimately the truth is what is going to redeem the world from hell. And that's where we're heading.

We are driven in many ways by the illusion of what makes us happy - instant gratification - exacerbated by the systems that encourage that behavior as well. That's not good for us mentally. Gandhi said, "It is health that is a real wealth and not pieces of gold and silver."

Rights are only won by those that make their voices heard. Hope is never silent.

CHAPTER 14

Pandemic Politics and America's COVID Cartel

Senator Ron Johnson

Senior United States Senator from Wisconsin

Ronald Harold Johnson is an American politician serving as the senior United States senator from Wisconsin, a seat he has held since 2011. A Republican, Johnson was first elected to the U.S. Senate in 2010. Senator Johnson served as Chairman of the Senate's Homeland Security and Governmental Affairs Committee from 2015-2021 and is now the ranking member for the Permanent Subcommittee on Investigations. He also serves on the Budget and Finance committees. In November 2022, he was elected to his third term as U.S. Senator for Wisconsin.

This essay is based upon an interview between US Senator Ron Johnson and Del Bigtree. It has been edited for clarity and length into an essay format. It is included in this book thanks to the generosity of Del Bigtree and The Highwire team.

Del Bigtree: This is the whole truth and nothing but the truth from a man who has been standing there all alone, Senator Ron Johnson, the United States Senator for Wisconsin.

Sen. Ron Johnson: I never thought I'd get involved in politics. I'm an accountant by education, I ran a manufacturing plant for 30 years, but I got involved in my community.

I was asked to give a speech at a Tea Party describing the harmful impact of government regulations on business. I'd never given a speech before in my life. What I talked about was the fact that President Obama was trying to sell his Obamacare plan, which I knew wouldn't work. I knew it wouldn't protect patients. I knew it wouldn't make care more affordable. But he was doing it by denigrating doctors. I remember him saying - I'm paraphrasing - that doctors are so greedy, they'll take out a set of tonsils, amputate a foot to make more money. "The doctor may look at the reimbursement system and say to himself, "You know what, I make a lot more money if I take this kid's tonsils out," said Obama.

I found that pretty offensive, because our first child, our daughter Kerry was born with a very serious congenital heart defect. One of those, according to President Obama, greedy, money grubbing doctors, came in at 1:30 in the morning and did a procedure on her heart that saved her life. And then eight months later, when her heart was the size of a small plum, in seven hours of open heart surgery, they completely re-baffled the upper chamber of her heart. Her heart operates backwards today, but she's 39 years old and has two children through surrogacy. I told that story in my speech. After this, people began to suggest I run for office.

I think the really important part of the story as it relates to COVID, is that during the experience with my daughter, I really came to understand what the term medical practice means. It's not a clinic. It's not a business. It's literally doctors using their skill to practice medicine. That's how we advance medicine. And so, when I heard President Obama denigrating doctors, people who had dedicated their lives to saving lives, it was obnoxious. When they passed Obamacare and started remortgaging our kids' future, I got involved in politics. It was 2009. I was elected in 2010.

I consider myself a citizen legislator. I had a full life, raised a family, and then at the age of 55, I decided to run for office and became a U.S. Senator. I knew I wouldn't be able to come here and save the world, but one of the things that inspired me was Jim DeMint saying we need more people coming here (to Washington) not to join the club, but to join the fight. But did I really understand the full dysfunction here? No, I didn't. This place is almost totally dysfunctional. What I have discovered is that there's basically four people in Washington, D.C. with power; the President, the Speaker of the House, and then as long as we maintain the filibuster, the majority and minority leader of the Senate. The rest of us can make noise, we can hold hearings, we can utilize our position and highlight things for the public, expose things. That's all.

Quite honestly, I came here to try to rein in deficit spending. When I came here we were $14 trillion in net debt. We're now over $30 trillion. On a bi-partisan basis, this place is very good at mortgaging our kids' future. I became chairman of the Senate Committee on Homeland Security and Governmental Affairs in 2015. That is the Senate Oversight Committee - Governmental Affairs. I didn't come here to do investigations, but I'm charged with oversight over the entire federal government and able to conduct an investigation into just about anything. After six years investigating things, I determined really how deep the Deep State is. I got a good sense of the level of corruption. It's got to be exposed. There aren't a whole lot of people like myself, who've been dedicated to exposing corruption.

There are a lot of good people here serving in Congress, but they're all faced with the same level of dysfunction. I think it's generally true that the top priority of many members is to get reelected. If you have that attitude, it affects your activity. From my standpoint, I'd be happy to go home and I would have done that, had Biden not taken over, Democrats got total control and promised to transform America and then proceeded to do so; with open borders, 41-year high inflation, record gasoline prices and rising crime. In 2022, we don't have enough baby formula to feed our infants in the United States of America. So in the end, what we find out is the "fundamental transformation" is basically fundamentally destroying it. I've never walked away from a problem in my life.

I first became aware of COVID in late January or early February 2020. I was doing other investigations, but all of a sudden there was this weird disease. We saw the pictures from China, people wearing moon suits. I still scratch my head and wonder, was that just a scare tactic on the part of the Chinese government? There's so much that doesn't make sense about COVID that I've got a pretty open mind trying to figure out what is going on here. I think the game plan always was to scare the American public so they can gain greater control. They did a pretty good job of it.

In mid-February 2020, I first became aware that in America we really don't produce pharmaceutical drugs. We do the research on it, but all the precursor chemicals and active pharmaceutical ingredients are primarily produced in China or India. We are really vulnerable. We've done nothing to correct that. For this reason, I was immediately focusing on therapies for COVID. Do we have drugs off the shelf? How quickly can we develop a cure for this?

I was completely opposed to shutdowns. I come from the private sector and I knew that you can't just shut the American economy down. People have to eat. I made the comment that we tragically lose 36,000 people a year on the highways, but we don't shut the highways down. Fauci called that a false equivalency, but it's actually a pretty accurate analogy. At the end of March 2020 I wrote an op-ed in USA Today opposing shutdowns. I was savagely attacked. "You want to kill people," they said.

The minute I heard the possibility of a drug like hydroxychloroquine for early treatment, my first thought was, if this works, can we produce enough of it? Do you remember in the early days when COVID was hitting Italy badly, then really hitting New York? We saw doctors go online after 12- 14- 16-hour shifts - these were people that President Obama had called greedy, these people just trying to practice medicine. They were practicing medicine, using their skills to try to figure out what was happening.

They were saying that this was different from the standard kind of lung issues they deal with. And therefore they had to try different things. But then those videos were being censored. I remember the video from two doctors in California. One of them was Dr. Dan Erikson, who said he thought that a lot of people had already had COVID. He was immediately shut down. Immediately censored. I was wondering, how are we going to allow doctors to practice medicine if we don't utilize what we have here in the year 2020 versus what we had in 1918? We have the Internet. We've got this marvelous information age where doctors can freely exchange information. They can practice medicine. They can share their experiences. We can get on top of this. But it was all being shut down.

I started reaching out to the manufacturers of hydroxychloroquine, the CEO of Novartis, which is one of the major manufacturers, and I found out they had already donated 30 million tablets to the national stockpile. Were those being distributed? Well I found out there was a big logjam there. So I tried to work with the administration to break that logjam, to get that distributed. I was dealing with people in the White House and it was like talking to a brick wall. But I had a pipeline to the CEO of Novartis, texting him all the time. He was saying, we've got a dozen trials that are going to be ready, between mid May and the end of June. They were excited about this.

All of a sudden, at about the end of April, silence; communication stopped. I've never talked to him since then. It's like a switch was turned. Boom. Obviously we never saw a trial come out of Novartis. What we did see were fraudulent trials coming from Surgisphere. Something happened there. I can't explain it, but it seems at some point in time, the cabal, I call them the COVID cartel, decided the solution was going to be a vaccine. Of course, that's one of the explanations of why they would want to tank and sabotage early treatment, because if you have an existing effective therapy, you're not going to get emergency use authorization on a totally novel therapy. They sabotaged hydroxychloroquine.

That's where you have to say, the buck stops with the President. I kept trying. President Trump kept trying. I remember one of those senate calls where literally Trump's on the phone and I was saying, "Mr. President, we've got to break this logjam on hydroxychloroquine. We have to make it available." The FDA had created this emergency use authorization, which made it way more restrictive. I remember President Trump on the phone with all these senators saying, "Mark, take care of Johnson's request". But we couldn't do it, just couldn't get it done.

You understand why when you know the support that Fauci still has in the media and you understand the power of the media. I don't care who you are. President of the United States, a U.S. Senator, it's difficult to buck the media. The media was so in the tank for Fauci that Trump couldn't contradict him. I hold them largely responsible for this. If we had an honest media, I don't think our response to COVID would have been as awful as it was.

I would go to Republican Senate lunches and go, "guys the solutions here, early treatment." It's not just one. It's not just hydroxychloroquine. There's literally a cornucopia of drugs. I didn't realize how large a cornucopia that was, but it turned out to be a multi-drug protocol and it works. The solution, the end of the pandemic was there for the taking. Now, this was before the vaccines had been approved. Crickets. It's still crickets.

The human tendency is that people don't like to admit they're wrong. So that's certainly part of what's happening here. We were savaged for suggesting that early treatment might stop the pandemic. We were vilified, ridiculed and called the "Snake Oil Salesman of the Senate."

I got a call from a former Green Bay Packer. Ken Ruettgers, who's a Hall of Fame lineman. His wife Sheryl, was vaccine injured and they were connected to a group of about 2000 vaccine-injured people on Facebook. He said, "I'm seeing what you're doing. I'm just calling to see if I can get help somewhere." These people, all they want is to be seen, heard and believed. That's all. Because they can't get treatment; nobody is acknowledging what they're suffering from. And some of them are suffering with these internal vibrations so severe they're committing suicide. "Can you help us out in some way, shape or form?" I said, "well, Ken, I don't have much power, but because I'm a U.S. Senator, I can garner attention. I can make myself a target. If I hold an event in Wisconsin, particularly if you come out, we can probably get some TV cameras and at least you can tell your story."

Hope springs eternal, so we held this event in June 2021 in Milwaukee, and we probably had at least a dozen TV cameras show up. We had Brianne Dressen. We had Maddie de Garay and her mother Stephanie. Maddie was in the Pfizer trial for children, Brianne Dressen in the Astrazeneca trial. We had the event and five individuals told their stories. I was hoping maybe some members of the media would show some measure of human compassion and interview these people, and put that on the news so people would be aware of the fact that it's not 100% safe. There are people being injured by it. But they didn't. Instead they attacked me. But I was proud that I at least gave these people a platform to tell their story. And I was appalled by their treatment by the media.

Right now it is definitely me against the media. It's all of us against the media. It's all of us against the COVID cartel; the administration, the health agencies, big pharma, the mainstream legacy media and big tech social media giants. That is the Covid cartel. They are the ones that keep telling people the lies. They can't afford to admit they're wrong at this point. The body count is so high. The problem is they've got the power to make it almost impossible to prove them wrong. It brings to mind the phrase, it's the victors that write the history. And they intend to be the victors.

I hold the media largely responsible. I first hold responsible radical leftists who took over our university systems in the sixties. They're the ones that have been cranking out teachers that indoctrinate our youth. Lawyers have become activist judges. Then journalists who aren't journalists, are advocates. They're also radical leftists. These people, these major networks, they don't do interviews with me. They argue with me. They're not journalists, they are advocates. So that's why I say they're part of the COVID cartel. They have every bit as vested interest in not being proven wrong now, because I believe these people have blood on their hands.

Hundreds of thousands of people are dead in America that didn't have to die. I am 100% thoroughly convinced of that. If the medical establishment had had an open mind toward early treatment and listened to people like Dr. Kory and Dr. McCullough and just tried it, given it to their patients who were begging them. They just wouldn't do it and I can't explain it. It makes me profoundly sad.

Let me make my appeal to doctors. If you're a doctor and you are awakened to what's happened, if you know that it's wrong don't sit by the sidelines anymore. Peter McCullough and Dr. Malone and Pierre Kory and all these courageous doctors who have stepped forward to warn the public, they need help. We literally need thousands of doctors who are aware of the problem to join together. There is safety in numbers; it's time to be honest and truthful with the American public. I'm begging doctors, I'm begging nurses to come forward, join together as one massive group and put an end to this insanity. Be loyal first to your patients and be the one to call the shots when it comes to how you care for your patients. I'm just begging doctors; you have to step up to the plate.

The truth is the way forward. It just is. It has its own power. I do try and counsel the people that are in this struggle with me, try not to marginalize yourself. I try not to use certain terms because I think it's important that those of us who are really fighting this battle don't make bigger targets of ourselves than we already are. And we're big targets. They want to, they want to destroy us. But I have hope.

https://thehighwire.com/videos/sen-ron-johnson-pandemic-politics-americas-covid-cartel

CHAPTER 15

The Criminal COVID-19 Vaccine Disaster

Dr. Peter A. McCullough

Practicing Internist and Cardiologist

Dr. McCullough is an internist, cardiologist, epidemiologist holding degrees from Baylor University, University of Texas Southwestern Medical School, University of Michigan, and Southern Methodist University. He manages common infectious diseases as well as the cardiovascular complications of both the viral infection and the injuries developing after the COVID-19 vaccine in Dallas TX, USA. Dr. McCullough has broadly published on a range of topics in medicine with > 1000 publications and > 685 citations in the National Library of Medicine. His works include "Pathophysiological Basis and Rationale for Early Outpatient Treatment of SARS-CoV-2 (COVID-19) Infection" the first widely utilized treatment regimen for ambulatory patients infected with SARS-CoV-2 in the American Journal of Medicine and subsequently updated in Reviews in Cardiovascular Medicine. Subsequently he published the first detoxification approach titled "Clinical Rationale for SARS-CoV-2 Base Spike Protein Detoxification in Post COVID-19 and Vaccine Injury Syndromes" in the Journal of American Physicians and Surgeons. He has dozens of peer-reviewed publications on the infection and has commented extensively on the medical response to the COVID-19 crisis in TheHill, America Out Loud, and on FOX NEWS Channel. Dr. McCullough testified multiple times in the US Senate, Texas Senate Committee on Health and Human Services, Arizona Senate and House of Representatives, Colorado General Assembly, New Hampshire Senate, Pennsylvania Senate, and South Carolina Senate concerning many aspects of the pandemic response. Dr. McCullough has had years of dedicated academic and clinical efforts in combating the SARS-CoV-2 virus and in doing so, has reviewed thousands of reports, participated in scientific congresses, group discussions, press releases, and has been considered among the world's experts on COVID-19.

Dr. McCullough is co-author of the best-selling book of **"The Courage to Face COVID-19: Preventing Hospitalization and Death While Battling the Biopharmaceutical Complex,"** by John Leake & Peter McCullough, MD, MPH. New York: Skyhorse Publishing, 2022.

(Updated) This essay is based upon testimony given by Dr. Peter A. McCullough at the De Madariaga room, European Parliament, Strasbourg, France, September 13, 2023. It has been edited for clarity and length into an essay format. It is included in this book thanks to the generosity and permission of Dr. McCullough.

There have been two waves of injury to the world. The first has been the SARS-CoV-2 infection, which preyed upon the frail and the elderly. The second wave of injury has now been the COVID-19 vaccines.

The role of the W.H.O. appears to be adverse in both of these. The W.H.O. appears to be operating within a biopharmaceutical complex, a complicated syndicate that has formed over time. It includes the W.H.O., the United Nations, the World Economic Forum, the Gates Foundation, Rockefeller Foundation, the Wellcome Trust, GAVI, UNITAID, CEPI (the Coalition for Epidemic Preparedness and Innovation) that the Gates Foundation and the W.E.F. formed. Also, the Department of State in the United States, the National Institutes of Health, the CDC, the FDA, the MHRA in the UK, the TGA in Australia, SAHPRA in South Africa, the EMA here in Europe. This grouping of non-governmental organizations with governmental public health agencies is operating as a unit. They're carefully coordinated and the impact has been adverse from the outset of the pandemic.

There was an investigation by the W.H.O. on the origins of SARS-CoV-2. That's when the beginning of the cover up began. Rear Admiral Brett Jarrar in the United States nominated three independent scientists to go to Wuhan and figure out what was going on. It has since come out in congressional hearings that Anthony Fauci, Francis Collins, Jeremy Farrar - previously at the Wellcome Trust, now the chief scientist at the W.H.O. - Kristian Andersen, PhD. at Scripps, Dr. Edwin Holmes in Sydney, Dr. Peter Daszak at the EcoHealth Alliance, all conspired in January of 2020 to cover up what they knew. Namely, that the virus was engineered in a joint US-Chinese collaboration in the lab in Wuhan, China., They deceived the world with 12 subsequent fraudulent papers in the peer reviewed literature. These papers were quarterbacked by Jeremy Farrar, who has been rewarded with a new job as the chief scientist at the W.H.O.. This is all documented in the series of reports in the House Select Committee in the United States by the US Congress, led by Representative Brad Wenstrup.

The W.H.O. has played an adverse role from the very beginning, deceiving the world on the origins of SARS-CoV-2. Doctors like us in clinical practice got behind on this because our governments and agencies weren't honest with us. Instead of helping us, or at least getting out of the way in terms of treating patients and saving lives, they got in the way and they impeded our ability to treat patients. They effectively created an entire environment of therapeutic nihilism.

There are only two things that prevent hospitalization and death. One was early treatment, then the second was to acquire natural immunity with the first episode of the infection. Nothing else worked. There were only two bad outcomes; hospitalization and death. To this day, the W.H.O. does not support, embrace or promulgate early treatment protocols for patients with acute COVID-19. That should tell you something. That should be a wake-up call. We're going on three years of this and still nothing to reduce human suffering from the W.H.O. Nothing. In fact, the W.H.O. has made efforts that enhance human suffering since the first wave was the illness.

I've testified in the US Senate multiple times. My position remains that the majority of hospitalizations and deaths were completely avoidable in the highest risk patients with early intervention, starting with virucidal nasal sprays and gargles, followed by intravenous and oral drugs administered at home to get people through the illness.

Now enter the vaccines. Since 2021, vaccines have ravaged the population in the world. Worldwide, two thirds of people took a vaccine; the United States Covid Community State study shows 75% of Americans took an ill-advised vaccine. Thankfully, 25% didn't. I was the only public health and public figure in the United States in writing to question the vaccines before they came out. And I did it as loudly as I could with an Op-Ed titled, "The Great Gamble of COVID-19 Vaccination," in *The Hill*.

Among those who accepted COVID-19 vaccines in the United States, 94% of Americans took a messenger RNA vaccine. It is the genetic code for the potentially lethal spike protein part of the virus. It was the worst idea ever to install the genetic code by injection and allow unbridled production of a potentially lethal protein in the human body for an uncontrolled duration of time.

Everything we've learned about the vaccines since they've come out is horrifying. There's not a single study showing that the messenger RNA is broken down, because its pseudouridine is made synthetically. It cannot be broken down. There's not a single study showing it leaves the body. We now have papers by Castriuta who demonstrates the messenger

RNA circulating for a month. That's as long as they've looked. We have the spike protein, the lethal protein from the vaccines found in the human body after vaccination, circulating at least for six months if not longer as shown by Brogna, Patterson, et al. If people take an injection in another six months, there's another installation circulating more, potentially-lethal protein accumulates in the body.

The spike protein is proven in 3400 peer-reviewed manuscripts to cause four major domains of disease. One is cardiovascular disease; heart inflammation or myocarditis. Every regulatory agency agrees the vaccines cause myocarditis. I'm a cardiologist. Before COVID, for years, we've had guidelines in cardiology when there is myocarditis, whether it's symptomatic or not. These guidelines include that people cannot exert themselves in athletics; it will cause cardiac arrest. And yet across Europe and across the United States, sports leagues were injecting young people who had no medical necessity, no clinical indication, with these vaccines. And we have seen a montage of cardiac arrests in young individuals. I'm telling you, as an expert cardiologist, these cardiac arrests are due to the COVID-19 vaccine, until proven otherwise.

Other cardiovascular diseases caused by the vaccine, proven: acceleration of atherosclerotic cardiovascular disease and heart attacks or cardiovascular arrest. Posterior orthostatic tachycardia syndrome or POTS, or people passing out due to low blood pressure. You have seen montages of people in the media, one after another passing out like you've never seen before. It is the vaccine, until proven otherwise. Aortic dissection. Atrial fibrillation. Other arrhythmias. Cardiac arrest in the absence of myocarditis has been described with the COVID-19 vaccines. The cardiovascular domain of damage in the human body from the vaccine is substantial, more than anything we've ever seen with cholesterol, high blood pressure or diabetes.

The second major domain is neurologic disease; stroke, both ischemic and hemorrhagic. Guillain-Barré syndrome, ascending paralysis that can lead to death, which has led to death with messenger RNA vaccines, agreed to by all of our regulatory agencies. Small fiber, neuropathy, numbness and tingling, ringing in the ears, headaches. These are common.

The third major domain is blood clots, blood clots the likes of which we've never seen before. The spike protein is the most thrombogenic protein we've ever seen in human medicine. It's found in the blood clots. The spike protein directly causes blood clots. Blood clots are larger and more resistant to blood thinners than we've ever experienced in human medicine.

I have patients with blood clots now going on two years and they are not dissolving with conventional blood thinners, due to these vaccines. We can't get these out of the body, we can't get the messenger RNA or the spike protein out of the body, as it is continually produced.

The fourth and last domain is immunologic abnormalities; vaccine induced thrombotic thrombocytopenia and multi-system inflammatory disorder are early acute syndromes, well-described and published. They have their own acronyms, all agreed to by the regulatory agencies.

So all of you are asking yourselves, will it be me, or my family member next with a fatal event? Is it my loved one who is going to drop after a vaccine? We've seen cardiac arrests and blood clots now two years after these shots. Two years, and it could be even longer.

I'm the senior author on the largest autopsy study ever assembled of death after COVID-19 vaccination worldwide. We searched the literature, 600 papers, and all the clinical findings. We reviewed them with contemporary knowledge experts in pathology and clinical medicine. Our conclusion, 73.9% of the deaths after vaccination are due to the vaccine. When the cause of death is suspected myocarditis and the body is submitted for autopsy, in a second paper of which I'm the senior author, cause of death is the vaccines 100% of the time. Death is due to the vaccine. Not COVID respiratory illness. The vaccine is the proximal cause of death.

We have heard three false narratives. The first false narrative was that the virus is unassailable. We have to stay in lockdown and be fearful. The second false narrative is to take the vaccine, it's safe and effective. The third false narrative now is that it's not the vaccine causing these problems, it's COVID. It's COVID that we saw back in 2020 causing all these problems in 2023. Don't fall for the false narratives. The medical literature at this point is compelling. The Bradford Hill criteria for causality have been fulfilled. The vaccines are causing this enormous wave of illness, *not* COVID-19 respiratory illness in the past, or at present, with mild variants.

Now, could it be you or your family member who will drop dead next?

A few important papers to finish my comments. One is by Schmeling and colleagues from Denmark, demonstrating that about 30% of people who have taken a vaccine have zero side effects. Nothing. Not even a sore arm, not even a sensation that anything happened with the injection. Those people appear to be fine, forever, as if they didn't take a shot. The data are the same in the United States in our VAERS system. The second group is about 70% of individuals and they have some moderate side effects, some trouble, but they don't seem to really have serious events. Then there's the small third batch group for 4.2% in the Schmeling data. It's through the roof. Myocarditis, cardiac arrest, blood clots, hemorrhagic stroke, disabilities, sudden death at home, in bed, and the data are the same in the United States. Four point two percent of people in Europe right now are in trouble. Because they were unlucky enough to get a high risk batch.

In the United States our CDC V-Safe data, which is self-reported data, by 10 million Americans, the number of people who have been unlucky enough to get a high-risk batch is 7.7%. Among these are people who got so sick with a shot they had to go to the hospital to be treated or be hospitalized. A Zogby survey from about a year ago, with a big representative sample in the United States, found 15% of those who took a vaccine have some medical problem that they're dealing with right now. So again, 4.2%, 7.7%, 15%. That's the penumbra of COVID-19 vaccine injuries, or worse, affecting vaccinated populations today. That is the Venn diagram that you're all going to be involved in the calculus for you and your family members.

What's the path forward? The path forward is clear for no one to take another shot. No one.

Now, on June 11th 2022, the World Council for Health, which is a multinational, evidence-based physician and health care provider organization, issued a pharmacovigilance report looking at 39 safety databases, including the W.H.O., V-Safe and EMA databases, the US databases. Their conclusion was to remove all the COVID-19 vaccines from the market for excess risk of death. I repeat, excess risk of death.

On the floor of the US Senate, on December 7th 2022, I co-moderated a session and our expert panel in the US Senate concluded all the COVID-19 vaccines should be removed from the market. All of them. No new boosters. Then on March 23rd 2023, the Association of American Physicians and Surgeons, a factual, fact based, evidence based, consensus driven organization, just like the two others, also concluded that the vaccines should be removed from the market. So I suggest to you that the COVID-19 vaccines and all of their progeny and future boosters are not safe for human use.

I implore you, as a governing body, the European Commission, and the European Medicine Agency, to apply all pressure and due urgency to remove the COVID-19 vaccines from the market.

In the United States it's going jurisdiction by jurisdiction, probably state by state, to remove them from the market if the federal government doesn't do so. It's going to happen all over the world. But the W.H.O. is standing behind these vaccines. They are far more of a problem than a help to the European Union.

It's my belief that the European Union, the United States and all major stakeholders should completely pull out of the W.H.O., to leave the W.H.O. to its own endeavors, so that this organization will not have any jurisdiction, authority, or dominion over what we do in health care. The W.H.O. will never have a say over what I do as a practitioner with the patients in my practice.

CHAPTER 16

How many deaths were caused by the COVID vaccines?

Dr. Norman Fenton

Professor of Risk, Queen Mary University of London

Norman Fenton is Professor Emeritus of Risk at Queen Mary University of London (retired as Full Professor Dec 2022). He is a mathematician by training with current focus on quantifying risk and uncertainty using causal, probabilistic models that combine data and knowledge (Bayesian networks). He has published seven books and over 350 peer reviewed articles. His works cover multiple domains including law and forensics (he has been an expert witness in major criminal and civil cases), and health. Since 2020 he has been active in analysing data related to Covid risk.

Summary

- Contrary to the claims made by COVID vaccine proponents there is hard evidence that most reports of vaccine deaths to the USA VAERS and UK Yellow Card systems are genuine. At most, 30% of these reports can be ruled as likely not to have been caused by the vaccine.

- There is also evidence that the reporting rates for deaths and adverse events to these systems is very low. It is likely that fewer than 10% of deaths and other adverse events ever get reported.

- With these minimal assumptions we estimate there have been:
  - approximately 120,000 deaths in the USA directly caused by the COVID vaccines (between Dec 2020 until 23 March 2023) and 16,000 in the UK (between Dec 2020 until 29 Sept 2022).
  - over 103 deaths per million doses of the COVID vaccines in the UK with big differences between the three main vaccines (187 for AstraZeneca, 68 for Pfizer and 35 for Moderna). For AstraZeneca that amounts to 1 death in every 5348 doses.

- Taking account of the small proportion of people reporting serious adverse reactions that may have subsequently led to early deaths, there are likely to have been an additional 70,000 deaths in the USA and 35,000 in the UK indirectly caused by the vaccines. This would mean deaths caused directly or indirectly by the vaccines account for about half the excess deaths in the UK since Jan 2021.

A personal story

At the beginning of January 2021 a friend's father was one of the early recipients of a covid vaccine in the UK. He was 90-years-old but, for his age, in reasonable health. He died less than 24 hours later. My suggestion of a possible link to the vaccination was treated with total incredulity by the family. In Jewish tradition he was buried the day after his death and, of course, no post mortem was ever considered. The vaccination was never mentioned again and it was assumed by all that his death was natural and inevitable.

Since then, I have lost several friends at relatively young ages from cancer and heart attacks. All were fully vaccinated. Two of the cancer victims had been in remission before the vaccinations. Again, not a single family member considered any possibility of a link to the vaccination and none of these cases were reported to the UK Yellow Card system for possible vaccine adverse reactions.

However, I know of one extremely serious and traumatic adverse reaction that followed shortly after the second dose of the AstraZeneca vaccine in April 2021 that *was* reported to the Yellow Card system. Here is the vaccination card with the batch numbers:

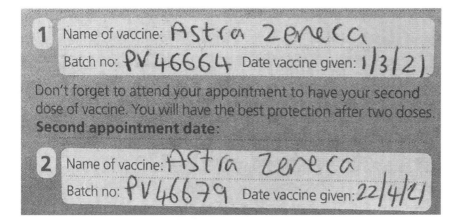

It is one I reported myself as it happened to a very close family member and the effects of this have been life-changing to the victim as well as myself.

I found the Yellow Card system extremely difficult to navigate and it did not allow me to input highly relevant specific information. It seemed designed not to collect such data. I suspect that many people attempting to navigate the system will have given up and not finalised and submitted their report. I have never received any confirmation or follow-up to my report. Furthermore, my GP and specialists involved in the case were dismissive of my claim of a vaccine link. A family member of this victim also suffered an adverse reaction which was reported to the Yellow Card system.

How many 'officially reported' deaths occurred?

Except for a tiny percentage of deaths occurring shortly after vaccination, doctors have been extremely reluctant to properly investigate claims of serious adverse reactions from covid vaccines by patients or their relatives. This reluctance to investigate happens even when deaths have been reported to the VAERS or Yellow Card systems. As such, only a tiny minority of cases have ever been subject to formal medical verification, and it is this tiny number that Governments are keen to promote to sustain the false argument that the benefits of vaccination far outweigh the harms. For example, in the UK only coroner-confirmed deaths qualify for the Government's £120,000 compensation payment scheme and (as of 3 March 2023) only 52 such deaths[1] were officially classified as having been caused by covid vaccines. This is despite the fact that as of 29 September 2022, there had been 2,272 COVID vaccine deaths reported[2] to the Yellow Card scheme.

In the USA things are even worse because, despite 17,315 deaths being reported to VAERS (as of 23 March 2023), it seems that no deaths have been 'officially' recognised as directly caused by COVID vaccines. And any attempt to use VAERS as the basis for estimating the true number of such deaths have been simply quashed by the 'fact checkers' as misinformation on the grounds that these are simply 'unconfirmed reports.'[3]

Fact Chokers ...not 'Fact Checkers'

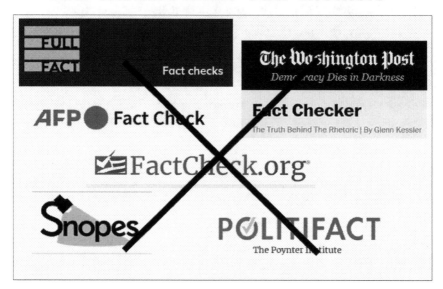

---

1   https://www.researchprofessionalnews.com/rr-news-uk-politics-2023-3-uk-pays-out-nearly-4m-in-covid-19-vaccine-damages/

2   https://yellowcard.ukcolumn.org/yellow-card-reports

3   https://apnews.com/article/fact-check-cdc-covid-vaccine-deaths-910677348223

Can we estimate the unreported number of deaths from VAERS and the Yellow Card systems?

We want to make the fewest assumptions possible to estimate the unreported number of deaths from those reported. To do this we need two measures:

1. The *reporting rate* (also often called, somewhat confusingly, the *under-reporting factor*): What proportion of vaccine deaths are actually reported to VAERS and Yellow Card? If, for example, only 10% of all vaccine deaths are reported then the reporting rate is 10%.

2. The *false positive rate*: What proportion of vaccine deaths actually reported to these systems are not caused by the vaccine. If, for example, 40% of all deaths reported as vaccine deaths were not caused by the vaccine then the false positive rate is 40% while 60% are true positives.

COVID vaccine sceptics claim that the reporting rate is very low due to a combination of:

- People having never heard of the reporting system or assuming someone else would complete it;
- Difficulty in completing the form;
- No surviving relative to complete the form;
- No surviving relative willing to complete the form;
- Failure to contemplate that the cause of illness or death may have been related to the vaccine.
- Compared to previous vaccines, the likely way in which harm is mediated by the mRNA vaccines means adverse events are much more spread out over both time and also the organs affected. This inevitably reduces attribution compared to previous vaccines and suggests under-reporting could be greater.

It has been claimed that (for all types of vaccines) as few as 1%[4] of vaccine injuries are reported to VAERS. A more recent analysis claimed[5] a figure of 1 in 41, i.e., 2.4%. I think that 10% is a conservative estimate, although I will consider a range of values. Whatever the actual underreporting figure is for VAERS, it is likely to be even lower for the Yellow Card scheme which is especially difficult to navigate to submit a report.

Vaccine 'proponents' often claim that the false positive rate for the VAERS and Yellow Card systems are very high because of either false/malicious reporting or the supposed lack of clinical knowledge of the reporters. However, when the first batch of deaths were reported in VAERS for the COVID vaccines, McLachlan et al. undertook a detailed analysis (with a 2023 update[6]) of a sample of 250 reports and concluded that less than 15% could be dismissed as invalid.

A reader has now alerted us to a much older paper[7] from 1982 published in the BMJ that provides further valuable insights into the false positive rate for reported serious vaccine adverse reactions. Although the sample size was small (57 reports to the Yellow Card scheme in the UK), it shows that 40 were true positives (77%) while none of the remaining 17 could be proved to be false positives. So, in the absence of evidence to the contrary, it seems reasonable to assume that at least 70% of death reports to the Yellow Card and VAERS systems are genuine, and it is reasonable to assume a false positive rate less than 30%

Estimate of direct deaths caused by the COVID vaccines

Taking account of the 30% false positive rate (70% of the reported vaccine deaths were caused by the vaccine), and different possible under-

---

4   https://openvaers.com/faq/what-is-underreporting-and-why-it-matters

5   https://jessicar.substack.com/p/the-under-reporting-factor-in-vaers

6   https://www.researchgate.net/publication/367030584_Extended_Analysis_of_CO-VID-19_Vaccine_Death_Reports_from_the_Vaccine_Adverse_Events_Reporting_System_VAERS_Database

7   https://www.ncbi.nlm.nih.gov/pmc/articles/PMC1495801/pdf/bmjcred00590-0033.pdf

reporting factors we get the following estimates of number of COVID vaccine deaths based on Yellow Card and VAERS for the UK and USA:

	UK	USA
	(up to 29 Sept 2022)	(up to 23 March 2022)
Number of deaths reported	2,272	17,315
True positives reported (assuming 70%)	1,590	12,121
Actual number of deaths assuming reporting rates		
1%	159,040	1,212,050
5%	31,808	242,410
10%	15,904	121,205
15%	10,603	80,803
20%	7,952	60,603
25%	6,362	48,482
30%	5,301	40,402

Hence, with a 10% reporting rate we estimate nearly 16,000 deaths in the UK and over 120,000 deaths in the USA. While these numbers may look high, they are only a tiny proportion of all deaths registered since Jan 2021 (when the vaccine programmes were fully rolled out). For example, in the UK there were over one million deaths in total registered between Jan 2021 and end of Sept 2022, so 16,000 covid vaccine deaths would, as far as excess deaths are concerned, barely be noticed (less than 1.6%).

But what about the impact of serious adverse events reported on indirect deaths?

The number of deaths reported to VAERS is just a small percentage of the total adverse events reported. As of 24 March 2023, the totals in the USA were 947,487 broken down as follows:

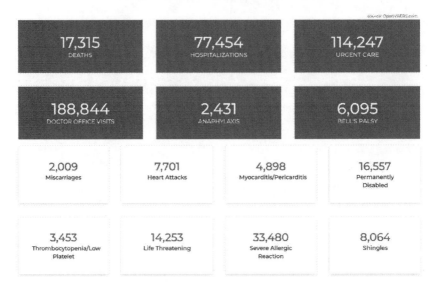

947,487 Reports Through March 24, 2023

Many of the more serious adverse reactions will increasingly contribute to early deaths that will never be directly attributed to the vaccines. Of course, whereas as noted above the number of deaths directly caused by the vaccines will barely make a dent on total excess deaths numbers, it has been hypothesised[8] that the large recent increases in excess deaths in highly vaccinated countries is due to the increasing number of deaths indirectly caused by the vaccines. What we really need to know is what proportion of those people reporting serious adverse events (approximately 200,000) have died earlier than they otherwise would have. If the figure is 5% then that would be 10,000 deaths. Based on the 70% true positive rate and 10% reporting rate that would mean an extra 70,000 deaths indirectly caused by the vaccines.

And serious adverse events reported in the UK?

This is where things become curious. In March 2023 the UK Government decided to stop properly updating the Yellow Card figures. In fact, the

---

8   https://wherearethenumbers.substack.com/p/the-devils-advocate-an-exploratory

latest report[9] does not even provide the updated death numbers. Nor does it provide the details of the proportion of reports that are classified as 'serious' in any easily searchable form. The only relevant numbers that are relatively easy to find are:

	Number of reports	Number of events	Number of doses	Reports per 1000 doses	Events per 1000 doses
Pfizer	177,925	511,776	84,700,000	2.1	6.0
AZ	246,866	874,912	49,159,700	5.0	17.8
Moderna	47,045	151,628	16,400,000	2.9	9.2
Other	2,182				

The total number of reports (summing the first column) is 474,018 which we can assume corresponds to different people reporting. If we assume that 20% of these 474,018 suffered at least one serious adverse event (as per VAERS proportion) then that would amount to 94,804 people. If 5% of these 'died early' then that would be nearly 5,000 deaths. Based on an assumed 70% true positive rate and 10% under-reporting factor that would mean an extra 35,000 deaths indirectly caused by the vaccines. Together with the above estimate of 16,000 deaths directly caused by the covid vaccines, a total of 51,000 would result. This is a significant proportion of the approximately 120,000 excess deaths recorded since Jan 2021.

What are the death rates per million doses?

Applying the same true positive rate and reporting rates to the data from the Yellow Card system (as of 29 Sept 2022) we get the death rate in the UK expressed in per million doses for all vaccines:

9   https://www.gov.uk/government/publications/coronavirus-covid-19-vaccine-adverse-reactions/coronavirus-vaccine-summary-of-yellow-card-reporting--2

	Number of deaths reported	Number of deaths based on 70% true positives and 10% under-reporting	Number of doses	Number of deaths per million doses
Pfizer	826	5,782	84,700,000	68.3
AZ	1,314	9,198	49,159,700	187.1
Moderna	82	574	16,400,000	35.0

In total we see 103 deaths per million doses, i.e., over 1 in 10,000, with big differences between the three main vaccines (187 for AstraZeneca, 68 for Pfizer and 35 for Moderna). For AstraZeneca that amounts to 1 in every 5348 doses. It is little surprise that the AstraZeneca vaccine was quietly and unofficially withdrawn in the UK as early as June 2021 (it had already been suspended[10] from many European countries as early as March 2021). That was before Dame Sarah Gilbert - who was in charge of the AstraZeneca development - received a standing ovation at Wimbledon Centre Court for her 'achievement.'

Conclusion

With a minimal set of conservative and reasonable assumptions we estimate that, since the end of Dec 2020 approximately 16,000 people in the UK have died directly from COVID vaccines, while in the USA the figure is approximately 120,000. An interesting validity check is that the US population is five times that of the UK. Taking account of the later date of the USA figures and the fact that the under-reporting is likely to be lower in the USA, the mortality rate is reasonably consistent between the two countries.

With respect to the additional number of those who may have died indirectly following serious adverse reactions, we have estimated 35,000 in the UK and 70,000 in the USA. This larger number (relative to

10 https://pharmanewsintel.com/news/european-countries-suspend-use-of-astrazenecas-covid-19-vaccine

population size) for the UK may be partly due to the widespread use of the especially problematic Astra Zeneca vaccine in the first half of 2021. Luckily for the Americans, this vaccine was not used in the USA. Three times as many adverse reactions per dose were reported for this vaccine than for the Pfizer vaccine and over twice as many per dose than for the Moderna vaccine. However, as reported on Twitter[11], all follow up reports are deleted from public VAERS, which means that many reports in VAERS are actually their least serious version. There are approximately 140,000 missing IDs, and each could be a deleted follow up report.

While AstraZeneca has effectively been discarded worldwide, the roll-out of yet more boosters of the other vaccines continues. Yet even before these vaccines were shown to be ineffective in stopping infection and transmission there were already sufficient safety signals that should have led to their suspension. In the USA, the CDC's own analysis[12] of the Pfizer and Moderna vaccines found hundreds of safety signals, while an analysis[13] of the original controlled trials data from these companies also revealed unacceptably high rates of serious adverse reactions. The recent Rasmussen poll[14] as well as the insurance data[15] from the USA provide strong evidence that the estimates we have made of deaths from the vaccines really are very conservative. With evidence of the increasingly low risk that COVID poses to any age group, there is no scientific basis for anybody to get another dose of a COVID vaccine.

This calamity needs to stop now.

11   https://twitter.com/OpenVAERS/status/1643402285228363778
12   https://childrenshealthdefense.org/defender/cdc-safety-signals-pfizer-moderna-covid-vac-cines-et/
13   https://pubmed.ncbi.nlm.nih.gov/36055877/
14   https://www.rasmussenreports.com/public_content/politics/public_surveys/covid_19_virus_deaths_vs_vaccine_deaths
15   https://www.google.com/url?q=https://valuetainment.com/new-vaccine-analy-sis-reveals-300000-excess-u-s-deaths-147-billion-in-damage/&sa=D&source=do-cs&ust=1688013284988413&usg=AOvVaw2HsoGwmlcBs9W2CkPh3R39

CHAPTER 17

The Day
Journalism Died

Rodney Palmer

A 20-year veteran of Canadian journalism
at the CBC & CTV

Rodney Palmer is a twenty-year veteran of Canadian journalism. He was an investigative reporter and producer for CBC Radio and Television. From 1996-2004 he was foreign correspondent for CTV News in India, the Middle East, and China.

On April 4, 2020 the top news anchor at the Canadian Broadcasting Corporation started speaking gibberish. Adrienne Arsenault, the highly respected and trusted co-host of The National started her news item looking at the cell phone in her hand and saying, "What do you do if this happens? A loved one, let's say it's your dad..." and she goes on to describe how to behave when your dear old dad sends you a wacky text falsely claiming this new virus was engineered in a Chinese lab.

I had reported on the SARS outbreak while stationed in Beijing as foreign correspondent for CTV News in 2003, and followed the snail's pace of the World Health Organization and its virus hunters who target patient zero. Back then it took about three months for the Chinese government to allow them into the country, and then they stalled them in Beijing while they tried to negotiate their way to Guangdong where the outbreak first emerged.

On April 4, 2020 the world was still only three months into the known emergence of the COVID-19 virus, and less than three weeks into the Canada-wide state of emergency. I knew the virus hunters hadn't begun to search for patient zero yet, because no one was getting in or out of Wuhan where it was first reported. But on this premature date, the CBC confidently reported that it would be so ridiculous to consider a leak from the Wuhan bat coronavirus laboratory, that only someone as archetypally clueless as your father would even suggest it. Arsenault's breaking story on the CBC National nightly news was an interview with Claire Wardle from "First Draft", a fellow member of the Trusted News Initiative, who instructed Canadians how to ensure their beloved dad gets put in his place without being too offensive. The interview portrayed a new social balancing act like an episode of Covid Miss Manners. A musical tension track played subtlety in the background. It wasn't news. It was fluff, with an underlying message of propaganda designed to misdirect any suspicion that this new virus might have come from a lab in Wuhan. But unlike most of Arsenault's audience, I happened to know it was too soon to rule that out.

Newsgathering: (*noun*) "The process of researching news items, especially those that will be broadcast on television or printed in a newspaper."

Misdirection is a common form of propaganda. Having worked in China I heard it on the state broadcaster daily. Especially when it related to Taiwan, Hong Kong, or the Falun Gong. When I worked in Israel, I learned how soldiers are trained to instantly identify misdirection, because their lives depend on looking away from it. Usually in the opposite direction. Arsenault's interview on April 4, 2020, the day journalism died, was a deliberate misdirection. It was designed to draw our attention away from the lab, where by all evidence we should have been looking.

Only ten days later, The Washington Post newspaper shone a spotlight of journalism onto the Wuhan lab. Their writer Josh Rogin described two communications cables sent from the US embassy in Beijing to Washington in 2018. The cables warned that the Wuhan Institute of Virology presented a high-level risk to global health due to unhygienic practices. The cables eerily predicted, "the lab's work on bat coronaviruses and their potential human transmission represented a risk of a new SARS-like pandemic," Rogin reported. The warnings were written in 2018 suggesting the Wuhan lab was the probable origin. Alternative origin stories were absurd and not worthy of attention compared to the likelihood of a predicted leak from the unhygienic lab that was working on this exact virus, and located in the city where it was first reported. By April 14, 2020 the international virus hunters had their prime suspect. But here in Canada? Adrienne Arsenault, one of the most recognizable faces in Canadian journalism, cheerfully and confidently told Canadians that it was beyond ridiculous to conceive of such a foolish notion.

Propaganda: (*noun*) Information, especially of a biased or misleading nature, used to promote or publicize a particular cause or a point of view."

What the CBC did was classic propaganda. An intentional misdirection. A year later Vanity Fair magazine flushed out the whole story. In June 2021, the magazine published a shocking and exhaustive investigation by journalist Katherine Eban. The story revealed that Shi Zhengli, the Director of Emerging Infectious Disease at the Wuhan Institute of Virology had been fondly nicknamed the Bat Lady by her colleagues. She had presented at scientific conferences recounting how she scraped bat guano from a mine in China in 2012 after she learned that some local miners grew fatally ill with a sudden onset respiratory virus. Back at the Wuhan lab, Shi isolated a deadly new virus already proven to jump from animals to humans – the miners. Vanity Fair's riveting deep dive into ten years of scientific publications outlined how the Wuhan team had injected a protein from this new and deadly virus into a sample of the SARS 2003 virus they had stored in the lab. The scientists in Wuhan had created a Frankensteinian new virus.

Then in 2019 around the time the US Embassy was sending warning cables to Washington, the Wuhan scientists published a new paper outlining how "genetically engineered rats with humanized lungs," were being grown in their lab.

Never was there a hotter smoking gun than the one sizzling off the pages of the 2019 scientific paper outlining how the Wuhan lab had engineered humanized lungs onto rats while experimenting with the new and deadly coronavirus it had engineered a few years earlier.

Vanity Fair cited peer reviewed publications, government emails and letters, and recorded public speeches by Shi and others who worked with her in Wuhan. This was real investigative journalism. The type we've come to expect from our best of the best, like the CBC. This is why journalism matters. It has the power to save the world.

Typically a big story like this, that is both true and easily verifiable, becomes the new standard by which all major news outlets begin to speak the same truth. However, this time Vanity Fair's explosive report was largely ignored. It was exhaustive and relevant to every human on the planet. It chronicled the Wuhan lab's decade-long effort to create a new and deadly coronavirus that was particularly contagious to human lungs. Yet it was not adopted as the new truth by our trusted messengers of news. Instead, they asked us to accept that a more likely scenario might be that two animals had engaged in interspecies copulation.

In the past, CBC was legendary for its journalism. Their top reporters got the wrongfully convicted freed from prisons. They exposed fraud in corporate Canada and acted as a government watchdog. Overnight they had transformed into the governments' lapdog.

Next, they engaged in fear mongering. Instead of reporting the pandemic deaths as a percentage of 100,000 people – the classic approach of epidemiologists – the CBC announced the number of sick and dead hourly. They gleefully began counting by the thousand while never examining the statistically flawed PCR test by which they counted them. While governments began closing schools, the reporters almost never identified that the age of most Canadians claimed by Covid was older than their expected lifespan, or that many were already dying in hospice or palliative care wards when they first tested positive for COVID.

Fear: (*noun*) "An emotional state evoked by a threat of danger"

Soon the CBC's other top anchors started speaking gibberish. Matt Galloway CBC Radio's big national morning man, the voice of the country; smart, curious, energetic, and self-woven into the fabric of Toronto, jumped on the misdirection bandwagon. He promoted the phrase "anti-vaxxer", identified what he called "misinformation" and one day even interviewed a man who said recommending natural medicines to stay healthy is the same as promoting hatred, and causing death. It was classic Orwellian doublespeak. The opposite of what he was saying was true.

Doublespeak (*noun*) "Language that is intended to make people believe something that is not true."

Even the legendary CBC Radio personality Brent Bambury, host of the always relevant Saturday morning current affairs show "Day 6", besmirched the reputation of film maker Stew Peters who produced a documentary called Died Suddenly about the recent onset of Sudden Adult Death Syndrome that is plaguing insurance companies and all-cause mortality statisticians across America. Bambury focused his coverage of this shocking subject on the irrelevant political views of the filmmaker, and besmirched his reputation. It's known as a smear job in the business. Its aim is to attack someone's character to distract the audience from what the person is claiming. Bambury smeared Peters for all of Canada to hear, instead of informing us that he's onto something. On the same day of his broadcast, Bambury or the journalists who work on his show, could have looked up on a Canadian government website to see that at least 427 Canadians were reported to have died suddenly after taking the "safe and effective" COVID vaccines that his network was vigorously promoting.

Similar data patterns are easily accessible on the US government's adverse event reporting system called VAERS, or the UK vaccine injury reporting system called Yellow Card. At the time of Bambury's smear job, these systems were listing tens of thousands of deaths and millions of injuries from the Covid vaccines alone. Bambury and the CBC chose to ignore this global trend, and instead attacked the character of a journalist who was pointing it out.

Con: (*Adj.*) "Swindling. Confidence with a sense of assurance based on insufficient grounds."

It's hard to rank the atrocities inflicted on the Canadian people by the CBC in the last three years, but disparaging a proven cure for COVID-19 has to be near the top. In October 2021 a Canadian doctor named Daniel Nagase started his shift at the emergency room in a hospital in rural Alberta. He found three patients growing progressively worse with symptoms of COVID-19. He administered ivermectin and all three patients improved in hours. One of them was over 90 years old and he was able to shake off the virus and get transferred back to his nursing home. After saving their lives, Dr. Nagase was fired from the hospital and has since had his medical license revoked. In its coverage of this story the CBC did not focus on the fact that Dr. Nagase had cured three hospitalized COVID patients with an inexpensive and common medicine that is proven to be effective in populations around the world. Instead, it reported that the doctor spread "misinformation" and was fired for it.

The CBC missed an opportunity to raise the pillar of journalism upholding our democracy by telling the truth about what happened. Instead, it assisted in the dismantling of our democracy by reporting only that we fired the doctor after he demonstrated we could cheaply and effectively dig ourselves out of this quagmire of lockdowns and mandatory masking.

As time crawled by it became evident to anyone who understands how news is written, that the CBC had embarked on the biggest pharmaceutical marketing campaign in the history of our country: COVID-19 vaccine promotion. The government is buying. The CBC is selling. They instructed us not to take the medicine that has been shown to work. Instead they said to take an experimental vaccine promising to prevent what you're already sick with. It was a double-speak, backward-think, con job that made no sense. And it was impossible to execute this charade without the most trusted voices of the CBC leading the attack.

Throughout 2020 and to this day, the CBC ignored the growing number of Canadians reported to be injured or killed by COVID vaccines. Thousands of them are listed by "serious" illness on an easily located government website. Even when 200 activist vandals plastered photos and symptoms of the injured and killed on the entranceway to CBC headquarters in Toronto one morning in January 2023, they still ignored the evidence. They derided Canada's most learned scientists who raised red flags. They suppressed them from alerting us about Pfizer's fine-print data which clearly predicted pericarditis and myocarditis reactions from the mRNA injections. The result was a wave of these cardiac injuries on the bodies of Canadians, mostly healthy young men, who trusted the CBC when they told us daily that these injections were completely safe, and completely effective.

I watched in horror as my national broadcaster belittled our elected Members of Parliament who stood together in opposition against coerced injections on behalf of themselves and their constituents. The CBC fomented fear and hatred against an increasingly identifiable group they labeled "anti-vaxxers" in a sustained campaign of derogatory propaganda. It must have been stomach-churning for those who could not comprehend what the CBC was perpetrating. Our gut understands a lie instantly, but our brain takes a moment to catch up.

The strongest messages were delivered by the big-name broadcasters who at one time represented decades of cumulative journalistic credibility. They are what Canada feels comfortable listening to because we've grown up with them, or we've grown old with them as they've matured in their careers. But when our government installed a malicious intent behind our most trusted level of talent and experience, they created a weapon. Like the stormtroopers in the Star Wars trilogy, CBC's announcers transformed overnight from trusted truth tellers into a propaganda machine hell bent on distracting us from the origin of the virus, igniting fear, advising us not to take medicine, and selling an unproven pharmaceutical potion as the only solution to our collective conundrum. During COVID-19, the CBC transformed into a weapon of the state, aimed at its citizens.

Weapon: (*noun*) "A thing designed or used to inflict bodily harm or physical damage."

There is as much abject reporting by other Canadian broadcasters, newspapers and magazines. And this is not unique to Canada. News media capture is in fact a global virus more deadly than COVID-19 because it succeeded in the genocidal annihilation of journalism. In the United States Pfizer conspicuously sponsors major news and current affairs programming. I have seen similar bullying tactics spoken by MSNBC's Rachel Maddow and CBS's Stephen Colbert. Both in a professional league of their own. Both weapons of the state when conducting a disinformation campaign aimed at their trusting audience.

Who is responsible for the toll of injured and dead from the vaccines, if not the people who bullied and tricked us into taking them?

Today, and since March 2020, we have observed a unification of our competing news agencies, a single source that silences critics. It is no longer journalism. It is propaganda. In this case it is largely pharmaceutical marketing disguised as journalism. This is why people who follow the news as gospel are currently in profound disagreement with their friends who seek their information elsewhere. A dictionary is an example of an agreed upon truth. The news is no longer an example of agreed upon truth. And in our democracies, we will never agree on what's right, if we can't first agree on what's true.

Without journalism we have no democracy. It is a critical pillar supporting the healthy function of an informed electorate. Right now, all we have is a distorted version of truth that has been carefully rebranded "Trust".

Trust: (*noun*) "Assured reliance on the character, ability, strength or truth of someone or something."

The standard bearer of news is now the Trusted News Initiative. A marriage of journalism and tech companies, it includes the BBC, CBC/Radio-Canada, Facebook, Google/YouTube, Twitter, Microsoft, AFP, Reuters, *Financial Times*, *The Wall Street Journal*, European Broadcasting Union (EBU), *The Hindu*, First Draft, and Reuters Institute for the Study of Journalism, among others. It works by the tech companies identifying online posts or stories that may harm pharmaceutical marketing, and recommending that the member news agencies label it "misinformation" and publish or broadcast counter narratives.

The members call it "fact-based journalism" which is more doublespeak because it seeks only to suppress facts.

There are others in the "Trust" pedaling racket including the "Journalism Trust Initiative" by Reporters Without Borders. Also the "Trust Project", another groupthink fact-suppressing agency that includes seventy major media members including CBC, CTV News, The Globe and Mail, The Canadian Press, as well as the BBC, The Economist magazine and dozens of others including such "independent" Canadian media outlets as The Walrus magazine. Project Verify is a recently launched venture of the BBC, designed to tell those who can't decide for themselves what that broadcaster has declared to be true or false. None of these organizations promise the truth, which would easily earn our trust. Instead they brand themselves with a promise of "trust".

Most of our trusted journalists have betrayed us, but not all of them. They're just not working for anyone you would recognize as a newsgathering organization anymore. The period that covered COVID-19 lockdowns and mass vaccination gave swift rise to alternative media websites, many of which are as reliable as what we now call the "mainstream media" used to be.

Millions more turn to Joe Rogan's podcast than listen to Canadian news broadcasters. Rogan interviews critical players in the world and lets them talk for hours. The Children's Health Defense electronically publishes a daily journal called The Defender which exceeds the standards of journalism at any current media outlet. In 2020 it quickly began publishing authoritative newsgathering about the World Health

Organization's growing dominance over our lives that was not being covered by CBC, or other Canadian media.

The rise of alternative media which hold verifiable truth as their north star is swiftly rendering CBC News and Current Affairs irrelevant. In Canada a little online media upstart called Rebel News catapulted from a right wing politically aligned thorn in the side of the Liberal government, to a news generating powerhouse fueled by a newfound hunger for truth in news reporting. Similar to Children's Health Defense, the Rebel News team began a campaign of lawsuits when it identified censorship, media favoritism and government overreach in its response to COVID-19. In addition to reporting daily news, it crowdfunded legal defense budgets for small businesses that were fined for staying open during the emergency. It asks for money in the body of every online story, usually taking a dig at the CBC's annual $1.2 billion government funded budget. Its daily diet of why we should be skeptical of Justin Trudeau grew relevant to more Canadians as they witnessed an escalating suspension of their right to free movement and free speech. There are many more relevant little upstarts such as Bright Light News, The Iron Will Report, Western Standard, and True North, but Rebel News more than any other has rushed in to fill the void created when CBC abandoned the truth, in favor of begging for our "Trust".

When the world-famous truckers' convoy in Ottawa was mis-portrayed as a Nazi rally, rather than the peaceful labor action that it was, Rebel News got to work. It sent reporter Alexa Lavoie to find the source of two mysterious photos of Nazi flags taken in odd locations. Lavoie was on the ground in the middle of the crowd for the entire three weeks of the protest. She was famously shot in the leg with a canister of teargas at harmfully close range when Trudeau sent the police to evict the peaceful protesters with force. Lavoie returned to the scene for a forensic investigation of the photos and through the most intrepid reporting this country has seen in the last three years, she plausibly connected the photographs to Trudeau's office, the office of his coalition government co-leader Jagmit Singh of Canada's New Democratic Party, and a CBC reporter who is a repeat offender of derogatory COVID-19 coverage. Anyone who watched could immediately understand the level of counter intelligence our government was capable of executing against its citizens. And none of it was possible without the compliance and participation of the CBC, our former watchdog.

On April 16 this year Elon Musk had Twitter add a banner to the CBC page that labeled it "Government Funded Media". The next day CBC announced that it was in a collective corporate huff and suspended its use of Twitter. It was mad and it was going to hold its breath until it got its own way. CBC's Editor in Chief Brodie Fenlon wrote a blog that said "We are beholden to no one. We report without fear or favour. We act only in the public interest."

However, it's easy to observe that Fenlon has overseen the weaponization of his on-air staff, and the betrayal of his country who trusted him to steer the CBC through the chaos and cacophony and deliver us the truth like we've come to expect it. Throughout its pandemic coverage, the CBC systemically disguised the identity of Trudeau government spokespeople. It regularly elevated the voices of a select group of Canadian "experts" affiliated with a newly formed organization called Science Up First that was founded in 2021 with a $1.75 million grant announced by Trudeau's Health Minister Patty Hajdu. The assignment was to promote vaccines and silence or ridicule what they deemed to be "misinformation" about COVID. These spokespeople were then interviewed dozens of times on the CBC, introduced to Canada as our national "experts" but it was never revealed that they are funded by the Trudeau government to promote COVID-19 vaccines. These "experts" spent the last three years misdirecting us from the failures of the vaccines. The most high-profile spokesman, a lawyer named Timothy Caulfield, is connected both to the Trudeau government funding, and to the private Trudeau Foundation, which was recently embroiled in a scandal accepting Chinese government money to influence the last Canadian election in Trudeau's favor.

The CBC has yet to identify any of these government funded "scientific advisors" in their role as government propagandists and pharmaceutical marketers. Instead, they are regularly misidentified in "news" items as Canada's top experts who we may trust without question.

We might be able to forgive a period of exception when the CBC broadcasting apparatus was considered useful as an instrument of government messaging, but that period is over and the CBC continues to advise us to wear masks and get vaccinated against COVID-19 despite the growing numbers of injured and dead listed from them on our government's website. The entire apparatus has donned propaganda as its new security blanket, even as its national audience shrinks because they've been forced to look elsewhere for the truth.

It is not comforting that in addition to the $1.2 Billion dollars the Canadian government spends to fund the CBC every year, it is now in the habit of spending more than $100 Million annually in grants to the rest of the private news media outlets across Canada, most of which continue to publish the government message about COVID. Coincidentally Rebel News does not receive any government funding. Despite all this financial support, the news media giants in Canada are in a freefall to becoming irrelevant. Across the country our guts are telling us something's not quite right when we listen, or watch, or read, and our brains are starting to catch up.

As we begin to look back at what went so horribly wrong worldwide, the news media appear increasingly culpable. It is reasonable to conclude that the most unsupportable and dictatorial aspects of government policies could not have been executed without their complicity. They duped their audiences by abandoning our expected standards of journalism, suppressing science, persecuting scientists, and ignoring Canadians who were unjustly injured or killed by this experimental gene therapy injection, the full damage of which is still unfolding. It is almost impossible to rebuild trust once it is lost. The only way to recover a whisper of truly earned trust in our news media might be a criminal investigation into why they knowingly disseminated false information which betrayed their audience and caused thousands of people to put themselves in harm's way. Only then might we find out who benefited from making journalism disappear.

Truth: (*noun*) "That which is true, or in accordance with facts or reality."

Have you gained important insight from this book? If so, we would like to hear your thoughts. Please rate and review on Amazon. Honest reviews help readers find the right books for their needs.

CHAPTER 18

COVID Exposed: A Corrupt Medical System

Dr. Paul Marik

Pulmonary and Critical Care Specialist & co-founder of the FLCCC

Dr Paul E Marik is a world-renowned Pulmonary and Critical Care Specialist, founding member and Chairman of the Frontline COVID-19 Critical Care Alliance (FLCCC) and co-developer of the highly effective treatment protocols for the prevention, treatment and recovery from Covid including vaccine injury. Dr. Marik is the second most published critical care physician, having authored over 500 peer-reviewed journal articles, 80 book chapters and 4 critical care textbooks.

This essay is based upon an interview between Dr. Paul Marik and Glen Jung at Bright Light News. It has been edited for clarity and length into an essay format. It is included in this book thanks to the permission of Dr. Marik and Bright Light News.

COVID has cast a really dark specter on medicine because I think everything they told us has been proven to be a lie. We knew it was a lie, but they really got away with it. Perhaps the only good thing to have come of this is that it's shone a bright light into the corrupt system, a fraudulent system that's been there for a long time. Many of us didn't see it. I didn't see it. For me, COVID has basically exposed the fraud, the corruption, the deception that's always been there. Now, once you see it, it's as bright as day, you can't unsee what you've seen.

There are two things that I think have been catastrophic. One is censorship; humanity and science and knowledge is based on an exchange of information, people talking, having a civil conversation. We may not agree with each other, but at least let's talk about it so that we can both understand each other better and we can grow. But that ability to have a conversation has been completely obliterated. People have dissenting points of view; that's been the history of mankind. That's how knowledge has been forged, by people discussing stuff. I think the censorship that we have experienced during COVID has had a terrible effect.

Second is the false narrative that's been propagated, "safe and effective." People get exposed to one point of view and one point of view over and over through captured mainstream media, social media and medical journals. In this way, people aren't exposed to dialog, and they are expose to the same narrative, which happens to be a false and deceptive narrative. In essence, it's what Mattias Desmet said, this is mass formation. Most of the population has been brainwashed.

Everything they told us was false, and these falsehoods were perpetuated. Many came from the CDC, the NIH, the W.H.O., the FDA. This wasn't by accident. This was a well-orchestrated plan with a nefarious agenda. At the outset, to question natural immunity was completely absurd. We've known about natural immunity ever since we understood immunity. To question that natural immunity doesn't exist is absurd because we know it's robust, we know it exists. To question the presence of natural immunity is like questioning the presence of the sun and the moon. It's such a basic fundamental concept in medicine and in science. The data is now clear and probably the best example is a study out of the Cleveland Clinic, a highly reputable, prestigious health care system in the U.S.

The Cleveland study has shown that the unvaccinated are at a lower risk of getting COVID than the vaccinated. Then each time you get a shot, one, two, three, four, it increases your risk of getting COVID. Consider that; the medical establishment is now recommending vaccination to prevent a disease which is actually causing the disease. While the medical establishment is claiming it protects you, their data is clear. Natural immunity is far better than anything the vaccine can induce. It's deceptive to have even suggested that natural immunity was less effective than the vaccine.

Then we have the masks. We know the masks didn't work. At the beginning, even Fauci said they didn't work. "Right now, there's no reason to be walking around with a mask. When you're in the middle of an outbreak, wearing a mask might make people feel a little bit better and it might even block a droplet. But it's not providing the perfect protection that people think that it is," he said.

We know the virus is infinitesimally smaller than the pores or holes in the mask. So to suspect that it would stop viral transmission or protect people is completely absurd. Now we have a Cochrane Review study - the gold standard - which definitively and categorically shows that masks simply do not work.

Next we have the lockdowns, which were one of the most detrimental policies ever. With all kinds of plagues and diseases threatening humanity through history, never have we ever locked people down. It simply doesn't work. We know that locking people down had terrible repercussions. The effect on childhood development, the combination of masks, lockdowns and social isolation has had a devastating effect on children. There's really good data looking at cognitive development and brain development, pre-COVID and post-COVID. We now have a generation of kids that are cognitively impaired from being exposed to all of these repressive, inhumane measures, and particularly masks, because facial recognition is very important. It's the way we communicate. It's so fundamental to human development.

The other thing which was insane is that we prevented children from playing in the park. Once again, complete absurdity because you don't get COVID outdoors. And kids, just because of their own innate immunity, have a far reduced risk. We prevented kids doing what kids do, playing outdoors. And we forced them to wear masks.

And so to the biggest hoax; the vaccination hoax. Safe and effective? We know now categorically, definitively, without question, that it is neither safe, nor effective. And Pfizer's own data and the CDC's own data proves that.

There was early treatment. That's how we got into this charade, right from the beginning, the W.H.O., the CDC, the NIH said there was no treatment. They basically told people stay at home until you go blue. Then when you go blue, you go to the hospital and they'll give you remdesivir. We know that remdesivir is a toxic compound. They tried to use it for Ebola but they had to stop the study because the Data Safety Monitoring Board deemed it a toxic, dangerous drug. We knew before COVID that it was toxic. But then they tried to use it again for COVID because of financial interests. We know, according to the W.H.O.'s own pharmacovigilance system data, that remdesivir increases risk of kidney failure 20-fold, and increases risk of death. So why in heaven's name would doctors use a drug which is ineffective against SARS-CoV-2 and increases the risk of death and adverse events?

There are many off-label interventions that are highly effective against SARS-CoV-2, but health policy makers don't want you to know about them. Because the first plan was a shot in every arm; that was the goal. If you had natural immunity, then they had a problem because how would they sift out who had and who didn't have natural immunity? So that's why they said natural immunity doesn't exist. End goal; everyone gets a vaccine. Then if there was safe, effective treatment, that again, would have interfered with their agenda for a vaccine in every arm. Therefore, safe, effective therapy in their eyes didn't exist. That was the propaganda they projected. We know that there are at least 20 well established interventions which limit the spread of COVID, limit hospitalization, limit death. These are simple interventions that are cheap and safe. But they didn't want anyone to know about them.

I think probably the biggest crime against humanity was vaccinating children. Their goal now is to get the COVID shot on the childhood vaccination program, which is abhorrent. It's pure evil because we know the risk of a child actually dying from COVID is negligible. Children without pre preconditions who are otherwise healthy, are at a greater risk of being struck by lightning. They are at a greater risk of drowning in their bathtub than ever of dying from COVID. The risks are infinitesimally small, yet we know the risks from the vaccine, which include myocarditis, which is a well-established complication in young kids and adolescents, as well as over 750 other reported diseases is common.

Next there's the problem of death. Young, healthy kids, just dying suddenly. There's overwhelming evidence that to vaccinate a child is a crime. And yet we continue to do it. It's interesting that some countries have woken up. For example, Sweden, Denmark and even the UK now have banned vaccinating people under the age of 50 because it is so cost ineffective, with so many adverse events. And yet we are still vaccinating children in the U.S.

Even more profoundly disturbing however, is vaccinating pregnant women. Pregnant women have always been considered highly vulnerable. You don't experiment with medications in pregnant women. We learned this from the thalidomide disaster. We know that using any medication in pregnancy, particularly the first and second trimester, is always a hazardous intervention. So here we were vaccinating women with an untested vaccine. The long term effects have never been established. Safety in pregnancy was never determined and yet the FDA and CDC continues to insist it's safe in pregnancy. Whereas we know from Pfizer's own data, the spontaneous miscarriage rate in vaccinated women was 84%. So the vaccine was more effective in terminating a pregnancy than the abortion tablet.

Recently, Dr. Thorpe did a really outstanding study based on CDC and FDA data. He compared complications with the COVID vaccine, with the influenza vaccine. The influenza vaccine was used as a control, and it's by no means completely safe. The data is stunning. It shows in terms of menstrual abnormalities in women that the risk with this COVID vaccine is increased 1000-fold. Not double, by 1000. The risk of spontaneous miscarriage, the risk of congenital abnormalities, the risk of eclampsia. It's just off the charts; the risks in women were so excessive. You can't hide that data. Fertility rates across the whole of Europe are plummeting; live births have gone down 20 to 25%. There's something really sinister going on.

One of the reasons many of us came to North America was we thought this was the seat of democracy, that one had freedom of speech, freedom of movement, freedom of expression, freedom of choice, freedom to decide what medical interventions you get. That's been taken away from us. Informed consent for a medical procedure is such a basic human right. It's part of the Helsinki Agreement. After the Nuremberg trials, it became such a fundamental concept that people should have informed consent that when it comes to their bodies, true informed consent, not deceptive consent where Big Pharma manipulates the consent form or is not truthful. Those rights have been eroded. That's the scariest part of this; that basic human dignity, human freedoms, human rights, human democracy are being eroded for some other nefarious agenda.

We're now facing a tsunami of vaccine injured people. This is not a conspiracy theory. We can look at the V-safe database. The V-safe database was an app which the CDC developed and they gave randomly to, I don't know, 10 million vaccinated people. They then tried to suppress the data because what happened was that people who were vaccinated could input their data; whether they had adverse events, whether they were hospitalized, whether they were treated. The CDC tried to hide that data, so ICAN and Aaron Siri (ICAN's lawyer) took them to court and had the data released. What did it show? Six point eight percent of people vaccinated had serious adverse events, 6.8%, which far exceeds the 1% of the threshold of the FDA. If a child car seat kills three kids, they'll take it off the market. But here we have a medical product that has maimed, killed and injured millions of people, and it's being promoted. If you extrapolate the data, we know that there are at least 18 million vaccine injured people in the U.S.

The problem is that the medical system doesn't recognize it, doesn't accept it and will not study it. These people suffer. They have no financial or medical support. Most of the doctors will say to these people, "it's psychological. It's in your head. You're making this up," largely because it's not been well-reported. Many of these patients have multiple symptoms, so it doesn't fit in with the usual paradigm of a specific medical condition.

In these patients, the average number of symptoms is 23. The spike protein goes to every single organ in the body. Arne Burkhardt's autopsy series from Germany shows the spike protein disseminates to every single organ in the body, most notably the brain, the heart, the kidneys and causes severe inflammation, clotting, all kinds of bad pathological things. That's why they have so many symptoms. And so this has become a massive humanitarian crisis.

We're facing this expanding population of severely injured people. There's no antidote. For these vaccines, they didn't come up with an antidote. So at the FLCCC we had to come up with what we think is the best way to deal with spike protein-induced disease. It's based on our best understanding of the disease. It's based on pathophysiology. It's based on our understanding of human physiology. We can't sit by and do nothing. So we've come up with a treatment protocol for the vaccine injured. This is available at FLCCC.net.

More recently, we have developed a treatment protocol for people who have been vaccinated and are worried about developing symptoms later on. People six or seven months post-vaccination are dropping dead. Thanks to the data of Arne Burkhardt and Ryan Cole, we know why this is happening. It's because of the spike protein. We've developed a protocol to help people reduce the risk. Ideally it would be something that the federal government should be interested in and we should be doing studies looking at some way to risk stratify those at greatest risk of complication, so that we could target those people. We have a general approach to what to do if you've been vaccinated and you're in the window of three- to four- months to maybe 12- to 14- months after vaccination, when you're at risk of dying suddenly and getting cancer. It will evolve with time.

COVID has shone a light on what was there before. Can you trust the medical system? Can you trust what they're telling us? I think you have to question everything because many of these narratives that we believe are the truth are not. When you dig deep into them, they are completely fabricated and false. The people who you thought you could trust, the medical agencies, the medical schools, the medical journals, are untrustworthy because you have to follow the money. That tells you the story. The goal is to make money. I think COVID has made this clear.

I think it's pretty obvious that the FDA, the CDC, the NIH are completely captured and you can't really trust them. The biggest problem is that the FDA regulates medicine, but they've taken it a step further. They think they are now in the business of telling doctors how to practice medicine, which is far beyond their charter. Part of the problem is the conflict of interest. There's this rotating door; people work for pharma, they go to FDA, they work for FDA, they go to Big Pharma. So the conflicts of interest between the FDA and Big Pharma is truly astonishing. The FDA hides data. There should be complete transparency. Research data should be available for everyone. But that's not the case. I mean, the fact that Pfizer and the FDA conspired to hide the data from the Pfizer trial for 75 years,, why would they have done that? They would only have done that if they wanted to hide the data. So the FDA is completely corrupt. I don't think it can be repaired.

The FDA should be funded 100% by the federal government. There needs to be a regulatory branch and a safety branch which act independently, not together because that's further conflict. But there's no incentive for Congress to change this as they get their money from Big Pharma. I think that's why we need to start with the state legislature and eventually, the American Congress has to do what they were elected to do, which is work for the people. Isn't that an amazing concept? They were elected to work for the people. They weren't elected to work for big pharma. They should do what they were elected to do. We need to reform, if not scrap the CDC, the FDA and the NIH, because they're all captured.

I think the bottom line is that people need to empower themselves. They can improve their health, not with medication, but with simple lifestyle changes. They can lead happier, more productive lives. That's what our goal is at the FLCCC.

CHAPTER 19

The Deadly Consequences of Censorship

Dr. Jay Bhattacharya

Professor of Medicine, Economics, and Health
Research Policy at Stanford University

Jayanta "Jay" Bhattacharya is an Indian American professor of medicine, economics, and health research policy at Stanford University. He is the director of Stanford's Center for Demography and Economics of Health and Aging. His research focuses on the economics of health care. Dr. Jay Battacharya was one of the original signatories to The Great Barrington Declaration in October 2020. The Declaration argued that targeted protection was the most reasonable reaction to COVID-19. It was pilloried and censored across big tech, by the media, by government, within the academic community and the medical profession.

This essay is based upon an interview between Dr. Jay Battacharya and Jan Jekielek. It has been edited for clarity and length into an essay format. It is included in this book thanks to the generosity and approval of Dr. Jay Battacharya and Jan Jekielek, his podcast American Thought Leaders and The Epoch Times.

It's one thing for me to be censored, because if this was just a story about me, that would be one thing. The problem is that me and many of my colleagues were trying to make an argument that the public health response we were following was incredibly misguided. It was going to lead to the harm of countless children and the starvation of millions of people around the world because of the economic harm from the lockdowns.

We were arguing that the diversion of attention from other vital medical priorities was quite shortsighted, and that there was an alternate strategy, focused protection, that could also have better protected older people from the disease. If we had been allowed to make that argument clearly, if we had not been suppressed by the government, by the university that I work at, or news organizations that basically put out propaganda, we would have won that argument. We had better science. We had the better argument regarding the balance of harms.

We had the better understanding of who was actually at risk of COVID. We would have won that argument and the world would have been better off. Many people that are dead would be alive today had we been allowed to make that argument. That's why to me, it's so important to tell this story about the suppression of science by the government, and the failure of academic institutions like my home university, Stanford, to stand up for academic freedom when it counted most.

Almost from the beginning of COVID, I faced tremendous backlash within my own home institution - Stanford - for speaking up. I wrote an op-ed in March of 2020 in the Wall Street Journal, the first op-ed I had ever written in my life. It said that we don't yet know how deadly COVID is. I just went through some evidence from the Diamond Princess data and said, "Look, the disease might be much more widespread than we initially believed."

And it called for a study. The conclusion of the piece was, "let's do a study." We had already locked down the world. It wasn't like we could go back in time. It just said, "What is the empirical basis for the policies that we are following? We don't even yet know how deadly the disease is."

That almost immediately led to my getting death threats. I started getting messages from friends. One of them eventually de-friended me on Facebook. It was petty little things. But the thing that was funny on campus was that it didn't lead to a broader discussion. Even though I had been at Stanford for 36 years, 20 as a professor, and 15 tenured, I felt like I was on the outside immediately. I had done something where I had breached some norm.

What happened was that I wrote the Great Barrington Declaration. I work in a medical school. I do health policy and infectious disease epidemiology for a living. We just put forward in the Great Barrington Declaration, in October 2020, a major proposal for an alternate strategy to the central policy problem facing the entire world.

It generated an incredible amount of attention, both positive and negative, and it certainly needed to be platformed at Stanford. What I mean by platformed is that one of the main things about the life of a university is that professors give talks about their ideas. It sounds so mundane and boring and most professors are saying, "Who cares?" about most of my talks.

But that is actually quite important. It tells the world, "Look, these ideas are things that are worth discussing, that are worth paying attention to, that are worth respecting even if you disagree with them, even if they turn out to be wrong." Normally, what would have happened when a professor at a major university makes a major proposal like that, is that there would have been invitations within the home institution of the university for debate and discussion.

Instead, what happened was essentially omerta, silence. Nothing. I was still getting death threats from various random sources. On campus, I started hearing the mutterings of people wanting to figure out how to deal with the Jay problem. The summer before, in 2020, there had already been an attack on my colleague, Scott Atlas, who was an advisor to President Trump. A hundred of my colleagues had signed a letter, which I believe was a deeply irresponsible thing to do, attacking him for things he didn't do.

The letter actually said that hand-washing was important, somehow implying that he didn't believe in hand-washing. Scott was trying to argue for focused protection of vulnerable people. He was trying to argue for opening schools. He was following the scientific evidence that actually supported all this, and that's what he was advising President Trump. These one hundred people that signed the letter didn't understand the evidence as well as Scott did. These were colleagues of mine, people I've written papers with, and people I respected.

I called one of them and asked him why he signed the letter. He said he hadn't taken a very close look at it. There was tremendous social pressure to sign, and even junior people who didn't have tenure were scared that if they didn't sign, what would happen to their tenure? That was the atmosphere at Stanford when the Great Barrington Declaration came out. I couldn't get any traction on trying to get my views aired on campus.

At one point, the former president of the university, John Hennessy, called me and asked me if I'd be willing to do a debate. This was in December of 2020. I was absolutely thrilled. I thought, "Okay, finally we have someone who's well respected in the Stanford community trying to organize something. I don't even know if he agreed with the Great Barrington Declaration. It didn't matter, right? What mattered was that there was going to be some discussion.

He couldn't get anybody on the other side to sign on. In my home department, the department chair essentially sent the proposal for a debate or a discussion off to a committee that he must have known was going to fail. There was no platforming. There was no time when Stanford said, "Okay, we're going to host a discussion about this."

I just want to emphasize why that was important. It's not because of me personally, although personally I did feel hurt. It was important, because if Stanford had done that, it would have been a major institution telling the world, "Look, this is a debate that's worth having."

We were already having legitimate people with legitimate credentials that didn't agree with the lockdown consensus. There wasn't a consensus. There was never a consensus. That was an illusion created by Tony Fauci and a small number of incredibly powerful people.

Four days after we wrote the Great Barrington Declaration - I learned this months and months later - Francis Collins, the head of the National Institute of Health, wrote an email to Tony Fauci calling me, Sunetra Gupta, and Martin Kulldorff, the three primary authors of the Great Barrington Declaration, fringe epidemiologists. I actually just laughed when I heard this because it's just funny.

Martin Kulldorff is probably the best biostatistician working in vaccine safety today. He designed the statistical infrastructure that the FDA and the CDC uses to track vaccine safety. I had used his methods before the pandemic, even before I met him or knew about him. Sunetra Gupta, is essentially the professor of theoretical epidemiology at Oxford University, an incredibly brilliant mathematician and epidemiologist. Just before the pandemic, she was working on developing a universal flu vaccine, a vaccine that you don't have to update every year. She is an incredibly impactful scholar who's had a career at the center of epidemiology.

I have a business card somewhere that says fringe epidemiology. A friend of mine sent it to me afterwards. It was a deeply irresponsible thing for Francis Collins to do. It was an abuse of his power. He's the head of the National Institute of Health. He sits on top of $45 billion of federal funding.

Stanford gets a half a billion dollars a year from the NIH. Not only does he control the money, he also controls the social status of scientists. If you don't get NIH grants as a biomedical researcher, it puts you down the social hierarchy within the social structure of academic medicine. I would not have gotten tenure at Stanford if I had not won NIH grants.

To say that these three people are fringe, why would he do that? It's because he didn't want to cope with our ideas. He didn't actually want to address the substance of our ideas. He just wanted to dismiss us, and socially, make us outsiders. He wanted to excommunicate us from the scientific community.

What is the message that top universities get when they hear this? They don't want their social status and their brand hurt by association with fringe epidemiologists or fringe figures. They don't want the possibility that maybe the funding sources that the NIH provides will get threatened, or that the social status conferred by the NIH to these institutions will get threatened. They brag about how much NIH funding they get.

So, you have a federal government figure abusing his power. Why? Because he couldn't stand the idea that there were prominent scientists that disagreed with him about pandemic policy. That's why he called for a devastating takedown of our premises. Initially, the best they could do was tendentious articles in Wired magazine. The substantive counterattack didn't exist.

When there finally was a substantial counterattack to the Great Barrington Declaration, it came in the form of pieces in prominent scientific journals, but with ridiculous scientific arguments like, "We don't know if there's any immunity after infection." There was a memorandum called the John Snow Memorandum signed by very prominent people, including the current CDC director, who signed her name in November of 2020.

The John Snow Memorandum was problematic because it misread the science. For instance, it said that you can't know for certain that there is immunity after infection. It acknowledged that there were some lockdown harms, but downplayed them. It pretended as if they were inevitable, as if the lockdowns were the only inevitable choice to make.

All of the harms that came from them were just downstream from this inevitable decision, as opposed to a thing that we decided to do.

It dismissed the possibility of focused protection, essentially sending a signal to the public health community, "Don't even try. The lockdowns will protect old people. That should be enough." But the result of that was essentially a corruption of the scientific process, a corruption of major institutions, governments, universities, and top scientific journals in service of a policy that almost everyone now agrees was entirely ineffective.

Even by the standards of COVID deaths alone, how many millions have died? Did the policy work? It essentially ignored the possibility there could have been alternate policy, which there was.

I joined Twitter in August of 2021. I only joined for one purpose and I figured I needed to make a very public case for the ideas in the Great Barrington Declaration for sane public health. Just writing scientific papers alone wasn't moving people within the scientific community. It was also clear to me that it was the public that had been most harmed by these lockdown policies—our kids out of school, poor people decimated by COVID, and the difficulty of working class people to make a living and feed their family.

I wanted to tell the public that there was this alternate policy. The purpose of joining Twitter was to reach people that hadn't heard my message, and perhaps disagreed with me. I could put the evidence that I had in front of them, and put the arguments they had in front of them.

With Twitter, you have your followers, you can send your message, and generally the followers will see it. Not always, but generally. Sometimes though, the posts go viral. They trend in the language of Twitter, so that the broader Twitter community, the millions and millions of people that read Twitter also see those messages from time to time. Not every message, but from time to time.

When Bari Weiss wrote that piece about the Twitter files and she put me at the top of it, she revealed that I had been placed on a trends blacklist. I love that term. It reminds me of the McCarthy era back in the 1950s. Actually, that's what this era feels like. It's like a strange suppression of dissidents by the government that is so sure that it's right, that it feels okay to do this. The trends blacklist made sure that whenever I did a Tweet, the broader Twitter audience wouldn't see it.

I felt like I was reaching an audience, because I had 100,000 followers, but I didn't know that I had no chance of actually accomplishing what I wanted to accomplish by going on Twitter, which is to tell the broader public that there was something deeply wrong with the COVID policy.

I got invited to visit with Elon Musk as a result of these revelations in the Twitter files. What I found out during my visit there at Twitter headquarters is that I was actually placed on the blacklist the very day I joined Twitter. Why did that happen? It's not Twitter 1.0 on its own that decided this.

That came about because government actors were involved at the highest levels of federal bureaucracy telling social media companies what ideas to censor and who to censor. Maybe the first or second post I did on Twitter was the Great Barrington Declaration. It is still my pinned tweet. You can go see it. And that is what led to the blacklisting.

There needs to be a bright wall of separation between government and media because there's a power imbalance. You can read the emails from Missouri versus Biden; the deposition testimony, the FOIAs, and all the discovery emails, and it looks like there's this collaborative buddy-buddy relationship. The government says, "These are the people to censor and these are ideas to censor." And Twitter says, or the social media companies say, "Oh great, we want to help you do this." It looks like a collaborative relationship, but at its heart, it cannot possibly be a collaborative relationship, because the government telling these companies to do this has an implied threat within it.

The government regulates these companies. The government has tremendous powers to make these companies succeed or fail. And so, when it gives these kinds of instructions, the implied threat is that we can destroy your company.

Normally, the U.S. Constitution would protect against these kinds of things. It was built into the very fabric of our government agencies that this would be something so far out of bounds they wouldn't do it. It's one thing if you have the government say, "This guy is an international criminal terrorist." You can understand how there may need to be some kind of line of communication around that.

But the line between that and suppressing scientific discussion, suppressing policy discussion should have been a bright red line that never should have been crossed. The government agencies essentially decided to treat scientific debate on COVID policy as if we were dissidents who were on the other side of the government, as if they were just like those international terrorists in some sense. They thought it was okay to suppress those kinds of people and those kinds of ideas.

As an American citizen, it's not right for the American government to have that kind of power. The basic fundamental American norm is free speech. I understand there are nuances around exactly what that means. Free speech is not the freedom to reach everybody, but at its very heart it is permitting a space for debate to take place among scientists and policy makers and concerned members of the public on vital policy issues.

The government decided through its actions that they didn't want to let that happen during the pandemic. Again, as a result, it's really not about me, it's about the fact that we would have won this debate about lockdown policy. So many people that were harmed would not have been harmed. These vaccine mandates would not have been in place.

People wouldn't have lost their jobs or careers over them. The schools would've opened earlier. The panic mongering would've been addressed, so the anxiety and depression problems that we are seeing might have been less. The economic devastation from the lockdown policies might have been avoided, at least to some degree.

From all of these consequences, the conclusion I take away from that is that this censorship activity killed people. Ironically, during the pandemic, we heard all these things like we can't have free speech during the pandemic. The constitution is not a suicide pact. Ironically, had the First Amendment actually been in place during the pandemic, it would have saved lives, would have led to less damage and destruction with fewer people dead.

Just take the damage to poor people around the world: There was an estimate that the World Bank put out that a hundred million additional people, as a consequence of the economic dislocation caused by just the early lockdowns, were thrown into dire poverty, living on less than $2 a day of income. Many of those people starved.

Many of them didn't send their kids to school. Actually in poor countries, they put their kids to work, and pulled their kids out of school entirely. Uganda is a good example of this. Four-and-a-half million kids never came back to school after two years of school closures. A lot of them, especially the young girls, were sold into sexual slavery because the families couldn't feed them. When you take an action as dramatic as a lockdown, you set in motion a whole domino set of effects.

On the subject of supply chains: The end point of a supply chain is some poor person in some poor country that's reorganized its economy to fit into the global economy. He loses his job, can't feed his family, and then he has to make a terrible choice between starving, or exploiting his kids so that they don't starve.

These are the kinds of things that policymakers really need to be thinking about when they make these decisions. They didn't think about them. They didn't think about them because the people that would've brought them up were being suppressed.

Lockdowns meant that some kids were out of school for a short time in the United States. Some kids were out of school for not just a short time, but a very long time. There's social science literature that precedes the pandemic that found even short interruptions to kids schooling has long-term consequences for the kids. They end up being poorer as adults, more likely to have chronic illness, and they live shorter lives. It's not equally distributed. It's the poor kids that suffer the most from this, because there's no making it up, or less of making it up. It's a generational driver of inequality that we created during the pandemic.

There have been a number of attempts to try to do an after-action report about the pandemic. The Democratic House, for instance, conducted one. There have been a couple of other COVID commissions, the idea of which is a good one in the sense that after natural disasters, after plane crashes, after terrible things, after a patient dies in a hospital, you come together with the experts that are involved, sometimes outside experts, and you do an honest assessment of what went wrong with the goal of reforming the process so that it doesn't happen again.

The problem is that these after-action reports have been conducted by people who made the decisions in favor of the lockdowns. As a result, they have not asked the critical questions that need to be asked to really do an honest after-action report. For instance, why was immunity after COVID infection ignored in basic decision-making? The science was really clear in 2020.

What were the forecasting models that were used to justify lockdown? There was a lot of evidence that those models were deeply inaccurate even at the time. Why was that evidence ignored? Why were the schools closed for such a long time when the evidence from around the world, especially in Europe, was showing that wasn't necessary?

Why did people think that vaccination would lead to permanent protection against infection, when there wasn't evidence from the randomized trials confirming that was true? These are both scientific questions and policy questions. Why were lockdown harms not considered? Normally, when you take an action, the regulatory agencies have to do a benefit-harm calculation. You can't just pretend there's only benefits, especially for a lockdown policy, which almost certainly causes deep harm.

If you don't consider the lockdown harms, then of course you can't consider how to mitigate them. These questions have to be asked and any honest COVID inquiry will ask those questions. It may be a question of who, but to me, the emphasis is on the what and why. If we answer those what and why questions, we will be in a much better position to make reforms so that the disaster of lockdowns does not recur. Nearly every prominent institution in the world that should have protected us failed. That disaster shouldn't be repeated.

But if we don't ask those questions, it will be repeated, because of what has happened in the commissions that have already come up. They have just whitewashed it. They have whitewashed the lockdowns. And they have institutionalized the lockdown strategy as the strategy that they will follow in future pandemics.

That's where we are currently. It's not a theoretical matter. These institutions, in order to avoid embarrassment, have said that they did a good job without ever asking the critical questions. This might have led people to conclude that they didn't do a good job.

For the questions that we put in the Norfolk Group document, there may be good answers to them. There may be answers where you say, "Okay, yes. They did a good job on this." You can understand why they did that. But if you don't ask those questions, you can't get good answers and you can't get good reform.

You can't get a good policy. Where we are now, when there's another respiratory virus pandemic, we will lock down again and we will use the vaccine-only strategy. The Biden administration actually put out a policy idea where the goal in the next pandemic will be to get a vaccine in 130 days.

There's a few things about that. If you are aiming at a vaccine in 130 days, what that means is you can't test the vaccine for very long, maybe for one month. You probably can't recruit very many people, so you're going to approve a vaccine in 130 days, and recommend it at scale with pretty inadequate testing.

What are you going to do for those 130 days? There is this deadly disease going around. At least that's what the authorities will say. And there's this promise that the science is going to produce the vaccine in 130 days. What we'll do is we'll lock down for four months in anticipation of the vaccine.

The de facto policy now for respiratory virus pandemics going forward into the future is the policy that we followed, this disastrous policy that didn't protect us against COVID, and that led to all the lockdowns. That is the current policy of the United States, and it's the current policy of many countries around the world.

We need an honest discussion, and an honest commission that actually asks the hard questions, which is what the Norfolk Group document is. It is providing an agenda for what those questions might be.

The danger is the power of groupthink married to power. You have a relatively small number of very powerful science bureaucrats who surround themselves with people that won't tell them that they've gone wrong. That's why that fringe epidemiology thing is so telling. You have these outside experts telling you you're wrong, "They must be fringe, because our group thinks it's right." They thought they were right. They thought they were so right that they could exclude outside voices.

There was a doubling down as the evidence started getting worse and worse about the policies they suggested, or that their reading of the science is wrong. It's very difficult for powerful people to say, "Yes, we got it wrong," and change their minds. I've seen a few, but it's very, very rare that it happens. The scientific establishment, especially the scientific bureaucracies in the World Health Organization and in the U.S. government and many other places just dug their heels in.

In 1500 in Europe, if you wanted to know the truth, you would look to your priests. There would be these trusted centers of authority that would tell you, "Here's what's true, here's what's false." Those centers of authority were rooted in the Christian religion. When those trusted centers of authority went outside of their real expertise, they got things very, very wrong. The persecution of Galileo was a good example of this.

In the modern world, the analogy of the Christian clerisy then, is the scientific bureaucracy and scientists now. If you want to know what's true and false, you follow the science. But science isn't like that. Science is complicated. At its heart, there's this deep humility that we're up against our ignorance about how the world actually works, and there is this method to try to develop it at the same time. So, you have this humble method that's trying to slowly expand our knowledge about the way the physical world works.

At the same time, you have the tremendous power from being at the top of this clerisy that can distinguish true from false unerringly. And then, based on that, policy gets made. People get excluded from society because they have an idea that is out of sorts with what the supposed consensus is.

It's the same problem that the Middle Ages faced. You have a high priest, and a clerisy that has divorced itself from the actual scientific method that gives it power, opining in places and making decisions in places where they don't actually know what is true or false. But in the minds of many, many people who don't know how to read science—like infectious disease epidemiology, it's a complicated subject—it's not surprising that so many people don't know how to read it.

There's nothing wrong with that. The problem is that you have someone like Tony Fauci going around on TV in a sort of avuncular way conveying to the world that he is some knowledgeable guru who can tell the difference between true and false unerringly, even when he changes his mind five minutes later, and even though the things that he's saying are not connected to actual science. It has a tremendous influence on the minds of people and we have to figure out systems not to allow that to happen.

The key mechanism to guard against what we've gone through is to allow a very large diverse set of voices to be heard, and not allow the government's power to render scientists that disagree with the government off to the fringe. We must permit dissent. The scientific process involves debate and discussion.

So I can say, "I have a hypothesis. It has some implications about what I expect to see in the data. You have a different hypothesis. You expect different things in the data." We don't fight. What we do is we go collect data and evidence and run experiments, and on the basis of that, the experiment may come out in the way they predicted, not my way.

Then, I can say, "Now, your hypothesis is more likely to be true than mine. Maybe someone else will come along and have a different idea about what's going on with implications that you didn't think about and now you run experiments." It's a conversation. It's a debate. It's a discussion. It often gets very heated because people are very attached to the way they think about the world. But that's fine. You want that debate and discussion.

Now, of course, there's a whole range of scientific topics. The earth is round, and there really isn't a debate on that. People who say the earth is flat, you can pretty much dismiss them because there's tremendous evidence that Earth is round. You don't have to refight that over and over again.

But on the most important scientific matters, things where it's not known what's true and false yet, because we're still in the midst of our ignorance over it, you have to have that debate. On the edge of scientific discussion and scientific knowledge is controversy and debate. If you don't allow that process to happen, science is dead.

Let people make their own decisions. That will be much more effective in the long run than if you make some pronouncement like, "If you get the COVID vaccine, you will not get COVID, you will not pass COVID on." It turned out to be false. Now all of a sudden, who's going to believe the person that said that?

The only real way for public health to be effective is to treat the people that they're supposed to represent, the people they're supposed to help, as reasoning adults with moral autonomy, not like chattel or children to be manipulated or nudged, or made to do exactly what public health wants them to do.

The responsibility for public health officials is to convey the science as it is, as honestly as possible. When there's uncertainty in the science, when there isn't a consensus, don't lie and say there is one. And when there actually is a consensus like smoking causes lung cancer, just convey that.

The problem during the pandemic was that public health abdicated responsibility to convey scientific ideas, ideas about benefit and harm in a reasonable way. They treated people like children, as opposed to treating people like adults and reasoning with them.

Right now the policy situation is actually quite grim due to how public health has looked at lockdowns. Most people have moved on. The compliance and the fear, a lot of that has just dissolved away. People mostly think that COVID is over in one sense or the other, at least as far as their own lives are concerned. They don't view it with the same kind of concern that they did in March 2020.

At the same time, governments have essentially institutionalized these policies. We haven't firmly repudiated them, and so we're in actually quite a dangerous place. Because as I said, if there's another respiratory virus pandemic, it will happen again. The legal authority, the regulatory precedent, and the fact that this power exists to impose the lockdowns is now institutionally part of government.

With a lot of the assessments, there has been a whitewash of what happened. There is this disconnect that needs to get fixed. I don't believe if the people actually knew how unnecessary the lockdowns were that they would ever want them again. Now, many, many people feel the harms of the lockdowns themselves. They feel it deeply, but they can't articulate exactly what went wrong or why it was unnecessary.

We have to have an honest discussion, and I would hope that it would be bipartisan. I don't see any reason why it needs to be inherently political, because it's a failure of public health in my view. Public health isn't supposed to be Democrat or Republican. It's just supposed to be public health. So, the polity has a responsibility to do the assessment in the bipartisan way of public health, which is supposed to serve the polity.

That's where we are now. We are in a situation where people feel like it's over. There's a lot of relief. Of course, COVID is still floating around. It will be here forever, so it's not over in that sense, but the danger it poses is gone. We don't want the disruptions to continue anymore in our lives. Public health authorities want to take a victory lap. They can't really, but they can whitewash their sins.

There was some focused protection policy that was good. In Germany I saw some cities that had organized free taxi rides for older people to go to the grocery store. There was an attempt to deliver food to older people in their homes. Governor DeSantis actually had this great idea for a policy where there was this therapy called monoclonal antibodies. You had to get it with an IV. Normally, you would have to go to the hospital to get it. He organized that people could actually just call and then the infusion site would come to them in their home, for older people and vulnerable people. There were some good policies. All the policies that were focused on protecting older people in ways that didn't destroy their autonomy were actually quite good.

It's not to say that everything we did was wrong. I don't agree with that, but I think that so much that we did was wrong. So much that we did in the name of public health was unethical, and so much that we did in the name of public health was so destructive.

You have to have an honest assessment or else the public is never going to trust public health again. Public health isn't going to deserve that. And yet, the government power to enforce public health ideas is going to remain in place. It's a recipe for disaster.

There has to be an honest assessment, whether the leaders of public health want it or not. Too many people have been hurt and too many people sense that there were huge mistakes made, at the very least, if you want to call them that.

So, there needs to be an assessment. The only question is the form of it. And for the folks at home, what can you do? You can ask your school leaders, "What was that two years of school closure about? What are you doing to address the gaps in knowledge that happened?"

You can go to the nursing home where your mom or dad is and say, "When they were depressed, why didn't you let me come and say hello? Why didn't you try to figure out some safe ways to allow humane treatment?" You go to the hospital where your parents died and say, "Look, why didn't you let me say goodbye?" You can push your elected leaders for reform so that things like this never happen again.

There are things that happened to you during the lockdown that were bad during the last two-and-a-half years as a result of the lockdown policies, and as a result of the fear mongering. You can constructively use that hurt to push leaders to acknowledge the harm and to make reforms. That's really the source of my hope—that all these people that were hurt, and the populace at large coming to understand what happened wasn't necessary, and we can do better.

In my deepest heart, I believe that will happen if we can just get the agenda in front of the people, saying, "Here are the questions to ask your leaders," and to actually ask for new leadership in those institutions that failed. I think that can happen. I think that will happen. I think it's inevitable that it will happen.

The only question is how can we help the process along, and make it as constructive as possible? I'm not interested in Nuremberg 2.0. That's tremendously destructive. What I'm interested in is deep institutional reform. This is still the United States, a country that responds to people, and that is driven by the people.

Government is for the people. Government is by the people. As corny as it sounds, it is still true. We just need to give the people a voice and a set of questions to ask. That's what I hope to be able to do.

CHAPTER 20

Speaking Truth in Letters

Dr. Joseph Ladapo

Florida Surgeon General and Professor of
Medicine at the University of Florida

Joseph A. Ladapo, MD, PhD, is the State Surgeon General of Florida and Professor of Medicine at the University of Florida. His research program has been supported by the National Institutes of Health and Robert Wood Johnson Foundation, and includes clinical trials of interventions for weight loss, smoking cessation, and cardiovascular disease prevention among people with HIV. Dr. Ladapo's studies have been published in leading medical journals, including *The Journal of the American Medical Association* and *Journal of the American College of Cardiology.* His writings about health policy and public health have appeared in the *Washington Post, Wall Street Journal,* and *USA Today.* Prior to joining the faculty of University of Florida, he was a tenured Associate Professor at UCLA. Dr. Ladapo graduated from Wake Forest University and received his medical degree from Harvard and PhD in Health Policy from Harvard Graduate School of Arts and Sciences.

This chapter reproduces the correspondence between Dr. Joseph Ladapo, the CDC and the FDA in the early part of 2023.

February 15, 2023

Robert M. Califf MD, MACC, Commissioner
U.S. Food and Drug Administration, 10903 New Hampshire Ave
Silver Springs, MD 20993

Rochelle P. Walensky, MD, MPH
Director
Centers for Disease Control and Prevention 2877 Brandywine
Rd, Room 2402 Atlanta, GA 30341

Drs. Califf and Walensky,

The COVID-19 pandemic brought many challenges that the health and medical field have never encountered. Although the initial response was led by a sense of urgency and crisis management, I believe it is critical that as public health professionals, responses are adapted to the present, to chart a future guided by data and common sense.

As Florida's Surgeon General, it was in the public's best interest to issue guidance for using mRNA COVID-19 vaccines in children and in young men based on the absence of a health benefit in clinical trials. This guidance followed preliminary data analyses by the Florida Department of Health. We continue to refine and expand these findings, including addressing methodological issues inherent to evaluating vaccine safety and efficacy.

In addition to Florida's analysis of mRNA COVID-19 vaccines, academic researchers throughout our country and around the globe have seen troubling safety signals of adverse events surrounding this vaccine. Their concerns are corroborated by the substantial increase in VAERS reports from Florida, including life-threatening conditions. We have never seen this type of response following previous mass vaccination efforts pushed by the federal government. Even the H1N1 vaccine did not trigger this sort of response. In Florida alone, we saw a 1,700% increase in reports after the release of the COVID-19 vaccine, compared to an increase of 400% in vaccine administration for the same period. The reporting of life-threatening conditions increased 4,400%.

This increase in adverse events, compared to the percent increase in vaccine use, further explains the significant uptick we are seeing in VAERS reports. These findings are unlikely to be related to changes in reporting given their magnitude, and more likely reflect a pattern of increased risk from mRNA COVID-19 vaccines. We need unbiased research, as many in the academic community have performed, to better understand these vaccines' short- and long- term effects.

According to a recent study, mRNA COVID-19 vaccines were associated with an excess risk of serious adverse events, including coagulation disorders, acute cardiac injuries, Bell's palsy, and encephalitis, to name a few. This risk was 1 in 550, much higher than other vaccines. To claim these vaccines are "safe and effective" while minimizing and disregarding the adverse events is unconscionable.

Communication between physicians and patients is a standard ethical practice that is fundamental to public health. Health care professionals should have the ability to accurately communicate the risks and benefits of a medical intervention to their patients without fear of retaliation by the federal government.

The State of Florida remains dedicated to responding to COVID-19 and other public health concerns through data-driven decisions. We will continue to shed light on the safety and efficacy of medications, including mRNA COVID-19 vaccines, that could be an imminent threat to those with preexisting conditions. We will also promote the importance of prevention by supporting good nutrition, exercise, and other healthy habits. As a father, physician, and Surgeon General for the State of Florida, I request that your agencies promote transparency in health care professionals to accurately communicate the risks these vaccines pose. I requestthat you work to protect the rights and liberties that we are endowed with, not restrict, and diminish them.

I look forward to your responses and appreciate your support of our collective efforts to serve the health and safety of Florida and our nation.

Sincerely,

Joseph A. Ladapo, MD, PhD

State Surgeon General

Florida Department of Health
Office of the State Surgeon General

March 10, 2023

Joseph A. Ladapo, M.D., Ph.D.
State Surgeon General
Florida Department of Health
4052 Bald Cypress Way, Bin A-00
Tallahassee, FL 32399-1701

Sent Via Electronic Mail Only

Dear Dr. Ladapo,

Thank you for your letter regarding COVID-19 vaccine safety. We appreciate this opportunity to address your questions and we would like to correct the associated misinterpretations and misinformation about the data from the Vaccine Adverse Event Reporting System[1] (VAERS), in the spirit of transparency and supporting and serving the health of our nation.

The U.S. Food and Drug Administration (FDA) and the Centers for Disease Control and Prevention (CDC) continue to diligently monitor a variety of data sources to identify any potential risks of the vaccines and to ensure that information is available to the public. That said, focusing on adverse events in the absence of causal association and without the perspective of countervailing benefits is a great disservice to both individuals and public health. Like every other medical intervention, there are adverse effects from vaccination. Serious adverse events from COVID-19 vaccines are rare and are far outweighed by the benefits of these vaccines for every age group.

The claim that the increase of VAERS reports of life-threatening conditions reported from Florida and elsewhere represents an increase

---

1   https://www.cdc.gov/vaccinesafety/ensuringsafety/monitoring/vaers/index.html

of risk caused by the COVID-19 vaccines is incorrect, misleading and could be harmful to the American public. The FDA-approved and FDA-authorized COVID-19 vaccines have met FDA's rigorous scientific and regulatory standards for safety and effectiveness and these vaccines continue to be recommended for use by CDC for all people six months of age and older. Both FDA and CDC have continued to collect outcome data from multiple sources that demonstrate the clear benefit of COVID-19 vaccines in preventing death, serious illness, and hospitalization from SARS-CoV-2 infection, along with indicating a modest benefit in the prevention of infection and transmission that wanes over time, even as new variants have emerged. Additional benefits include a reduced risk of known complications from SARS-CoV-2 infection, including post-COVID conditions, COVID-19-associated stroke and heart disease, and COVID-19-induced venous thromboembolism.

Reports of adverse events to VAERS following vaccination do not mean that a vaccine caused the event. Since December 2020, almost 270 million people have received more than 670 million doses of COVID-19 vaccines in the U.S., with over 50 million people having received the updated bivalent vaccine. The Emergency Use Authorizations (EUAs) for the COVID-19 Vaccines require sponsors and vaccine providers to report certain adverse events through VAERS, so more reports should be expected. Recent concerns about increased reports of cardiovascular events provide an instructive example of the need to do further analysis when increased reporting of an event occurs. Despite increased reports of these events, when the concern was examined in detail by cardiovascular experts[2], the risk of stroke and heart attack was actually *lower* in people who had been vaccinated, not higher.

---

2   https://www.ncbi.nlm.nih.gov/pmc/articles/PMC9939951/

FDA and CDC physicians continuously screen and analyze VAERS data for possible safety concerns related to the COVID-19 vaccines. For signals identified in VAERS, physicians from FDA and CDC screen individual reports, inclusive of comprehensive medical record review. Most reports do not represent adverse events caused by the vaccine and instead represent a pre-existing condition that preceded vaccination or an underlying medical condition that precipitated the event.

Adverse events must be compared to background rates in the population. This VAERS review methodology allows for successful identification of rare adverse reactions related to specific COVID-19 vaccines (e.g., Guillain-Barré Syndrome, thrombosis with thrombocytopenia syndrome , and immune thrombocytopenia following use of the Janssen COVID-19 Vaccine or myocarditis, pericarditis and anaphylaxis following use of the Pfizer-BioNTech and Moderna COVID-19 vaccines). Information about these adverse reactions is included in the fact sheets[3] for healthcare providers administering vaccine and vaccine recipients and caregivers. FDA and CDC also continue to post summaries of the key safety monitoring findings[4] and present the data publicly at regularly scheduled advisory committee meetings.

In addition to VAERS, FDA and CDC utilize complementary active surveillance systems to monitor the safety of COVID-19 vaccines. Active surveillance involves proactively obtaining and rapidly analyzing information occurring in millions of individuals recorded in large healthcare data systems to verify safety signals identified through passive surveillance or to detect additional safety signals that may not have been reported as adverse events to passive surveillance systems.

---

3   https://www.fda.gov/emergency-preparedness-and-response/coronavirus-disea-se-2019-covid-19/covid-19-vaccines

4   https://www.cdc.gov/coronavirus/2019-ncov/vaccines/safety/adverse-events.html

FDA is conducting active surveillance using the Sentinel BEST[5] (Biologics Effectiveness and Safety) System and collaborating with the Center for Medicare and Medicaid Services (CMS) and Department of Veterans Affairs (VA). These efforts complement those of CDC's Vaccine Safety Datalink[6] (VSD) and the v-safe text-based monitoring system for conducting surveillance of adverse events, as well as the Clinical Immunization Safety Assessment[7] (CISA) Project. FDA and CDC are also collaborating with other non-federal partners, including state and local health departments.

Based on available information for the COVID-19 vaccines that are authorized or approved in the United States, the known and potential benefits of these vaccines clearly outweigh their known and potential risks. Additionally, not only is there no evidence of increased risk of death following mRNA vaccines, but available data have shown quite the opposite: that being up to date on vaccinations saves lives compared to individuals who did not get vaccinated. Multiple well conducted, peer-reviewed, published studies[8] [9] demonstrate that the risk of death, serious illness and hospitalization is higher for unvaccinated individuals for every age group. Because we are not the only country in the world using COVID-19 vaccines, we also benefit from the experience of other countries. More than 13 billion doses of COVID-19 vaccines have been given around the world, including hundreds of millions of doses of mRNA vaccines and hundreds of millions of doses to children. Consistent with our data, these multiple international partners have

---

5   https://www.fda.gov/vaccines-blood-biologics/safety-availability-biologics/cber-biologi-cs-effectiveness-and-safety-best-system

6   https://www.fda.gov/vaccines-blood-biologics/safety-availability-biologics/cber-biologi-cs-effectiveness-and-safety-best-system

7   https://www.cdc.gov/vaccinesafety/ensuringsafety/monitoring/cisa/index.html

8   https://www.cdc.gov/mmwr/covid19_vaccine_safety.html

9   https://www.bmj.com/content/377/bmj-2021-069317

robust monitoring for both safety and effectiveness. They find little evidence of widespread adverse events, also detect rare events as we do, and conclude that the benefits of the vaccines generally far outstrip their risks.

While many studies could be cited, a retrospective cohort study[10] using the CDC's Vaccine Safety Datalink found no increased risk of death for the mRNA and Janssen vaccines across age, sex, and race/ethnicity groups. They found that crude non-COVID-19 mortality rates among COVID-19 vaccine recipients were lower than those among unvaccinated comparators. Another study[11] using mathematical modeling estimated that the vaccines saved an estimated 14 million lives from COVID-19 in 185 countries and territories between December 8, 2020, and December 8, 2021. Vaccination is also associated with a reduction of post-acute sequelae of COVID-19[12]. The data supporting the benefits of the COVID-19 vaccines have been critically reviewed and accepted by the medical and public health community, including state and local public health agencies and academic and professional organizations.

The most recent estimate[13] is that those who are up to date on their vaccination status have a 9.8 fold lower risk of dying from COVID-19 than those who are unvaccinated and 2.4 fold lower risk of dying from Covid-19 than those who were vaccinated but had not received the updated, bivalent vaccine. Roughly 90% of deaths from COVID-19, as carefully classified[14] by the CDC, in recent months have occurred among those who were not up to date on their vaccines. Furthermore, as stated

---

10   https://www.ncbi.nlm.nih.gov/pmc/articles/PMC9763207/

11   https://www.thelancet.com/journals/laninf/article/PIIS1473-3099(22)00320-6/fulltext

12   https://www.thelancet.com/journals/eclinm/article/PIIS2589-5370(22)00354-6/fulltext

13   https://covid.cdc.gov/covid-data-tracker/#rates-by-vaccine-status

14   https://www.cdc.gov/coronavirus/2019-ncov/covid-data/covidview/past-reports/012723.html

above, emerging reports indicate a possible reduction in the risk of post-COVID conditions in vaccinated people who survive an infection.

As the leading public health official in state, you are likely aware that seniors in Florida are under-vaccinated, with just 29% of seniors having received an updated bivalent vaccine, compared to the national average of 41% coverage in seniors. It is the job of public health officials around the country to protect the lives of the populations they serve, particularly the vulnerable. Fueling vaccine hesitancy undermines this effort.

We agree that communication between patients and their health care providers is critical, and fully support clear, accurate communication about the benefits and risks of medical products. It is inaccurate to suggest that the federal government will "retaliate" against any health care provider for communicating with their patients about the benefits and risks of a particular medical product.

Over the course of the pandemic, FDA and CDC have held numerous public meetings to discuss the safety and effectiveness of the COVID-19 vaccines where detailed safety data are shared with outside experts and public comment is encouraged. Further, FDA publishes the full regulatory action package containing hundreds of pages summarizing clinical studies and review for each COVID-19 approval on FDA's website[15] (see "COVID-19 Vaccines Authorized for Emergency Use or FDA Approved") and CDC publishes an extensive amount of information on their clinical use in Interim Clinical Considerations[16]. Complete information about both benefits and risks helps health care providers better care for their patients.

---

15   https://www.fda.gov/emergency-preparedness-and-response/coronavirus-disea-se-2019-covid-19/covid-19-vaccines

16   https://www.cdc.gov/vaccines/covid-19/clinical-considerations/covid-19-vaccines-us.html

Unfortunately, the misinformation about COVID-19 vaccine safety has caused some Americans to avoid getting the vaccines they need to be up to date. This has led to unnecessary death, severe illness and hospitalization. These tragic outcomes not only have a devastating effect on individuals and their families, but they also create a tremendous strain on our healthcare systems and clinicians, potentially compromising care for other patients.

We stand firmly behind the safety and effectiveness of the mRNA COVID-19 vaccines, which are fully supported by the available scientific data. Staying up to date on vaccination is the best way to reduce the risks of death and serious illness or hospitalization from COVID-19. Misleading people by overstating the risks, or emphasizing the risks without acknowledging the overwhelming benefits, unnecessarily causes vaccine hesitation and puts people at risk of death or serious illness that could have been prevented by timely vaccination.

Sincerely,

Robert M. Califf, MD
Commissioner
U.S. Food and Drug Administration

Rochelle P. Walensky, MD, MPH
Director
Centers for Disease Control and Prevention

May 10, 2023

Robert M. Califf, MD, MACC Commissioner
U.S. Food and Drug Administration 10903 New Hampshire Ave
Silver Springs, MD 20993

Rochelle P. Walensky, MD, MPH
Director
Centers for Disease Control and Prevention 2877 Brandywine
Rd, Room 2402 Atlanta, GA 30341

Drs. Califf and Walensky,

Your ongoing decision to ignore many of the risks associated with mRNA COVID-19 vaccines, alongside your efforts to manipulate the public into thinking they are harmless, have resulted in deep distrust in the American healthcare system. Beginning with Operation Warp Speed, and possibly to be continued with an additional $5 billion investment in Project NextGen, the federal government has relentlessly forced a premature vaccine into the arms of the American people with little to no concern for the serious adverse ramifications.

It is critical to acknowledge and address the negative global impact caused by the emergence of COVID-19. Nonetheless, after two years, your collective decisions to deny that natural immunity confers comparable or superior protection to COVID-19 vaccination, push mRNA COVID-19 boosters for the young and healthy, and delay acknowledging the risks of vaccine- induced myocarditis have only sowed doubt between the American people and the public health community.

Data are unequivocal: After the COVID-19 vaccine rollout, the Vaccine Adverse Events Reporting System (VAERS) reporting increased by 1,700%, including a 4,400% increase in life-threatening conditions.

We are not the first to observe such a trend. Dismissing this pronounced increase as being solely due to reporting trends is a callous denial of corroborating scientific evidence also pointing to increased risk and a poor safety profile. It also fails to explain the disproportionate increase in life-threatening adverse events for the mRNA vaccines compared to all adverse events.

Based on the Centers for Disease Control and Prevention's (CDC) own data, rates of incapacitation after mRNA vaccination far surpass other vaccines. This is illustrated in a recent Lancet publication, Rosenblum H et al, *Lancet.* 2022, that reports up to one third of individuals being "unable to perform normal daily activities, unable to work, or [receiving] care from a medical professional" in the days following mRNA vaccination.

The study, Fraiman J et al, *Vaccine.* 2022, also found an excess risk of serious adverse events of special interest for 1 in 550 after mRNA vaccination. As you are aware, this is extraordinarily high for a vaccine. In comparison, the risk of serious adverse events after influenza vaccination is much lower (Lusigan S, *Lancet Regional Health - Europe,* 2021). For you to claim that serious adverse events such as these are "rare" when Pfizer and Moderna's clinical trial data indicate they are not, is a startling exercise in disinformation.

I want to reemphasize that these questions could have been answered if you had required vaccine manufacturers to perform and report adequate clinical trials. Although Project NextGen has been launched under another administration, I anticipate with regret, that you will repeat past mistakes and prematurely promote new therapies to Americans without accurately and truthfully weighing data on risks and benefits.

In light of your stated commitment to transparency and the communication of the risks and benefits associated with these therapies, I am asking that you publicly:

1. Report why randomized clinical trials were not required prior to the approval of mRNA COVID-19 boosters, including the new bivalent booster.

2. Explain why adverse events first detected in the Food and Drug Administration's (FDA) safety surveillance system in 2021 were not published in scientific literature until December of 2022. (Hui-Lee Wong et al, *Vaccine*. 2023)

3. Report the FDA and CDC's interpretations of the study performed in Thailand, which showed a 3% incidence of myocardial injury in young boys, and the Swiss study, which also showed a 3% incidence of myocardial injury in adults after receiving the bivalent booster. (Mansanguan S, *Tropical Medicine and Infectious Disease*. 2022; NCT05438472)

4. Explain why the Pfizer deadline for reporting their subclinical myocarditis study was delayed until December of 2022, despite the CDC promoting vaccination to millions of young people, and then postponed again until June of 2023.

5. Report the results of the VAERS proportionality analyses that you performed.

6. Explain why 26 of the 31 published studies using the V-Safe system only report symptoms within the first seven days of vaccination when it is recognized that most serious events occur after this time.

7. Disclose the rates of adverse events in V-Safe that vaccine recipients believe are related to their COVID-19 vaccine at 12 month follow up.

8. Explain why the patient reporting fields provided for adverse events in V-Safe are limited to those considered "non-serious" by the CDC and why there is an absence of reporting fields for serious adverse events, such as stroke, myocarditis, shingles, etc.

9. Report the number of adolescents that have died within days of receiving a second dose or booster of the mRNA COVID-19 vaccine. (Gill J et al, *Archives Pathology and Laboratory Medicine.* 2022)

10. Explain why you have not publicly reported on the studies indicating a likely increased risk of COVID-19 infection after four to six months from receiving mRNA COVID-19 vaccines. (Chemaitelly H, *Lancet Infectious Disease.* 2023; Altarawneh HN, *New England Journal of Medicine.* 2022; Lin DY, *New England Journal of Medicine.* 2022).

11. Explain why you have not required Pfizer to report results of its randomized trial in pregnant women (NCT04754594), which was completed in July of 2022

12. Comment on studies illustrating an increased risk of dysautonomia and postural orthostatic tachycardia syndrome after mRNA COVID-19 vaccination. (Kwan AC et al, *Nature Cardiovascular Research.* 2022).

Your organizations are the main entities promoting vaccine hesitancy – Florida promotes the truth. It is our duty to provide all information within our power to individuals so they can make their own informed health care decisions. A lack of transparency only harms Americans' faith in science.

I, Floridians, and people around the world await your response.

Sincerely,

Joseph A. Ladapo, MD,

PhD State Surgeon General

CHAPTER 21

Introducing 5th-Gen Warfare: Terms and Tactics

Drs. Robert & Jill Malone

Scientist/physician and the original inventor of
mRNA vaccination as a technology

Dr. Robert Malone is a scientist/physician and the original inventor of mRNA vaccination as a technology, DNA vaccination, and multiple non-viral DNA and RNA/mRNA platform delivery technologies. He holds numerous fundamental domestic and foreign patents in the fields of gene delivery, delivery formulations, and vaccines: including for fundamental DNA and RNA/mRNA vaccine technologies. He is also author of a new book *"Lies My Government Told Me: And the Better Future Ahead."*

Congratulations. You and the rest of the world have managed to survive the largest, most globally coordinated psychological warfare operation in the history of mankind: the COVIDcrisis.

During this period, on a daily basis, we had to experience the US Government and many western nations deploying highly refined, military-grade fifth generation warfare technologies and PsyWar weapons against their own citizens. For those who avoided the genetic vaccine jabs, which are now proven to be neither safe nor effective in preventing infection, replication, or spread of SARS-CoV-2, and do not prevent disease or death attributed to COVID-19 disease, you deserve a medal for your ability to see through the fog of information warfare. For those, like me, who trusted the FDA and took the initial jabs only to suffer the adverse effects of same, perhaps a purple heart for being wounded in battle is in order. For the millions of battlefield dead, the excess mortality documented by Ed Dowd and so many others, a moment of silent mourning is in order. Then there are the countless children, who have endured masking and social distancing in school for years on end. How do they recover developmentally? How do we ensure that this never happens again?

This essay focuses on how to stop the military grade psyops from happening on a global or even national scale in the future. Or at the very least, how to learn to not be a target of these techniques and to be able to use them yourself to fight back "against the machine". Governments are currently planning for the next "pandemic" ("Plandemic") and they have no intention of scaling back their weaponized public health policies, used to control us all. This control is not only limited to COVID-19 policies; the ability to control populations through the use of psy-ops and 5th-Gen warfare is just too tempting for governments and international organizations (such as the United Nations and The World Economic Forum), not to deploy in the future. The use of military-grade PsyWar methods on civilian populations to alter election outcomes, to weaponize fear, and to influence or control (literally) all information, beliefs and emotions of civilian populations is just too lucrative and enticing for those for whom the ends justify the means.

So, what is 5th-Generation warfare and why does it matter?

"The deliberate manipulation of an observer's context in order to achieve a desired outcome."

"The basic idea behind this term [fifth-generation warfare] is that in the modern era, wars are not fought by armies or guerrillas, but in the minds of common citizens."
(from the: *The Handbook of 5GW: A Fifth Generation of War* Abbott, 2010)

5th-Gen warfare is an extension of Asymmetric and Insurgent Warfare strategies and tactics, whereby both conventional and unconventional military tactics and weapons are incorporated and deployed, including exploitation of political, religious and social causes. This new gradient of warfare uses the internet, social media and the 24-hour news cycle to change cognitive biases of individuals and/or organizations. It can be conducted by organized or unorganized (ergo decentralized) groups; it may be led by nation states, non-nation state actors and organizations, non-governmental organizations or even individuals. A key characteristic of 5th-Gen warfare is that the nature of the attack is concealed. The goal is to disrupt and defeat opponents by creating new cognitive biases.

The most effective 5th-Gen warfare strategies employed by those lacking integrity are not purely based on pushing false narratives, mis-dis- or mal- information. The most effective strategies mix truth with fiction, and act to increase confusion and disorder in the thoughts and minds of those being targeted, so that they are not sure what or whom to believe.

"The very nature of Fifth Generation Warfare is that it is difficult to define." ("*Handbook of 5GW*", Abbott, 2010).

Some have written that the term 5th-Gen warfare should only be applied to those opponents with fewer resources (asymmetric warfare), but this is not consistent with current practice. Large and small governments, transnational corporations, globalist non-governmental organizations (such as the Bill and Melinda Gates Foundation) and the UN, WTO, WHO and their affiliates which seek to govern world affairs, and even ordinary citizens, have learned how effective the 5th-Gen toolkit is, and deploy 5th-Gen warfare tactics to their advantage.

"Any sufficiently advanced technology is indistinguishable from magic -Arthur C. Clarke."

With this chapter, my goal is to teach the reader how to begin to recognize 5th-Gen warfare tactics and to learn to use these tools for him or herself in surviving the information warfare to which they are being subjected. Only after realizing the broad scope of what is being done to all of us, can each of us begin to master these methods and become truth warriors in the 5th-Gen battles that lie ahead.

Just to be clear, the concept of 5th-Generation warfare as being traditional "warfare" is not accurate. When the term "war" is applied, the concept of a physical war as a battle for territory using kinetic weapons looms large. This is not the case with 5th-Gen warfare.

For my own use, I find the term fifth generation psyops or PsyWar as more accurately characterizing what is currently happening across the world-wide web. 5th-Gen warfare is a more general term. When a collaborative or synchronized 5th-Gen psyops program is being referred to, then I will use that term when appropriate.

There is also the small point that although "5GW" or 5G warfare is commonly used, this term can often confuse those first encountering 5th-Gen warfare terminology, who may confuse 5th-Gen warfare with 5G communication technologies (cell phone tower tech). For this reason, I avoid using the "5GW" acronym. This may all seem esoteric, but words and definitions matter.

The *"Handbook of 5GW"* (Abbott, 2010) defines fifth generation warfare as:

- A war of information and perception
- Targets existing cognitive biases of individuals and organizations
- Creates new cognitive biases
- Is different from classical warfare for the following reasons:

- Focuses on the individual observer / decision maker
- Is difficult or impossible to attribute
- Nature of the attack is concealed

Below is a general summary list of common 5th-Gen warfare weapons, tactics, and technologies.

- Misinformation (Data Driven)
- Deepfakes: Deepfakes are audio and visual media in which a person in an existing image or video is replaced with someone else's likeness. With AI, even matching audio voice overs can be generated. While the act of creating fake content is not new, deepfakes leverage powerful techniques from machine learning and artificial intelligence to manipulate or generate visual and audio content. It is predicted that deep fakes will soon be so real, that even "experts," will be unable to tell the differences. Digital certificates (or footprints) are being developed to differentiate real from fake media
- Cyberattacks
- Honeypots: (not the sexual entrapment kind). Honeypots mimic typical victim-targets of cyberattacks, such as vulnerable networks or individual email accounts. A honeypot can be used to attract, detect, and thereby deflect hacks from potentially vulnerable high-value systems or targets.
- Social engineering: Social engineering is any manipulation technique that exploits human behavior and error in order to gain access to sensitive or confidential information. Where some scammers would steal someone's personal information, social engineers convince their victims to willingly hand over the requested information like usernames and passwords. "Nudge" technology is actually applied social engineering.
- Social media manipulation (Data Driven)

- Decentralized and highly non-attributable psychological warfare fake/deepfake information (memes, fake news, planted stories): Often elements of truth will be woven into the narrative, to confuse and change the biases of the individual(s) being targeted. Evolving artificial intelligence/machine learning-based information technologies can be deployed to generate convincing deepfake documents and videos. It is already trivial to construct fake tweets and other forms of disinformation and then distribute these fakes into social media discussions. This will eventually require development of methods to differentiate fake from real documents, but until that time it will continue to be viewer beware as chaos agents and disruptors generate and distribute synthetic disinformation via a wide range of methods.

- Controlled opposition, disruptors and chaos agents: Historically, these tactics involve a fake protest movement that is actually being led by government agents - otherwise known as false-flag operations. Nearly all governments in history have employed this technique to trick and subdue their adversaries, going back at least as far as Sun-tzu and his classic monograph titled *"The Art of War"*. However, in 5th-Gen warfare, controlled opposition often may come in the form of disruptors and chaos agents. Either real people or bots that generate outrageous claims intended to delegitimize a movement; examples currently may be, snake venom in the water, or everyone who took the vaccine is going to die within two years. Another tactic is the placement of agents of chaos into key positions within otherwise legitimate organizations, or enablers of protest movement leaders. The job of the chaos agents is to disrupt organizations and events. This may also come in the form of reporters who assert fake or highly exaggerated news stories, and who most likely are funded by the opposition. Undermine the order from the shadows is the tactic here.

- Bad jacketing, cyberstalking, gang stalking, flash mob and Astroturf organizations are common tools used by organizations or agents deploying 5th-Gen warfare tactics and strategies.

- Mass surveillance, including data fusion operations which integrate social media, other cyber surveillance tools, and high resolution geospatial tracking and imaging technologies, such as cell phone and Gorgon stare technologies. Gorgon stare is video capture technology developed by the U.S. military.

- Open-source intelligence: Open-source intelligence (OSINT) is the collection and analysis of data gathered from open sources (covert and publicly) to produce actionable intelligence.

- Tracking surveillance software: COVID trackers and cell phone keyword searches.

- Commercially available social media analytics.

- The use of publicly available raw data and surveys to sway public opinion by use of memes, essays and social media posts.

- Grey and dark market data sets: A grey market or dark market data set is derived from the trading of information through distribution channels that are not authorized by the original manufacturer or trade mark proprietor.

- Commercially available satellite / SA imagery

- Commercially available electromagnetic intelligence

- Cryptographic backdoors: This is any method that allows an entity to bypass encryption and gain access to a system. Often these are placed purposefully but sometimes an unintentional backdoor can be located, allowing a system to be hacked.

- Open-source encryption/ DeFi (decentralized finance)

- Community technology: Community technology is the practice of synergizing the efforts of individuals, community technology centers and national organizations with federal policy initiatives. This may include the use of broadband, cell phones, information access, radio, education and economic development.
- Low-cost radios that can escape normal surveillance techniques.
- Traditional protest tools combined with 5th-Gen warfare: An example would be a large rally combined with social media tools to create synergy or opposition for a movement.
- The synergistic use of mixed media to build excitement or to create outrage.
- Decentralized leadership or leaderless movements that use the above technologies.

So, although the list is extensive, the truth is that only a subset of these tools are readily available to poorly-resourced individuals and groups. However, these groups may compensate for the deficit by leveraging populism.

The asymmetric warfare battlescape

Asymmetric warfare is a conflict in which the opponents' resources are uneven or not balanced. When it is the people against a government or governmental policy, the people may have numbers behind them, but typically fewer technology, financial, and physical assets such as vehicles, kinetic weapons, intelligence-gathering capabilities. Late 20th century (Viet Nam, for example) and the current 21st century (Taliban, Al-Qaeda et al) warfare clearly demonstrates that by coordinating their efforts, very effective asymmetric battlefield campaigns can be deployed by forces and organizations that confront more powerful opponents which otherwise have strategic and tactical advantages.

The good news is that some of the most effective 5th-Gen warfare tools are the ones that cost the least. Decentralized and highly non-attributable psychological warfare and community synergy are two methods that can be utilized by individuals and groups to make a difference.

Another recent example of the use of 5th-Gen warfare on an asymmetric battlefield involves activists being able to shift the general narrative about COVID-19 vaccines to acknowledge that post-COVID vaccination myocarditis occurs in athletes and children. In this example, when a new case is identified, posts and media are shared both openly and via semi-private direct messages to influencers. The information about the victim is spread and often goes viral via the world-wide web. These posts reach not only those who already believe that there is a problem, but those who are unaware of myocarditis adverse events.

The counter strategy deployed by mainstream media/big tech in response to this activity was swift. Their response included clamping down via censorship, shadow banning of posts, videos and influencers. Even direct messaging can be targeted by governments or big tech intent on controlling the narrative. An example includes T-Mobile not forwarding DMs relating to messages contradicting the approved COVIDcrisis narrative during the pandemic. Unfortunately, at the operational heart of these anti-free speech policies we often find agents of the US government.

Astroturf organizations are fake grassroots-based citizen groups, non-profits or coalitions typically created by or funded by corporations, political interests, public relations firms or even the government. These are designed to create the impression of widespread support of a platform or position. These fake groups are used to mislead the public that there is widespread support for the views being promulgated.

The Epoch Times has recently published an article based on whistleblower evidence that the United States Government, Centers for Disease Control and Prevention, has used its congressionally-approved non-profit (called the CDC Foundation) to contract with at least one company to perform cyberstalking and gang stalking attacks (via astroturf organizations) on licensed physicians accused of spreading misinformation about COVID public health policies including genetic vaccines (*"CDC Partners With 'Social and Behavior Change' Initiative to Silence Vaccine Hesitancy"*, The Epoch Times, April 7, 2023) https://www.theepochtimes.com/cdc-partners-with-social-and-behavior-change-initiative-to-silence-vaccine-hesitancy_5175172.html) . These attacks included getting physicians banned from social media platforms like Twitter, having physicians fired from their jobs and convincing state and medical specialty boards to retract licenses and specialty certifications.

According to the Epoch Times, we have the CDC Foundation - which receives funding from a wide range of donors including Merck, Pfizer, PayPal, Fidelity, Blackrock, the Imperial College of London, Emergent Biosolutions, the Robert Wood Johnson Foundation (as in J&J) and many other major corporate and state donors - which has been funding cyberstalking and gang stalking of licensed physicians. Cyberstalking is both a federal crime and a crime in many states. This article documents (via FOIA-ed emails) a large number of social media physician and scientist influencers involved in this project to cyberstalk and gang stalk physicians who spoke counter to the COVID narrative regarding pseudo-mRNA vaccines, mandates, lockdowns and masks.

Cyberstalking involves the use of technology to make someone else afraid or concerned about their safety. Generally speaking, this conduct is threatening or otherwise fear-inducing, involves

an invasion of a person's relative right to privacy, and manifests in repeated actions over time. Most of the time, those who cyberstalk use social media, Internet databases, search engines, and other online resources to intimidate, follow, and cause anxiety or terror to others. (From the Cyberstalking Research Center).
https://cyberbullying.org/cyberstalking)

Gang stalking is a form of cyberstalking or cyberbullying. Apparently, unproven accusations of physicians spreading "misinformation" were considered by the CDC Foundation sufficient for engaging in state-sponsored cyberstalking. What does this weaponized term "misinformation" actually refer to? Misinformation in the context of current public health is defined as any speech which differs from the official statements of the World Health Organization or local health authorities (ergo CDC, FDA, NIH). So, any physician who says, writes or highlights opinions or information which differs from the (current) CDC position is defined as spreading misinformation. Disinformation is such speech which is provided for political purposes.

A tactic utilized by the World Economic forum (WEF) uses influencers and social media to exploit the non-scalable nature of the internet and social media. The WEF has enlisted almost 10,000 "global shapers" to help spread their messaging. The global shapers are a group of high-profile young people that volunteer for the WEF to share and create enthusiasm for the WEF agenda worldwide. This agenda includes visions for a new world order based on transnational corporations working together with the UN, to effect climate change solutions through agenda 2030, and stakeholder capitalism. This messaging is particularly compelling to younger people, who view many of the global shapers as heroes. Understanding 5th-Gen warfare is critical in fighting effectively in this battlespace of minds, ideas and memes.

With a 5th-Gen warfare campaign, it is easy to get involved. Just follow the social media posts, news stories from alternative sources, trends and jump in! Anyone can play. Just be aware of false flag operations.

Because the U.S. government (or WHO, or WEF) identifies and censors messaging content from alternative sources, the messages and keywords must change rapidly in asymmetric 5th-Gen warfare. These actors enjoy a tactical advantage with their automated censoring and shadow banning apparatus. Therefore, it is often necessary to misspell words and phrases, or in the case of video, use slurring or blanking out words to get past the automated censors.

The focus on decentralized action, of a leaderless battlespace, effectively forces those that seek to advance and insert a false narrative into susceptible minds to play whack-a-mole. With many autonomous actors working in a decentralized fashion, there is no one target to attack. In this case, as one person is taken down, another rises. This is where being a shape-shifter is adaptive. Be ready to change social media platforms, handles, email accounts, etc. This is how I survived and thrived when de-platformed from Twitter, Facebook and Linked-in, and defamed by almost every single mainstream media corporation.

It can be helpful to keep a separate identity from your social media accounts. Use emails that aren't tied to your personal affairs for social media.

But we also have to be smart. Which is to say don't be stupid. For instance, don't play that quiz game based on your name and date of birth, don't respond to emails that need personal information, etc. No Nigerian Prince is going to send you millions of dollars. So learn to recognize pfishing and other strategies employed by con artists.

Challenge authority when it is wrong. Don't allow yourself to be bullied. Don't give up, and don't get depressed.

We are fighting now not only for our medical freedom, but for our very sovereignty. We are fighting to prevent ourselves and our children from becoming indentured servants to self-appointed centralized global masters of the Universe.

There is no end in sight. Digital spying will continue to be relentless. Look up and learn about the "Pegasus" and "Pegasus II" spyware, and let yourself think through what that means to you in a practical sense, and how you chose to respond to these threats.

Our job is to understand the terrain, the tools and the tactics.

The term for 5th-Gen warfare is war. This is not a game, with rules to which we all agree. There are no rules in 5th-Gen warfare, only tactics and strategy. Nothing is fair, and your mind, thought and emotions are the battlefield.

However, I choose to have a set of ethical boundaries for myself, and expect those that I work with to adhere to a similar moral code. I stand by my ethics. I don't lie. I don't cheat and I don't break the law. I seek to maintain personal integrity, and respect others, and act to heal and build community wherever I can. If I break these rules for myself, I will never be able to claim victory.

This is a war for my mind, your mind, our children's minds, and our collective minds. Stay true. Stay sovereign. Don't be a victim. Be a 5th Gen warrior for truth, and for the sake of our children, and for their children. The Truth is like a Lion. Set it free, and let it defend itself.

CHAPTER 22

A State of Fear: Covid-19 and Lockdowns

Lord Sumption

Retired Senior UK Supreme Court Judge

Lord Sumption is a British author, mediaeval historian and former senior judge who sat on the Supreme Court of the United Kingdom between 2012 and 2018. "In 2019, he delivered the BBC Reith Lectures, later published under the title Trials of the State.

This is the text of a lecture delivered to the Menzies Institute, Melbourne Australia, in November 2021 by Lord Sumption. Special thanks to Lord Sumption for the permission to publish here.

Sir Robert Menzies was an Australian liberal conservative, an individualist and a believer in the middle class virtues of ambition, family loyalty and self-reliance. In all these respects Menzies was a man of his time, very much in the same mould as contemporary European statesmen, such as Harold Macmillan in Britain and Konrad Adenauer in Germany.

I was born the year before Menzies began his second premiership in 1949. In my adult lifetime, there have been radical changes in our world, which have undermined many of the values that Menzies and his contemporaries held dear. The west's share of the world's resources and output, which Menzies took as a given, has been much reduced. Today, western economies are being challenged by low-wage economies. The west's technological lead is less durable than it was. We face problems of faltering growth, relative economic decline, redundant skills and capricious patterns of inequality. At the same time, there has been a dramatic rise in public demands on the state: as the provider of amenities, as a guarantor of minimum standards of economic security and as a regulator of an ever-widening range of human activities. As a result, the language of government has become much more authoritarian. In many ways the intellectual goalposts have shifted. It is more difficult to be a liberal conservative and an individualist in those conditions.

Perhaps the most striking manifestation of these changes has been the response of most states to the pandemic. I am not going to embark on a denunciation of lockdowns as a way of dealing with Covid-19, although I am on record as objecting strongly to them, for a mixture of principled and pragmatic reasons. I am concerned with a different question, namely what this episode in our history tells us about current attitudes to the state and to personal liberty. On that larger canvass, lockdowns are only the latest and most spectacular illustration of a wider theme.

At the root of the political problems generated by the pandemic was the public's attitude to the state and to risk. People have a remarkable degree of confidence in the capacity of the state to contain risk and ward off misfortune. An earlier generation regarded natural catastrophes as only marginally amenable to state action. The Spanish flu pandemic of 1918-1921 is the event most closely comparable to the Covid-19 pandemic of 2020. It is estimated to have killed 200,000 people in the United Kingdom at a time when its population was about two thirds what it is now. Estimates of global mortality range from 20 to 100 million people at a time when the world's population was about a sixth of what it is now. Australia was largely protected by distance and quarantine. In Europe, where Spanish flu took a much heavier toll, governments took no special steps to curtail its transmission, apart from isolating the infected and the sick, which had been the classic response to epidemics from time immemorial. No one criticised them for this. The related pathogens behind Asiatic flu pandemic of 1957 and Hong Kong flu in 1968 had an infection and mortality rate roughly comparable to Covid-19. No special steps were taken to control transmission. In the

US a deliberate decision was made not to take such steps because of the disruption that they would have had on the life of the nation. Instead there was heavy investment in therapies and vaccine development.

Covid-19 is a more infectious pathogen than Spanish flu, but it is significantly less mortal. It is also easier to deal with because it mainly affects those over 65 or suffering from one of a number of pre-existing clinical conditions. A high proportion of these people are economically inactive. By comparison, Spanish flu had a particularly devastating impact on healthy people aged under 50. Yet in 2020 Britain, in common with Australia and almost all western countries, ordered a general lockdown of the whole population, healthy or sick, old or young, something which had never been done before in response to any disease anywhere. These measures enjoyed substantial public support, at any rate initially. In Melbourne, lockdown was enforced with a brutality unequalled in liberal countries, but the Lowy Institute poll conducted in 2021 found that 84% of Australians thought that their government had handled it very well or fairly well. Australians thought even better of New Zealand's approach, with 91% in favour.

In the intervening century between Covid-19 and Spanish flu, something radically changed in our collective outlook. Two things in particular have changed. One is that we now expect more of the state, and are less inclined to accept that there are limits to what it can do. The other is that we are no longer willing to accept risks that have always been inherent in life itself. Human beings have, after all, lived with epidemic disease from the beginning of time. Covid-19 is a relatively serious epidemic but historically it is well within the range of health risks which are inseparable from ordinary existence. In Europe, bubonic plague, smallpox, cholera and tuberculosis were all worse in their time. Worldwide, the list of comparable or worse epidemics is substantially longer, even if they did not happen to strike Europe or North America.

The pandemic, serious as it was, was well within the broad range of mortal diseases with which human beings have always had to live. It is certainly within the broad range of diseases with which we must expect to live with in future. The change is in ourselves, not in the nature or scale of the risks that we face.

Epidemic disease is not the only peril from which we crave the protection of the state, There are other risks which are inherent in life itself, and from which we look to the state for salvation: financial loss, economic insecurity, crime, sexual violence and abuse, sickness, accidental injury. This is not irrational. It is in some ways a natural response to the remarkable increase in the technical competence of mankind since the middle of the nineteenth century, which has considerably increased the range of things that the state can do. As a result, we have inordinately high expectations of the state. We are less inclined to accept that there are things that it cannot or should not do to protect us. For all perils, there must be a governmental solution. If there is none, that implies a lack of governmental competence.

Attitudes to death provide a striking example. There are few things as routine as death. "In the midst of life, we are in death," says the Book of Common Prayer. Yet the technical possibilities of modern, publicly financed medicine have accustomed us to the idea that except in extreme old age, any death from disease is premature, and that all premature death is avoidable. Starting as a natural event, death has become a symptom of societal failure.

In modern conditions, risk-aversion and the fear that goes with it, are a standing invitation to authoritarian government. If we hold governments responsible for everything that goes wrong, they will take away our autonomy so that nothing can go wrong. The quest for security at the price of coercive state intervention is a feature of democratic politics which was pointed out in the 1830s by the great political scientist Alexis de Toqueville in his remarkable study of American democracy, a book whose uncanny relevance to modern dilemmas still takes one by surprise even after nearly two centuries. His description of the process cannot be bettered. The protecting power of the state, he wrote, "extends its arm over the whole community. It covers the surface of society with complicated rules, minute and uniform, through which the most original minds and the most energetic characters cannot penetrate, to rise above the crowd. The will of man is not shattered. But it is softened, bent, and guided. Men are seldom forced to act, but they are constantly restrained from acting. Such a power does not destroy, but it prevents existence; it does not tyrannise, but it compresses, enervates, extinguishes. It stupefies a people until each nation is reduced to nothing better than a flock of timid and industrious animals, of which the government is the shepherd."

Most regulation is designed to limit risk by limiting freedom. Governments do this not in order to protect us from risk, but mainly in order to protect themselves from criticism. During the pandemic, regulations addressed the risk of infection by Covid, because governments identified that as the thing that they were most likely to be criticised for. Governments were willing to accept considerable collateral damage to mental health resulting from the lockdown, and large increases in deaths from cancer, ischaemic heart disease and dementia, because they believed that they were less likely to be criticised for those.

People who are sufficiently frightened will submit to an authoritarian regime which offers them security against some real or imagined threat. Historically, the threat has usually been war. In the two world wars of the twentieth century Britain transformed itself into a temporary despotism with substantial public support. Wars, however, are rare. The countries of the west have generally conducted their wars at a distance. They have not faced an existential threat from external enemies since 1940. However, the real threat to democracy's survival is not major disasters like war. It is comparatively minor perils which in the nature of things occur more frequently. This may seem paradoxical. But reflect. The more routine the perils from which we demand protection, the more frequently will those demands arise. If we confer despotic powers on the government to deal with perils which are an ordinary feature of human existence, we will end up doing it most or all of the time. It is because the perils against which we now demand protection from the state are so much more numerous than they were, that they are likely to lead to a more fundamental and durable change in our attitudes to the state. This is a more serious problem for the future of democracy than war.

In the first of my 2019 Reith lectures, I drew attention to the implications of public aversion to risk for our relationship with the state. I referred to what I have called, then and since, the Hobbesian bargain. The seventeenth-century English political philosopher Thomas Hobbes argued that human beings surrendered their liberty completely, unconditionally and irrevocably to an absolute ruler in return for security. Hobbes was an apologist for absolute government. In his model of society, the state could do absolutely anything for the purpose of reducing the risks that threaten our wellbeing, other than deliberately kill us. Hobbes's state was an unpleasant thing, but he had grasped a profound truth. Most despotisms come into being not because a despot has seized power, but because people willingly surrender their freedoms in return for security. Our culture has always rejected Hobbes's model of society. Intellectually, it still does. But in recent years it has increasingly tended to act on it. The response to Covid-19 took that tendency a long way further. I could not have imagined in 2019 that my concerns would be so dramatically vindicated so quickly.

Until March 2020, it was unthinkable that liberal democracies should confine healthy people in their homes indefinitely, with limited exceptions at the discretion of government ministers. It was unthinkable that a whole population should be subject to criminal penalties for associating with other human beings and answerable to the police for the ordinary activities of daily life. In the UK, the man mainly responsible for persuading the government to impose a lockdown was Professor Neil Ferguson, an epidemiological modeler based at Imperial College London. In an interview in February 2021, Professor Neil Ferguson explained what changed. It was the lockdown in China. "It's a communist one party state, " we said. "We couldn't get away with it in Europe, we thought... And then Italy did it. And we realised we could." It is worth pausing to reflect on what this means. It means that because a lockdown of the entire population appeared to work in a country which was notoriously indifferent to individual rights and traditionally treats human beings as mere instruments of state policy, they could "get away with" doing the same thing here. Entirely absent from Professor Ferguson's analysis was any concept of the principled reasons why it had hitherto been unthinkable for western countries to do such a thing. It was unthinkable because it was based on a concept of the state's authority over its citizens which was morally repellent, even if it worked.

It is not simply the assault on the concept of liberty that matters. It is the particular liberty which has been most obviously discarded, namely the liberty to associate with other human beings. Association with other human beings is not just an optional extra. It is fundamental to our humanity. Our emotional relationships, our mental wellbeing, our entire whole social existence is built on the ability of people to come together. Historically, the response to an epidemic like this would have been a matter for individuals to make their own risk assessments, in the light of their own vulnerability and those of the people around them.

The substitution of a governmental decision applicable to the whole population irrespective of their individual situation, is an extraordinary development in the history of our society and of other western countries which have done the same thing.

The way that this one-size-fits-all approach has been justified adds to the totalitarian flavour of the day. One is to say that uniform rules applied to people with different levels of vulnerability are necessary for the sake of social solidarity. There are two kinds of solidarity: the solidarity of mutual support, and the solidarity of intolerant conformism. There has, perhaps, been too much of this last kind. The other argument was that it would be too difficult to enforce rules that differentiated between different people according to their degrees of vulnerability. In other words, the rules were couched in indiscriminate terms to make life easier for the police.

All of this marks a radical change in the relationship between the citizen and the state. The change is summed up in the first question that was asked of the UK Prime Minister when No. 10 press conferences were opened up to the public. "Is it OK for me to hug my grand-daughter?" Something extraordinary has happened to a society if people feel that they need to ask the Prime Minister if it is OK to hug their grand-daughter. I would sum up the change in this way. What was previously a right inherent in a free people, has come to depend on government licence. We have come to regard the right to live normal lives as a gift of the state. It is an approach which treats all individuals as instruments of collective policy.

All of this was made possible by fear. Throughout history fear has been the principal instrument of the authoritarian state. Fear and insecurity were the basis on which Hobbes justified the absolute state. That is what we have been witnessing in the last two years. A senior figure in the UK government told me during the early stages of the pandemic that in his view the liberal state was an unsuitable set-up for a situation like this. What was needed, he said, was something more "Napoleonic." That says it all. Napoleon was a despot.

At least as serious as the implications for our relations with the state are the implications for our relations with each other. The pandemic generated distrust, resentment and mutual hostility among citizens in most countries where lockdowns were imposed. The use of political power as an instrument of mass coercion fuelled by public fear, is corrosive. It is corrosive even, perhaps especially, when it enjoys majority support. For it tends to be accompanied, as it has been in Britain, by manipulative government propaganda and vociferous intolerance of the minority who disagree. Authoritarian governments fracture the societies in which they operate.

It is widely assumed that this is a phase which will pass when Covid-19 disappears (if it ever does). I am afraid that this is an illusion. We have turned a corner, and it will not be easy to go back. I say that for several reasons.

The first and most obvious is that governments rarely relinquish powers that they have once acquired. In Britain, wartime controls were kept in place for years after the end of the war. Food rationing was kept in place in the name of social solidarity until 1952, long after it had disappeared in Germany and in the European countries which Germany overran. Regulations requiring people to carry identity cards, which had been introduced in 1940 to control spies and fifth columnists, remained in force until the mid-1950s. Many wartime regulations had a sunset clause which provided for their repeal as soon as His Majesty declared by Order in Council that the war was at an end. The clause was circumvented by the simple device of not putting such an Order in Council before His Majesty. During the Falklands war, the government was still trying to requisition property with limited compensation under wartime regulations, on the basis that in law the Second World War had not yet ended.

My second concern is that I see no reason why politicians should want or need to respect basic liberal values, if the public is happy with a more authoritarian style of government. Public support for mass coercion was high throughout the pandemic, and at the outset was almost unanimous. There will be other pandemics, which will provoke the same reaction. But public support for Napoleonic government is not simply a response to epidemic disease. It is a response to a much more general feeling of insecurity, combined with a profound faith in the ability of government to solve any problem with sufficient talent and money. It is a symptom of a much more general appetite for authoritarian government, as the price for greater security, what I have called the Hobbesian bargain. And it is accentuated by a growing feeling that strong governments are efficient and get things done while deliberative assemblies like Parliament are just a waste of time and a source of inefficiencies. Strongmen get things done. They do not waste time in argument or debate. Historical experience should warn us that this idea is usually wrong. Government by decree is usually bad government. The concentration of power in a small number of hands and the absence of wider deliberation and scrutiny enables governments to make major decisions on the hoof, without proper forethought, planning or research. Within the government's own ranks, it promotes loyalty at the expense of wisdom, flattery at the expense of objective advice. The want of criticism encourages self-confidence, and self-confidence banishes moderation and restraint. Authoritarian rulers sustain themselves in power by appealing to the emotional and the irrational in collective opinion.

You might say: Well, if the public is happy, isn't that democracy in action. I answer that that is how democracies destroy themselves. Democracies are systems of collective self-government. It is of course possible for democracies to confer considerable coercive power on the state without losing their democratic character. But there is a point beyond which the systematic application of coercion is longer consistent with any notion of collective self-government. The fact that it is hard to define where that point lies, does not mean that there isn't one. A degree of respect for individual autonomy seems to me to be a necessary feature of anything which deserves to be called a democracy.

My final reason for believing that we have turned a corner on liberal democracy, is perhaps the most fundamental. Aristotle regarded democracy as an inherently unstable form of government, because it was too easily transformed into despotism by the natural tendency of people to fall for an appealing tyrant. What has spared most western democracies from this fate for the century and a half during which they have existed is a shared political culture. Governments have immense powers, not just in the field of public health but generally. These powers have existed for many years. Their existence has been tolerable in a liberal democracy only because of a culture of restraint which made it unthinkable that they should be used in a despotic manner. It has only ever been culture and convention which prevented governments from adopting a totalitarian model. But culture and convention are fragile. They take years to form but can be destroyed very quickly. Once you discard these, there is no barrier left. The spell is broken. If something is unthinkable until someone in authority thinks of it, the psychological barriers which were once our only protection against despotism have vanished.

There is no inevitability about the future course of any historical trend. But the changes in our political culture seem to me to reflect a profound change in the public mood, which has been many years in the making and may be many years in the unmaking. We are entering a Hobbesian world, the enormity of which has not yet dawned on our people.

CHAPTER 23

The Nanny State's a Bitch

To defeat COVID collectivism, reject the administrative state

Professor Bruce Pardy

Professor of law at Queen's University and
Executive Director of Rights Probe

Bruce Pardy is professor of law at Queen's University and executive director of Rights Probe, a law and liberty thinktank. He warned of dire consequences as soon as COVID-19 lockdowns were imposed in spring 2020, and is one of the authors of the Free North Declaration, a call to arms to protect civil liberties from COVID irrationality and overreach.

Do you approve of the nanny state? Nearly everybody does.

One can't blame people for their devotion. Most of them have lived their lives under the nanny state – or the "administrative state," as it is more formally known. They think that government exists to manage society and solve social problems for the common good. What else is government for?

But now some people are not so sure. The COVID-19 train wreck unfolded before their eyes. One senseless government diktat followed another. Close your business. Keep your kids home from school. Stay out of the park. Wear a mask to go into the store. Take a vaccine to keep your job. These edicts have destroyed lives. They caused vaccine injuries and deaths, cancelled jobs and education, and tore families apart. They eviscerated civil liberties. Society unravelled.

But not everyone can see that our own government did this. Some are blinded by their faith in the benevolence of state authorities. Others struggle with cognitive dissonance. Traumatized, they sift through the ashes of the past three years, looking for explanations. Why did government fail?

It did not fail. The administrative state excelled beyond its wildest dreams. The COVID regime has been its pinnacle achievement, at least so far.

To defeat COVID collectivism, we must reject the nanny state.

Separation of powers

"Give me liberty or give me death" declared Patrick Henry in 1775, urging the Second Virginia Convention to deliver troops for the Revolutionary War. Henry wasn't decrying a tax that should have been lower, or benefits that should have been higher. He and his compatriots were fighting the oppression of the British Crown. Today our oppression comes not from foreign lands but from our own state, which dominates our lives in every conceivable way. Instead of challenging its authority, we criticize its policies.

American revolutionaries would not comprehend the extent to which the state now controls our lives. Its tentacles are everywhere. COVID is merely the leading case. Our technocratic overlords regulate fishing rods, dog food, cow flatulence, and the holes in Swiss cheese. They supervise our speech, employment, bank accounts, and media. They indoctrinate our children. They control the money supply, the interest rate, and the terms of credit. They track, direct, incentivize, censor, punish, redistribute, subsidize, tax, license, and inspect.

It wasn't supposed to be this way. The King once ruled with absolute power over England. Centuries of struggle and social evolution eventually produced a radically different legal order in Anglo-American countries. The constitutional architecture of the United Kingdom, United States, Canada, Australia and New Zealand does not feature an all-powerful executive. Instead, to achieve "the rule of law," their state authorities are divided into three parts: legislatures, administration or executive branch, and judiciary.

These three branches do distinct jobs. Legislatures pass rules. The administration enforces and executes those rules. Courts apply the rules to specific disputes. This "separation of powers" is the foundation of the rule of law. Keeping them apart protects us. If each branch can do only its own job, power cannot concentrate in any one. No single person or authority can apply their own preferences. As Friedrich Hayek put it, "It is because the lawgiver does not know the particular cases to which his rules will apply, and it is because the judge who applies them has no choice in drawing the conclusions that follow from the existing body of rules and the particular facts of the case, that it can be said that laws and not men rule."

With few exceptions, the administrative branch has power to do nothing except that which a statute specifically provides. Government bodies – that is, everything not legislature or court, including cabinets, departments, ministries, agencies, public health officials, commissions, tribunals, regulators, law enforcement, and inspectors – are supervised by the other two branches. "I know of no duty of the Court which it is more important to observe, and no powers of the Court which it is more important to enforce, than its power of keeping public bodies within their rights," wrote Lindley M.R. in an 1899 UK case. "The moment public bodies exceed their rights they do so to the injury and oppression of private individuals."

The Unholy Trinity of the Administrative State

But that was then. Slowly but inexorably, the legal ground has shifted beneath our feet. Separation of powers has eroded. We have moved away from the rule of law back towards rule by fiat. Control resides not in a monarch but in a professional managerial aristocracy.

Legislatures, instead of enacting rules, pass statutes that delegate rule-making authority. They empower the administration to make regulations, orders, policies, and decisions of all kinds. The legislature has abdicated its responsibility. The administrative branch, not the legislature, is now making the bulk of the rules.

Instead of curbing this practice as a violation of the separation of powers principle, courts have long said, "No problem." And courts now tend to defer to administrative action, even when the officer or agency in question colors outside the lines of the statute's mandate. Judges don't want to look too closely to see if officials are acting strictly within the limits of their formal authority, because after all, goes the story, officials and technocrats are the ones with expertise. Courts now defer to public authorities to do as they think best in the "public interest".

Instead of the rule of law, we have the Unholy Trinity of the Administrative State: ***delegation*** from the legislature, ***deference*** from the courts, and ***discretion*** for the administration to decide the public good. Instead of separation, we have concentrated power. Instead of checks and balances between the three branches, they are all on the same page, cooperating to empower the state's management of society. Officials and experts place individual autonomy aside in the name of public welfare and progressive causes. Broad discretion in the hands of a technocratic managerial class has become the foundation of our modern system of government.

Unlike COVID, which transformed society with a fury, the administrative state triumphed slowly over many decades. Its exact origins and timing are matters of debate. In the US, the New Deal paved the way, legitimized by the Great Depression. The UK, battered by World War Two, doubled down on state control when the war was done. In Canada, state paternalism has long been part of the national identity. Whatever its historical roots, the managerial nanny state is ascendant in the Anglo-American world.

Discretion is the premise. The premise dictates the conclusion

Consider an elementary example of deductive reasoning. Cats have tails. Felix is a cat. Therefore, Felix has a tail. The premise (cats have tails), plus evidence or minor premise (Felix is a cat), produces a conclusion (Felix has a tail). The conclusion presumes that the premise is correct.

The same simplistic reasoning applies to the administrative state. The premise: officials have discretion to decide the public good. Evidence: officials mandated a vaccine. Conclusion: the vaccine mandate is for the public good. The conclusion follows from the premise.

Note the nature of the evidence, which is not about the vaccine. It does not speak to its efficacy or safety. It is not evidence about whether the vaccine is in the public good. Instead, the evidence shows what officials decided. Officials have the discretion to decide the public good. No argument can challenge the conclusion without attacking that premise. Objecting to government policies by proffering evidence that they are not in the public good is a fool's errand.

Put another way: "Public good" is not an objective measure. Like beauty, it lies in the eyes of the beholder. Since the administrative state rests on its discretion to decide the public good, it alone can define what public good means. Policies make trade-offs. Trade-offs reflect values. Values are political, not factual. Evidence may be relevant but never determinative. An avalanche of data showing that electric cars provide no comparable environmental benefit will not nullify rules that mandate the sale of electric vehicles. Through their own ideological lens, governments decide where the public interest lies.

Arguments challenging COVID policies abound. Lockdowns caused more harm than good. Masks did not prevent the spread of the virus. The mRNA vaccines were not vaccines, and their risks outweigh their benefits. Propaganda caused unnecessary fear. Medical censorship prevents doctors from speaking the truth. These objections miss the plot. They argue, using evidence of bad outcomes, that public good was not achieved. But state officials don't have to show that their policies achieved public good, since the meaning of public good is up to them.

Paradoxically, criticizing the state's policies legitimizes its control. Alleging that lockdowns are bad because they cause harm implies that they are good if they work. Challenging vaccine mandates because vaccines are dangerous attacks the vaccines, not the mandates. If policies are bad only because they don't work, they are good when they do.

When COVID madness descended, people thought the law would save them. Some found lawyers to challenge the rules. Some defied restrictions and disputed their tickets. These efforts failed to turn the ship around. Courts did not repudiate the pandemic regime. That is not surprising, since courts helped to establish the administrative state in the first place, long before there was a virus.

The administrative state is its own purpose

The nanny state is neither neutral nor benign. It exists to exist. It controls to control. The public has been persuaded that public administration is indispensable. Modern life is too complex, they think, not to be managed by an expansive and knowledgeable bureaucracy. They have been taught to confuse authority with substance. As Catholic philosopher Ivan Illich wrote, people have been schooled to confuse the existence of institutions with the objectives that the institutions claim to pursue. "Medical treatment is mistaken for health care, social work for the improvement of community life ... Health, learning, dignity, independence, and creative endeavor are defined as little more than the performance of the institutions which claim to serve these ends."

The state's "pandemic management" hurt more than it helped. As Professor Denis Rancourt put it to the National Citizens Inquiry in Ottawa, if governments had done nothing out of the ordinary, had not announced a pandemic, and had not responded to a presumed pathogen in the way that it did, there would have been no excess mortality. But the nanny state's performance is never reviewed or compared to the alternatives because none are thought to exist. That is the real triumph of the administrative state. It dominates the room yet is regarded as simply part of the furniture.

Free people act without regard for public good. Those who cringe at that notion have succumbed to our brave not-so-new world of subservience, collective impoverishment, and concurrent beliefs. Of course, on balance, acting freely in our own self interest enhances the welfare of the whole. The free market's invisible hand produces prosperity in a way no collection of policies ever could. But neither safety nor prosperity is what makes freedom right. Liberty is not merely the means to welfare and good outcomes, even if it happens to work out that way. As Friedrich Hayek observed, "Freedom granted only when it is known beforehand that its effects will be beneficial is not freedom."

With few exceptions, the problem is not the content of policy but its very existence. If lockdowns had succeeded, they would still have restrained people against their will. If COVID vaccines were safe and effective, mandates still take medical decisions away from individuals. These policies were wrong for the coercion they imposed, not the goals they failed to achieve.

The conceit of our functionaries has become intolerable. Most public policy, good or bad, is illegitimate. No doubt there are subjects – foreign relations, public infrastructure – where government policy may be necessary. But these are exceptions to the general rule: people's lives are their own.

The King's absolute power served him, not his subjects. People who believe that the administrative state is different have been hoodwinked. By debating the niceties of policy, we quibble in the margins and surrender the battlefield. "Give us liberty," we might say, "or just do what you think best." Patrick Henry would not be impressed.

CHAPTER 24

The Most Egregious Violation of Medical Ethics in the History of Medicine

Drs. James & Maggie Thorp

Board-certified in obstetrics and gynecology (OB/GYN) as well as a specialist in maternal-fetal medicine

Dr James Thorp MD is an actively practicing, extensively published 70-year-old physician from Florida. He is board-certified in obstetrics and gynecology (OB/GYN) and also in maternal-fetal medicine and has 44 years of clinical experience in obstetrics.

Few things are more illustrative of government corruption during the COVID-19 pandemic than the clandestine capture of private medical organizations by the U.S. Department of Health and Human Services (HHS), in what would eventually be exposed as a covert propaganda campaign to push experimental mRNA shots into every arm. Of all the lessons learned from the pandemic, this lesson is among the most important for those who envision the U.S. as a free democracy protected by the First Amendment.

In addition to protecting the right to express opinions without government censorship and control, the First Amendment also protects Americans' right to call out government corruption and abuse of power and petition the government for redress of grievances. These protections were stripped away during the COVID-19 pandemic by a government that recruited and bribed private entities and individuals to do its dirty bidding.

There is still no government acknowledgment of harms caused by reckless pandemic policies which sent sick people home to die in the treatable first stage of the disease, while silencing and maligning medical professionals who advocated for the use of safe, repurposed medicines. There is still no meaningful redress for millions in this country who are COVID-19 "vaccine" injured, who have lost a loved one to the "vaccine," and who continue to endure silencing by their government, their physicians, and corporate media.

To avoid further erosion of the First Amendment, it is essential that Americans come to understand how all this unfolded: How could upwards of 75% of the country be persuaded into taking experimental gene therapy injections with no informed consent and zero long-term safety data? If the U.S. government's illicit pandemic strategy is not exposed for the betrayal it was, then make no mistake – the same clandestine and totalitarian techniques will be deployed again on unsuspecting Americans.

This essay will delve into the shady techniques used by the HHS to convince Americans that the experimental shots were "safe, effective and necessary" in pregnancy – despite evidence to the contrary. Even Pfizer's own 90-day 5.3.6 post marketing experience, which both Pfizer and the FDA had in early 2021, showed its mRNA vaccine to be the most lethal drug ever rolled out, with 1223 deaths in the first 90 days (page 7), a multitude of adverse pregnancy outcomes (page 12) and nine pages of "Adverse Events of Special Interest" (Appendix).[1] However, the government had an unstoppable mRNA agenda, and so the band played on.

Enlisting "Trojan Horses" to do the CDC's Ugly Bidding: HHS launches <u>COVID-19 Community Corps</u>

Pfizer's 5.3.6 ninety-day post marketing experience report, which tracked adverse event data from December 1, 2020 to February 28, 2021, showed its COVID-19 mRNA "vaccine" to be the deadliest drug ever rolled out in U.S. history. Instead of hitting pause on rollout of the vaccines, however, on April 1, 2021 the HHS launched *COVID-19 Community Corps*[2] – a colossal COVID-19 vaccine propaganda machine designed to exploit "trusted" private entities and individuals across the country, turning them into covert government agents to push the vaccines. As part of the strategy to get a shot in every arm, HHS used *COVID-19*

Community Corps to recruit private, non-government "trusted" sources to push the CDC's message that the novel mRNA genetic injections were safe (despite clear evidence to the contrary) – but *without* directly disclosing that these messages were actually from the government.[3]

Under the guise of *COVID-19 Community Corps*, HHS awarded billions of federal dollars to recruit what HHS referred to as "trusted community leaders" who could push the "vaccines" within our most private relationships.[4] Much like modern-day trojan horses, these "trusted messengers" would be unique in their ability to permeate all facets of private life.[5] Essential to successfully deploying its strategy on the public, HHS sought to identify credible and influential community leaders, enlist them to join its *COVID-19 Community Corps*, and then exploit these "trusted sources" to convince those around them to take the COVID-19 vaccines.[6] The focus was on finding people with not just local, but also uniquely *interpersonal* influence. As Harvard public health professor Jay Winsten,[7] who has advised previous administrations, reportedly explained to *CBS News* in a December 2020 article about the HHS' monumental effort, "You want to go for the low hanging fruit, those that are easiest to pick and harvest."[8] Noting that the focus should be on finding locally influential people to push the vaccines, Winsten added, "People trust their own doctors, their own nurses, their own pastors, their own social networks. That's very, very different from a distant figure."[9] And indeed it was.

American College of Obstetricians and Gynecologists (ACOG): A "Trusted Messenger"

Along with 275 other organizations, twenty-five of which were health and medical organizations, the American College of Obstetricians and Gynecologists (ACOG) jumped on board as a founding member of *COVID-19 Community Corps*,[10] ultimately receiving millions in federal grant money.[11] Shortly thereafter, on July 30, 2021 ACOG began recklessly endorsing COVID-19 vaccination in pregnancy, even though the clinical trials failed to include pregnant women.

Perhaps no other medical organization had as much potential to persuade Americans into taking these experimental injections as did ACOG. A pregnant patient's relationship with her ob-gyn is arguably one of the most intimate and sacred physician-patient relationships in all of medicine. This is not without reason – as one patient and writer notes, "They're right next to you for the most momentous occasion of your life."[12] Pregnant mothers trust their ob-gyn doctor with the most intimate and sensitive information about their own bodies, their sex lives, and, if pregnant, about the new life growing inside of them. Some individuals have even reported the development of a non-romantic affection for their ob-gyn that rivals that of the baby's father in some ways, due to the "complete vulnerability" many women reportedly experience with their gynecological and pregnancy specialists.[13]

Government capture of ACOG would capitalize on this unique and sacred doctor-patient relationship, using ob-gyn doctors – with their unparalleled physician influence – as pro-vaccine "trusted messengers." Additionally, convincing pregnant women to take novel mRNA shots would yield an exponential harvest of "low hanging fruit." This is because women reportedly make a full 90% of all healthcare decisions about their household and have long been considered "A Brand's Powerhouse" by professional marketers.[14] Convincing pregnant women to take the COVID-19 shots was almost a guarantee that they would become pro-vaccine "trusted messengers" within their own families.

Moreover, the optics were exceptionally good for persuading other "vaccine" hesitant Americans to roll up their sleeve for the experimental shots – if the COVID-19 "vaccines" were considered safe enough to administer to pregnant patients (and thereby trans-placentally to their unborn babies) – certainly they were safe enough for everyone. If HHS and CDC could pull off government capture of ACOG and convince its ob-gyn members to push the shots on their patients, this would be a bonanza for reaching the "vaccine" hesitant – what HHS Deputy Assistant Sec. Mark Weber referred to as the "moveable middle."[15]

As it would turn out, the HHS' grand marketing strategy worked. The methods utilized by HHS to push the COVID-19 "vaccines" – including the creation of *COVID-19 Community Corps* – were so vastly different from any other HHS effort that an academic article was published in *Journal of Health Communication* in April of the following year, detailing the process and commending its success.[16] Featuring now-retired HHS Deputy Assistant Sec. Mark Weber as lead author, the article confirms that HHS did, in fact, target interpersonal relationships. [17] Weber's and his colleagues "vaccine" marketing efforts were so successful that, after retiring from HHS, Weber apparently formed his own private company aimed at "Achieving bold goals at the Federal Level"[18] – in revolving door fashion.

Today the HHS campaign to push the COVID-19 "vaccines" is far from over. Having entered its third phase in 2022, according to Weber and his co-authors it has evolved into a highly targeted approach using both paid and "earned" media strategies. As explained in Weber's article, the HHS campaign:

> focuses more on precision marketing to identify subgroups with vaccine hesitancy, working directly with communities and using trusted messengers in those communities **to deliver messages without the Federal government being directly involved (even though the information may come from a Federal source)**.[19]

Notably, the article neglects to fully explain – or even recognize – that what HHS has engaged in is arguably exploitative, deceptive and unethical. This is because HHS used persons and methods targeting trust within interpersonal relationships to push messages that the "vaccines" were safe and effective – but often government involvement behind the messaging was not fully disclosed.

ACOG: A Revealing Case Study of Government Capture of Medical Non-Profit Organizations

On February 1, 2021, ACOG had been awarded the first of what would eventually be three HHS and CDC "Cooperative Agreement" grants made during the pandemic.[20] Under these three Cooperative Agreement grants, ACOG would receive over $11 million in federal money over coming years.[21] But there was a catch: Documents obtained in a Freedom of Information Act (FOIA) request made in connection with these three Cooperative Agreement grants has recently exposed that ACOG relinquished independent control over its COVID-19 recommendations for patients to the CDC when it accepted the federal grant money.[22] Receipt of grant money by ACOG was contingent on ACOG's full compliance with CDC guidance on COVID-19 infection and control.[23] Eerily similar to what former HHS Deputy Assistant Sec. Mark Weber writes about, the FOIA documents reveal that HHS and CDC seemed to be using ACOG to "deliver messages without the Federal government being directly involved (even though the information may come from a Federal source)."[24]

Although they were heavily redacted, the FOIA documents revealed startling information about the extent of control CDC wielded (and still wields) over ACOG. For example, the FOIA documents show that CDC grants totaling $3,300,000 were awarded to ACOG on Sept. 2, 2021 for two separate programs, entitled *"Engaging Women's Health*

Care Providers for Effective COVID-19 Vaccine Conversations," and "*Improving Ob-Gyns' Ability to Support Covid-19 Vaccination, Mental Health, Social Support.*"[25] As part of receiving funds under these awards, ACOG is required to "comply with existing and or future directives and guidance from the [HHS] Secretary regarding control of the spread of COVID-19."[26] The award is also expressly contingent on ACOG's agreement "to comply with existing and future guidance from the HHS Secretary regarding the control and spread of COVID-19."[27] In addition, ACOG must also "flow down" these terms to any person or entity who receives a "subaward."[28] Moreover, the CDC is expressly authorized to terminate any award due to material failure to comply with "the terms and conditions of the federal award."[29]

If this sounds like government capture of ACOG – it is. Disturbingly, the FOIA documents show CDC working *through* ACOG, in essence exploiting ACOG's authority and sway to influence not only doctors and patients, but also a host of others, including public health entities and "partner organizations." [30] The FOIA documents obtained make it difficult to tell where ACOG ends and CDC begins.

CDC Recommends COVID-19 Vaccines for Pregnant Women on April 23, 2021

Fast forward to April 23, 2021. On this day, CDC Director Dr. Rochelle Walensky announced during a highly publicized White House COVID-19 press briefing the CDC's new recommendation that all pregnant individuals receive the COVID-19 "vaccine."[31] Pointing to a flawed CDC study published just two days before, which study featured CDC Immunization Safety Office Director Tom Shimabukuro, MD as lead author,[32] Walensky publicly declared that the vaccines appeared to be safe for pregnant women. However, Walensky neglected to mention that the Shimabukuro article was another mRNA marketing product of the CDC. In addition to serving as Director of the CDC's Immunization Safety Office, over the course of the pandemic, Shimabukuro has been deeply entrenched in the CDC. He has reportedly served as VAERS "team lead" (raising valid questions about why the CDC seems to be ignoring the VAERS database) and "acting team lead" of the Vaccine Safety Datalink (VSD) team.[33] He has also served on the CDC "COVID-19 Vaccine Coordination Unit."[34] With Shimabukuro's deep ties to the CDC and pro-COVID-19 "vaccine" stance, his serving as lead author on this critically timed and flawed study constituted a flagrant conflict of interest and never should have been allowed.[35]

ACOG Follows CDC's Lead

Following the lead of CDC, on July 30, 2021 ACOG, along with the Society for Maternal Fetal Medicine (SMFM), recklessly began endorsing COVID-19 vaccination in pregnancy,[36] even though the clinical trials failed to include pregnant women. Now bound under terms and conditions of the Cooperative Agreements grants (which ceded control to CDC for programs involving COVID-19 grant funding), ACOG seemingly had no choice, and thus played right into the hands of the HHS' strategy to enlist "trusted messengers" to push the COVID shots. As ACOG explains on its website, a pregnant patient's ob-gyn had the potential for enormous influence: "Pregnant people need to feel confident in the decision to choose vaccination, and a strong recommendation from their obstetrician-gynecologist could make a meaningful difference for many pregnant people."[37] In this case, ACOG seems to say the quiet part out loud – a recommendation from an ob-gyn could be a game changer for convincing pregnant women to take the COVID-19 "vaccines." Sadly, the targets of the experimental "vaccine" campaign would be society's most vulnerable – pregnant mothers and their unborn babies.

ACOG's July 30, 2021 announcement strongly recommending COVID-19 "vaccination" in pregnancy was a sharp about-face from ACOG's previous stance on the issue. Website archives show that for the months of the pandemic preceding July 30, 2021 (Dec. 2020 through July 21, 2021), ACOG's official recommendation was to allow pregnant women the freedom to choose, stating throughout the first half 2021: "In the interest of patient autonomy, ACOG recommends that pregnant individuals be free to make their own decision regarding COVID-19 vaccination."[38] Yet, ACOG's recommendation abruptly changed on July 30, 2021.[39] In place of patient autonomy, independent clinical judgment, and informed consent about the known and unknown risks of the COVID-19 "vaccines," ACOG's recommendations would now follow CDC's guidance, announced by CDC director Walensky on April 23, 2021, that novel, experimental gene therapy "vaccines" with zero long term safety data were somehow safe in pregnancy.

Multiple Sources Flash Danger

Multiple sources, including the government's *own* data contained in VAERS, [40] casts doubt on the veracity of the claim that the COVID-19 vaccines are safe in pregnancy. One published investigational study, led by ObGyn and Maternal Fetal Medicine physician James A. Thorp, looked at adverse events reported in VAERS following COVID-19 "vaccination" in pregnancy compared to adverse events reported following Influenza vaccines since 1998.[41] The results of this VAERS investigational retrospective study are catastrophic: the FDA and CDC use a 2-fold increase as a breach in the safety signal, yet the study led by Thorp found a 57-fold increase in miscarriage, and a 38-fold increase in fetal death (stillbirth) following COVID-19 vaccination when compared to Influenza vaccines. A total of 18 separate adverse events, including abnormal menses and 17 other major pregnancy complications, all exceeded CDC and FDA safety signals.

Most recently, *The Defen*der, a publication which is affiliated with Children's Health Defense (an organization which advocates for greater vaccine safety founded by Robert F. Kennedy Jr.), reports alarming data. Calling into question the veracity of CDC's and ACOG's recommendations that the vaccines are safe in pregnancy, the data reported on by *The Defender* suggest that authorities knew of health risks with the mRNA shots, but assured pregnant mothers it was safe anyway.[42] According to a recent troubling report from Naomi Wolf's organization, DailyClout, the April 2023 batch of Pfizer clinical documents released under court order demonstrate that both Pfizer and FDA knew the mRNA shots caused serious harm to both fetuses and infants – yet CDC pushed the shots anyway.[43]

A Troubling Relationship between ACOG and CDC

ACOG's July 30, 2021 page recommending the COVID-19 "vaccines" for pregnant individuals does not disclose that ACOG – a membership funded non-governmental organization – was operating under the purview of the HHS and CDC regarding its COVID-19 guidance for pregnant women at the time that recommendation was made.[44] Which begs multiple questions: When ACOG changed its official COVID-19 "vaccination" position on July 30, 2021 – choosing to follow CDC's April 23, 2021 recommendations that COVID-19 "vaccines" be given to pregnant women – why didn't ACOG simply disclose it was following the CDC's recommendations? Was ACOG's July 30, 2021 recommendation also its own independent recommendation? If so, what exactly was ACOG's independent recommendation based upon? How many of the 275 medical and other founding members organizations of the *COVID-19 Community Corps* perhaps sold their souls – trading free speech, the protections of the First Amendment, bodily autonomy, and informed consent– for money, power or both? Without FOIA requests for each of the founding members, it is impossible to know for sure. But what we do know about the HHS *COVID-19 Community Corps* and the FOIA documents involving ACOG should make us wary.

Finally, ACOG's capture by HHS and CDC regarding COVID-19 vaccination recommendations in pregnancy is troubling for yet another reason – potential conflict of interest via the CDC's nonprofit support entity, the CDC Foundation.[45] Donation records show that the CDC Foundation has, in past years leading up to the pandemic, received donations from Pfizer, Inc.,[46] the Bill and Melinda Gates Foundation,[47] and a host of other pharmaceutical companies and private entities.[48]

As government capture of ACOG strikingly illuminates – at the heart of the HHS' vaccine propaganda campaign was exploitation of our trust, built upon age-old marketing tricks – and not anything approaching actual medical "science." HHS, working with the Biden administration, injected itself into our most private relationships, utilizing trusted leaders who were viewed as the golden ticket to reach government vaccination goals. The US government cherry picked groups and individuals because of their capability to engender widespread influence and confidence. Some of these included hospitals, administrators physicians, nurses, pastors, local celebrities, business leaders, academic institutions, and many more viewed as voices which resonated trust. Literally no facet of life or society was left untouched. The government's strategy: to exploit those identified by "communication science" as highly "trusted,"[49] using them to infiltrate the most sensitive, personal and intimate areas of our lives. The government's goal: To convince the "low hanging fruit, those that are easiest to pick and harvest"[50] to take part in novel and experimental therapy injections rebranded as vaccines.

While some have tried to explain what happened by arguing that there was a kind of mass hypnosis that took hold, that explanation falls short. Rather, in a disturbing and intentional campaign for control typically characteristic of totalitarian dominator societies, the US government co-opted our most intimate relationships and the voices we trusted into a vast covert government operation, unleashed on the unsuspecting public at the height of fear and isolation. Understanding the breadth and depth of the government's illicit actions can assist us in never letting such a grab for totalitarianism control happen again.

Endnotes

[1] Pfizer 5.3.6 Post Market Data, December 1, 2020 to February 28, 2021. https://phmpt. org/wp-content/uploads/2022/04/reissue_5.3.6-postmarketing-experience.pdf. Accessed May 19, 2023.

[2] U.S. Department of Health and Human Services (HHS). 2021. "U.S. Department of Health and Human Services Launches Nationwide Network of Trusted Voices to Encourage Vaccination in Next Phase of COVID-19 Public Education Campaign." (Screen Snapshot captured on April 1, 2021, at 22:51:02, by Internet Archive Wayback Machine. Accessed May 1, 2023). https://web.archive.org/web/20210401225102/ https://www.hhs.gov/about/news/2021/04/01/hhs-launches-nationwide-network-trusted-voices-encourage-vaccination-next-phase-covid-19-public-education-campaign. html.

[3] See Thorp, Maggie and Jim Thorp. 2022. "Tentacles of a Covert and Exploitative Propaganda Machine Compliments of the US Government." *America Out Loud*, October 28, 2022. Accessed May 1, 2023. https://www.americaoutloud.com/tentacles-of-a-covert-and-exploitative-propaganda-machine-compliments-of-the-us-government/

[4] U.S. Department of Health and Human Services (HHS). 2021. "U.S. Department of Health and Human Services Launches Nationwide Network of Trusted Voices to Encourage Vaccination in Next Phase of COVID-19 Public Education Campaign." (Screen Snapshot captured on April 1, 2021, at 22:51:02, by Internet Archive Wayback Machine. Accessed May 1, 2023). https://web.archive.org/web/20210401225102/ https://www.hhs.gov/about/news/2021/04/01/hhs-launches-nationwide-network-trusted-voices-encourage-vaccination-next-phase-covid-19-public-education-campaign. html.

[5] U.S. Department of Health and Human Services (HHS). 2021. "U.S. Department of Health and Human Services Launches Nationwide Network of Trusted Voices to Encourage Vaccination in Next Phase of COVID-19 Public Education Campaign." (Screen Snapshot captured on April 1, 2021, at 22:51:02, by Internet Archive Wayback Machine. Accessed May 1, 2023). https://web.archive.org/web/20210401225102/ https://www.hhs.gov/about/news/2021/04/01/hhs-launches-nationwide-network-trusted-voices-encourage-vaccination-next-phase-covid-19-public-education-campaign. html.

[6] U.S. Department of Health and Human Services (HHS). 2021. "U.S. Department of Health and Human Services Launches Nationwide Network of Trusted Voices to Encourage Vaccination in Next Phase of COVID-19 Public Education Campaign." (Screen Snapshot captured on April 1, 2021, at 22:51:02, by Internet Archive Wayback Machine. Accessed May 1, 2023). https://web.archive.org/web/20210401225102/ https://www.hhs.gov/about/news/2021/04/01/hhs-launches-nationwide-network-trusted-voices-encourage-vaccination-next-phase-covid-19-public-education-campaign. html.

[7]   Harvard T.H. Chan: School of Public Health. 2023. "Jay A. Winsten, Ph.D." Accessed May 6, 2023. https://www.hsph.harvard.edu/jay-winsten/.

[8]   Kates, Graham. "Inside the $250 Million Effort to Convince Americans the Coronavirus Vaccines are Safe." *CBS News*, December 23, 2020. Accessed May 2, 2023. https://www.cbsnews.com/news/covid-vaccine-safety-250-million-dollar-marketing-campaign/.

[9]   Kates, Graham. "Inside the $250 Million Effort to Convince Americans the Coronavirus Vaccines are Safe." *CBS News*, December 23, 2020. Accessed May 2, 2023. https://www.cbsnews.com/news/covid-vaccine-safety-250-million-dollar-marketing-campaign/.

[10]   You can find HHS' "Full List of COVID-19 Community Corps Founding Members: Public Health & Medical Organizations" on this page: U.S. Department of Health and Human Services (HHS). 2021. "U.S. Department of Health and Human Services Launches Nationwide Network of Trusted Voices to Encourage Vaccination in Next Phase of COVID-19 Public Education Campaign." (Screen Snapshot captured on April 1, 2021, at 22:51:02, by Internet Archive Wayback Machine. Accessed May 1, 2023). https://web.archive.org/web/20210401225102/https://www.hhs.gov/about/news/2021/04/01/hhs-launches-nationwide-network-trusted-voices-encourage-vaccination-next-phase-covid-19-public-education-campaign.html.

[11]   USASPENDING.gov. 2023. "Spending by Prime Award." Accessed May 3, 2023. https://www.usaspending.gov/search/?hash=2b9bbf7349e6c520a55164cbe34c6321.

[12]   Pickworth, Carin. "I'm in Love with my Obstetrician, and I'm not Alone." News.com.au. *KidSpot*, April 5, 2018. Accessed May 2, 2023. https://www.kidspot.com.au/pregnancy/labour/im-in-love-with-my-obstetrician-and-im-not-alone/news-story/1fc5007077f517444c29fe53acecce56.

[13]   Pickworth, Carin. "I'm in Love with my Obstetrician, and I'm not Alone." News.com.au. *KidSpot*, April 5, 2018. Accessed May 2, 2023. https://www.kidspot.com.au/pregnancy/labour/im-in-love-with-my-obstetrician-and-im-not-alone/news-story/1fc5007077f517444c29fe53acecce56.

[14]   WCA_FemalePowerhouse_Infographic_2018.pdf. https://womenschoiceaward.com/wp-content/uploads/2018/01/WCA_FemalePowerhouse_Infographic_2018.pdf. (Pg. 8).

[15]   Kates, Graham. "Inside the $250 Million Effort to Convince Americans the Coronavirus Vaccines are Safe." *CBS News*, December 23, 2020. Accessed May 2, 2023. https://www.cbsnews.com/news/covid-vaccine-safety-250-million-dollar-marketing-campaign/.

[16]   Mark A. Weber, Thomas E. Backer & April Brubach. "Creating the HHS COVID-19 Public Education Media Campaign: Applying Systems Change Learnings." April 25, 2022. *Journal of Health Communication*, 27:3, 201-207, DOI: 10.1080/10810730.2022.2067272.

[17]   Mark A. Weber, Thomas E. Backer & April Brubach. "Creating the HHS COVID-19 Public Education Media Campaign: Applying Systems Change Learnings." April 25, 2022. *Journal of Health Communication*, 27:3, 201-207, DOI: 10.1080/10810730.2022.2067272.

[18] LinkedIn. 2023. "Mark Weber (He/Him): "Your success is my success!" Accessed May 1, 2023. https://www.linkedin.com/in/mark-weber-595918a/.

[19] Mark A. Weber, Thomas E. Backer & April Brubach. "Creating the HHS COVID-19 Public Education Media Campaign: Applying Systems Change Learnings." April 25, 2022. *Journal of Health Communication*, 27:3, 201-207, DOI: 10.1080/10810730.2022.2067272 (emphasis added).

[20] USASPENDING.gov. 2023. "Spending by Prime Award." Accessed May 3, 2023. https://www.usaspending.gov/search/?hash=2b9bbf7349e6c520a55164cbe34c6321.

[21] USASPENDING.gov. 2023. "Spending by Prime Award." Accessed May 3, 2023. https://www.usaspending.gov/search/?hash=2b9bbf7349e6c520a55164cbe34c6321.

[22] Centers for Disease Control and Prevention (CDC). 2023. Documents responsive to FOIA Request. 2023. https://centersfordiseasecontrol.sharefile.com/d-sa6cdb04fbfef4 f579490cc942fe74945 . Accessed May 3, 2023. See pp. 569-575. Specifically, p. 573 states in connection with a COVID-19 related grant awarded to ACOG on July 13, 2022: **Substantial Involvement by CDC**: This is a cooperative agreement and CDC will have substantial programmatic involvement after the award is made. Substantial involvement is in addition to all post award monitoring, technical assistance, and performance reviews undertaken in the normal course of stewardship of federal funds. (Emphasis in original.)

[23] Centers for Disease Control and Prevention (CDC). 2023. Accessed May 3, 2022. Documents responsive to FOIA Request can be accessed at https://centersfordiseasecontrol.sharefile.com/d-sa6cdb04fbfef4f579490cc942fe74945. (See, e.g., Page 440.)

[24] *See* Mark A. Weber, Thomas E. Backer & April Brubach. "Creating the HHS COVID-19 Public Education Media Campaign: Applying Systems Change Learnings." April 25, 2022. *Journal of Health Communication*, 27:3, 201-207, DOI: 10.1080/10810730.2022.2067272 (emphasis added).

[25] Centers for Disease Control and Prevention (CDC). 2023. Accessed May 3, 2022. Documents responsive to FOIA Request can be accessed at https://centersfordiseasecontrol.sharefile.com/d-sa6cdb04fbfef4f579490cc942fe74945. (Pages 436-441, 439.)

[26] Centers for Disease Control and Prevention (CDC). 2023. Accessed May 3, 2022. Documents responsive to FOIA Request can be accessed at https://centersfordiseasecontrol.sharefile.com/d-sa6cdb04fbfef4f579490cc942fe74945. (Page 439.)

[27] Centers for Disease Control and Prevention (CDC). 2023. Accessed May 3, 2022. Documents responsive to FOIA Request can be accessed at https://centersfordiseasecontrol.sharefile.com/d-sa6cdb04fbfef4f579490cc942fe74945. (Page 440.)

[28] Centers for Disease Control and Prevention (CDC). 2023. Accessed May 3, 2022. Documents responsive to FOIA Request can be accessed at https://

centersfordiseasecontrol.sharefile.com/d-sa6cdb04fbfef4f579490cc942fe74945. (Page 440.)

[29] Centers for Disease Control and Prevention (CDC). 2023. Accessed May 3, 2022. Documents responsive to FOIA Request can be accessed at https://centersfordiseasecontrol.sharefile.com/d-sa6cdb04fbfef4f579490cc942fe74945. (Page 441.)

[30] Centers for Disease Control and Prevention (CDC). 2023. Accessed May 3, 2022. Documents responsive to FOIA Request can be accessed at https://centersfordiseasecontrol.sharefile.com/d-sa6cdb04fbfef4f579490cc942fe74945. (Page 1000.)

[31] Coleman, Justine. "CDC Recommends Pregnant People Get COVID-19 Vaccine." *The Hill*, April 23, 2021. Accessed May 2, 2023. https://thehill.com/policy/healthcare/549965-cdc-declares-it-recommends-pregnant-people-get-covid-19-vaccine/.

[32] Shimabukuro TT, Kim SY, Myers TR, Moro PL, Oduyebo T, Panagiotakopoulos L, Marquez PL, Olson CK, Liu R, Chang KT, Ellington SR, Burkel VK, Smoots AN, Green CJ, Licata C, Zhang BC, Alimchandani M, Mba-Jonas A, Martin SW, Gee JM, Meaney-Delman DM; CDC v-safe COVID-19 Pregnancy Registry Team. "Preliminary Findings of mRNA Covid-19 Vaccine Safety in Pregnant Persons." N Engl J Med. 2021 Jun 17;384(24):2273-2282. doi: 10.1056/NEJMoa2104983. Epub 2021 Apr 21. Erratum in: *N Engl J Med.* 2021 Oct 14;385(16):1536. PMID: 33882218; PMCID: PMC8117969. https://www.nejm.org/doi/full/10.1056/nejmoa2104983.

[33] Google. 2023. "Tom T. Shimabukuro. MD, MPH, MBA: Centers for Disease Control and Prevention." Accessed February 6, 2023. https://www.eventscribe.com/2018/NFIDFallCVC/ajaxcalls/PresenterInfo.asp?efp=SUhOV09EUVQ0MjE2&PresenterID=491468&rnd=2.500141E-02%20h%0D.

[34] Centers for Disease Control and Prevention (CDC). "COVID-19 Vaccine Safety Updates: Primary Series in Children Ages 5-11 Years." Advisory Committee on Immunization Practices (ACIP). May 19, 2022, slide 1. https://www.cdc.gov/vaccines/acip/meetings/downloads/slides-2022-05-19/03-covid-shimabukuro-508.pdf.

[35] *See* Thorp, Maggie and Jim Thorp. 2022. "Pushing COVID-19 Shots in Pregnancy: The Greatest Ethical Breach in the History of Medicine." *America Out Loud*, February 12, 2023. Accessed May 3, 2023. https://www.americaoutloud.com/pushing-covid-19-shots-in-pregnancy-the-greatest-ethical-breach-in-the-history-of-medicine/.

[36] The American College of Obstetricians and Gynecologists (ACOG). 2023. "ACOG and SMFM Recommend COVID-19 Vaccination for Pregnant Individuals." Accessed May 1, 2023. https://www.acog.org/news/news-releases/2021/07/acog-smfm-recommend-covid-19-vaccination-for-pregnant-individuals.

[37] The American College of Obstetricians and Gynecologists (ACOG). 2023. "ACOG and SMFM Recommend COVID-19 Vaccination for Pregnant Individuals." Accessed May

1, 2023. https://www.acog.org/news/news-releases/2021/07/acog-smfm-recommend-covid-19-vaccination-for-pregnant-individuals.

[38] The first appearance of ACOG "Conversation Guide for Clinicians" page was Dec. 31, 2020. From the first appearance of this *url* ACOG through mid-July of 2021, ACOG recommended that pregnant individuals should be able to make their own decision.

- Dec. 31, 2020 ACOG recommendation: "ACOG recommends that pregnant individuals should be free to make their own decision **in conjunction with their clinical care team**." https://web.archive.org/web/20201231213634/https://www.acog.org/covid-19/covid-19-vaccines-and-pregnancy-conversation-guide-for-clinicians . (Screen Snapshot captured on Dec, 30, 2020, by Internet Archive Wayback Machine. Accessed May 3, 2023) (emphasis added).

- Feb. 28, 2021 ACOG recommendation: "In the interest of patient autonomy, ACOG recommends that pregnant individuals be free to make their own decision regarding COVID-19 vaccination." https://web.archive.org/web/20210228211947/https://www.acog.org/covid-19/covid-19-vaccines-and-pregnancy-conversation-guide-for-clinicians. (Screen Snapshot captured on Feb. 28, 2021, by Internet Archive Wayback Machine. Accessed May 3, 2023).

- Mar. 31, 2021 ACOG recommendation: In the interest of patient autonomy, ACOG recommends that pregnant individuals be free to make their own decision regarding COVID-19 vaccination. https://web.archive.org/web/20210331111624/https://www.acog.org/covid-19/covid-19-vaccines-and-pregnancy-conversation-guide-for-clinicians. (Screen Snapshot captured on Mar. 31, 2021, by Internet Archive Wayback Machine. Accessed May 3, 2023).

- Apr. 26, 2021 ACOG recommendation: In the interest of patient autonomy, ACOG recommends that pregnant individuals be free to make their own decision regarding COVID-19 vaccination. https://web.archive.org/web/20210426181952/https://www.acog.org/covid-19/covid-19-vaccines-and-pregnancy-conversation-guide-for-clinicians. (Screen Snapshot captured on Apr. 26, 2021, by Internet Archive Wayback Machine. Accessed May 3, 2023).

- May 21, 2021 ACOG recommendation: In the interest of patient autonomy, ACOG recommends that pregnant individuals be free to make their own decision regarding COVID-19 vaccination. https://web.archive.org/web/20210521184756/https://www.acog.org/covid-19/covid-19-vaccines-and-pregnancy-conversation-guide-for-clinicians. (Screen Snapshot captured on May 21, 2021, by Internet Archive Wayback Machine. Accessed May 3, 2023).

- June 18, 2021 ACOG recommendation: In the interest of patient autonomy, ACOG recommends that pregnant individuals be free to make their own decision regarding COVID-19 vaccination. https://web.archive.org/web/20210618020731/https://www.acog.org/covid-19/covid-19-vaccines-and-pregnancy-conversation-guide-for-clinicians. (Screen Snapshot captured on June 18, 2021, by Internet Archive Wayback Machine. Accessed May 3, 2023).

- July 16, 2021 ACOG recommendation: In the interest of patient autonomy, ACOG recommends that pregnant individuals be free to make their own decision regarding COVID-19 vaccination. https://web.archive.org/web/20210716225120/https://www.acog.org/covid-19/covid-19-vaccines-and-pregnancy-conversation-guide-for-clinicians (Screen Snapshot captured on July 16, 2021, by Internet Archive Wayback Machine. Accessed May 3, 2023).

[39] The American College of Obstetricians and Gynecologists (ACOG). 2023. "ACOG and SMFM Recommend COVID-19 Vaccination for Pregnant Individuals." Accessed May 1, 2023. https://www.acog.org/news/news-releases/2021/07/acog-smfm-recommend-covid-19-vaccination-for-pregnant-individuals.

[40] Thorp, Maggie and Jim Thorp. 2022. "Pushing COVID-19 Shots in Pregnancy: The Greatest Ethical Breach in the History of Medicine." *America Out Loud*, February 12, 2023. Accessed May 3, 2023. https://www.americaoutloud.com/pushing-covid-19-shots-in-pregnancy-the-greatest-ethical-breach-in-the-history-of-medicine/.

[41] Thorp JA, Rogers C; Deskevich, MP, Tankersley S, Benavides A, Redshaw, M.D.; McCullough, P.A. COVID-19 Vaccines: The Impact on Pregnancy Outcomes and Menstrual Function. Journal of the American Physicians & Surgeons Spring 2023; 28(1) https://www.jpands.org/vol28no1/thorp.pdf.

[42] Bell, David, MD. "COVID Vaccines Were Never Sage for Pregnant Women, Pfizer's Own Data Show." *the Defender: Children's Health Defense News &Views*, April 28, 2023. Accessed May 3, 2023. https://childrenshealthdefense.org/defender/pfizer-covid-vaccine-pregnancy/ .

[43] Kelly, Amy. "Report 69: Bombshell – Pfizer and FDA Knew in Early 2021 that Pfizer mRNA COVID "Vaccine" Caused Dire Fetal and Infant Risks, Including Death. They Began an Aggressive Campaign to Vaccinate Pregnant Women Anyway." *DailyClout*, April 29, 2021. Accessed May 3, 2023. https://dailyclout.io/bombshell-pfizer-and-the-fda-knew-in-early-2021-that-the-pfizer-mrna-covid-vaccine-caused-dire-fetal-and-infant-risks-they-began-an-aggressive-campaign-to-vaccinate-pregnant-women-anyway/.

[44] The American College of Obstetricians and Gynecologists (ACOG). 2023. "ACOG and SMFM Recommend COVID-19 Vaccination for Pregnant Individuals." Accessed May 1, 2023. https://www.acog.org/news/news-releases/2021/07/acog-smfm-recommend-covid-19-vaccination-for-pregnant-individuals. This page states:
ACOG encourages its members to enthusiastically recommend vaccination to their patients. This means emphasizing the known safety of the vaccines and the increased risk of severe complications associated with COVID-19 infection, including death, during pregnancy," said J. Martin Tucker, MD, FACOG, president of ACOG. "It is clear that pregnant people need to feel confident in the decision to choose vaccination, and a strong recommendation from their obstetrician–gynecologist could make a meaningful difference for many pregnant people." (Emphasis retained).

See also, The American College of Obstetricians and Gynecologists (ACOG). 2023. "COVID-19 Vaccines and Pregnancy: Conversation Guide - Key Recommendations and Messaging for Clinicians." Accessed May 1, 2023. https://www.acog.org/covid-19/covid-19-vaccines-and-pregnancy-conversation-guide-for-clinicians. This page states: The American College of Obstetricians and Gynecologists (ACOG) strongly recommends that pregnant individuals be vaccinated against COVID-19. Given the potential for severe illness and death during pregnancy, completion of the initial COVID-19 vaccination series is a priority for this population.

[45] The CDC Foundation. 2023. "Supporting CDC and Public Health." Accessed May 3, 2023. https://www.cdcfoundation.org/supporting-cdc.

[46] The CDC Foundation. 2023. "Corporations, Foundations & Organizations: Fiscal year 2018 Report to Contributors." Accessed May 3, 2023. https://www.cdcfoundation.org/FY2018/organizations. https://www.cdcfoundation.org/FY2018/organizations. (Screen Snapshot captured on June 9, 2019, at 02:46:13, by Internet Archive Wayback Machine. Accessed May 6, 2023).

[47] The CDC Foundation. 2023. "Corporations, Foundations & Organizations: Fiscal year 2018 Report to Contributors." Accessed May 3, 2023. https://www.cdcfoundation.org/FY2018/organizations. https://www.cdcfoundation.org/FY2018/organizations. (Screen Snapshot captured on June 9, 2019, at 02:46:13, by Internet Archive Wayback Machine. Accessed May 6, 2023).

[48] American Society of Hematology. 2023. "CDC Pressed to Acknowledge Industry Funding." Accessed May 3, 2023. https://ashpublications.org/ashclinicalnews/news/4797/CDC-Pressed-to-Acknowledge-Industry-Funding.

[49] Kates, Graham. "Inside the $250 Million Effort to Convince Americans the Coronavirus Vaccines are Safe." CBS News, December 23, 2020. Accessed May 2, 2023. https://www.cbsnews.com/news/covid-vaccine-safety-250-million-dollar-marketing-campaign/.

[50] Kates, Graham. "Inside the $250 Million Effort to Convince Americans the Coronavirus Vaccines are Safe." CBS News, December 23, 2020. Accessed May 2, 2023. https://www.cbsnews.com/news/covid-vaccine-safety-250-million-dollar-marketing-campaign/.

CHAPTER 25

The Pain of Listening to Twitter Censorship Testimony

Dr. Naomi Wolf

Author of 7 nonfiction bestsellers.

Cofounder/CEO, DailyClout.io

Dr. Naomi Wolf is a bestselling author, columnist, and professor; she is a graduate of Yale University and received a doctorate from Oxford. She is co-founder and CEO of DailyClout.io, a successful civic tech company. Since the publication of her landmark international bestseller, *The Beauty Myth*, which The New York Times called "one of the most important books of the 20th century," Dr. Wolf's other seven bestsellers have been translated worldwide. The End of America and Give Me Liberty: A Handbook For American Revolutionaries, predicted the current crisis in authoritarianism and presented effective tools for citizens to promote civic engagement. Dr Wolf trains thought leaders of tomorrow, teaching public presentation to Rhodes Scholars and co-leading a Stony Brook University that gave professors skills to become public intellectuals. She was a Rhodes scholar herself, and was an advisor to the Clinton re-election campaign and to Vice President Al Gore. Dr. Wolf has written for every major news outlet in the US and many globally; she had four opinion columns, including in The Guardian and the Sunday Times of London. She lives with her husband, private detective Brian O'Shea, in the Hudson Valley.

Nasty, Ill-Dressed Technocrats, I Want My Life Back

As I type, I am undergoing the excruciating experience of listening to C-SPAN, which is airing "Twitter's Response to Hunter Biden Laptop Story."

The larger issue is: who censored Twitter, and why, and whether there was illegal collusion (there was) between Twitter and the US government.

So I finally am seeing them — up close, in real life, in person. I am finally able to look at the faces of the heretofore faceless technocrats who took it upon themselves to try to destroy my life and ruin my name. I am witnessing, as I see them seated primly in rows in a Congressional hearing room, the very faces — the somber, ill-cut but costly blue suits, the bad wire-rimmed glasses, the judgmental expressions — of those who were personally responsible for the misery, trauma, reputational damage, shattered dreams, and loss of income, in my one life, over the curse of last two and a half years.

Here at last are the very people who took it upon themselves, or who oversaw their colleagues, to single me out, to collude with the White House, and with Carol Crawford of CDC, and with DHS perhaps, to suspend me — following an accurate tweet of mine that warned women of menstrual harms following mRNA injection.

The positions of these people, the views of them — their self-regarding, self-satisfied, smug certainty that their rightness is the only rightness that could ever be — do not remind me of the testimony or views of actual Americans. They remind me rather of the affect of functionaries in a Stalinist show trial, or of the nameless bureaucrats in Kafka's *The Trial*.

There, onscreen, present at last, is Yoel Roth, "Former Twitter Head of Trust & Safety" - with that oddly prim, pursed mouth that these technocrats all seem to have; with those fingertips touching each other, presenting himself as if he is the moderator of reality itself, and as if he finds himself in the presence of something that smells bad. There are his glazed defiant blue eyes, his balding pate; there is the sneering downward cast of his mouth. I try not ever to make critical personal remarks, but the ugliness, sorrow, loss, isolation and pain I sustained, and still sustain every day, at the hands of these until-now-faceless, certain-that-they-are-right people, tend to make me see them aversively; or perhaps I see the moral ugliness of their decisions, as if manifested in their faces and body language.

Sorry — not sorry.

There he is: Mr Roth, wrongly claiming that, "paradoxically," more speech equals more danger and not more safety for society. There he is, this person so sure that he is so right, having tweeted that Republicans are "NAZIS." And here he is, sorry about that tweet now - that is, now that he is being asked about it — by those same Republicans.

There is Anika Collier Navaroli, "Former US Safety Policy Team Senior Expert," talking about "dangerous speech." There is her pale-gray jacket, her earnest if not bullying posture, as she leans forward, passionately describing the terrifying nature of freedom of speech. She describes a Twitter policy to address "coded incitement to violence" and to "address dog whistles." Overt threats of violence are of course already illegal, and they are the province of law enforcement, not of social media functionaries. Yet based on these "coded" tweets, rather than on actual threats of violence, Navaroli calls for more censorship. Thus she is already staking out and defending the Orwellian province of "thought crimes" or "pre-crime." It was never Ms. Navaroli's role to decide if "dog whistles" would lead to violence; that is the role of police and of the FBI. Why is she claiming that a *social media platform* is supposed to take on the role of maintaining physical public safety, that belongs to law enforcement?

Ms. Navaroli ends her aggressive introductory peroration with a pious, condescending conclusion that her mission is to make communication online "safe." Her evidence of the crimes committed by speaking on Twitter, include this 1984-level sentence: "The President said he liked to send out his tweets like "little missiles"; and to me that sounded like weaponization of a platform.'" Has the woman never taken an English class or learned about metaphors?

Here is Rep. Andy Biggs, asking Yoel Roth about marking certain speech as "unsafe."

There is Rep Eleanor Holmes Norton, a leader whom I used greatly to respect, fulminating about "conspiracies." There she is using the dangerous language of "incitement," a meaningless word that serves only to criminalize first amendment protected speech.

There is former Twitter counsel Ms Vijaya Gadde, with her slightly more polished look and her sapphire-colored jacket, a package that proves however only that pure evil can be as well dressed and coiffed as not. There Ms. Gadde is, prevaricating when Rep Nancy Mace (R-SC) asks her directly if Twitter ever censored Americans pursuant to demands from the Government. At Ms. Gadde's mumbling gibberish in response, phrased haplessly in the passive voice, Rep Mace thanked Gadde for admitting that Twitter had become a "subsidiary" of the FBI in illegally violating the First Amendment rights of Americans.

There is Rep. Summer Lee wrongly stating that it is her job to "protect the American people from misinformation," — a role that is identified literally nowhere in the Constitution or the Bill of Rights.

It is so painful for me to see these faces. I have a very intimate relationship to these people.

They tried to destroy me, and did a fair job of it, by some measures.

These are the people — "my" people, paradoxically; people educated like me, people who shared my political views until 2020; these are people who vacationed where I used to vacation, who hang out with people I know — who were the agents behind full- on Stalinist-type persecution of innocent Americans; of me; these are the people who ruined my life, or sought to do so, and destroyed my career, or sought to do so. These emotionally ugly, these nasty, these self-satisfied folks, so sure that they are right, so very, very wrong; are here at last; right here on C-Span.

They persecuted not just me, but Dr Martin Kulldorff; Dr Jay Bhattacharya; Dr Paul Alexander; Dr Peter McCullough. So many others. They scrubbed and manipulated the discourse of a platform that has no right to be any more censorious than a telecom company, because they were willing to collude illegally with the government to decide what can be said in America. The messaging from the FBI via "the super-secret James Bond teleportal," as Rep Jim Jordan so brilliantly and rightly put it, reached the voices of Americans and strangled Americans' rights; but Twitter and their political friends went further than mere silencing. These smarmy people ultimately hurt, and may have helped to injure and kill, many thousands.

These are the people who decided to remove a true tweet of mine — an accurate tweet — about menstrual symptoms, subsequent MRNA vaccines, that could have saved millions of women from the current menstrual agony and infertility that they now endure. These are the people who obeyed the instructions of their colleagues in government to censor me (I looked at the bios of the people cc'd on Twitter's communications with the White House about my accurate tweet; they were a lot of young functionaries at the US Bureau of the Census, at least two of them, oddly, educated at the University of Delaware).

These are the people who thought it was fine to destroy the career and try to shred the reputation of someone who had written seven international bestsellers, who had been a Rhodes scholar and an advisor to a Presidential campaign and to a Vice President; who had gone back to school at midlife and had worked for seven years successfully to complete a DPhil at Oxford University; who had been invited onto every major platform and written for every major newspaper and was a commentator on every major news network for 35 years, and who, for those decades, by those same platforms and news sites, had been identified as a global leader in the worldwide feminist movement.

These *nothing* people in front of me, these hacks, these people of zero cognitive distinction, these essentially trivial-minded humans, used their unearned, thug-like, intellectually meaningless power — the intellectually two-dimensional power of a *social media platform* — to announce to the world that I was crazy, unhinged; to present what appears to have been a file, to *The Guardian,* the *BBC,* to *NPR,* to *The New York Times - to my own former colleagues* —- seeking to represent me as crazy.

For the two years subsequent to my deplatforming, news outlets — including those where I used to be a columnist, such as *The Guardian* and the *Sunday Times of London* — did not need to claim let alone prove that I was *wrong* in some actual, concrete way; all they had to do now — and they did this repeatedly, clearly as we see at the behest of the governments involved - was to repeat the phrase now replicated around the world, and now also embedded in posterity on my Wikipedia bio:

"Naomi Wolf was banned from Twitter for misinformation."

"Misinformation" is never in quotes; the accurate caveat — "what Twitter called "misinformation"" — is never added, in describing me, in spite of this phrasing being actually the journalistically ethical and correct phrasing. This damning but really meaningless summary then is to what 35 years of labor, a status as a feminist leader, two degrees, eight bestsellers, thousands of footnotes, and the publication of essays in every major news site in North America, as well as most of Western Europe — got reduced.

It is incredible to me as someone who was raised in an American meritocracy, and who has until very recently believed in American meritocracy, that a group of nonentities in Twitter, in collusion with nonentities at CDC (hi there, Carol Crawford), the White House and the US Dept of the Census — were able thus so simply, and at such immediate, nuclear scale, to destroy the reputation of someone identified since 1990 as a major American writer and voice in feminism.

These ill-dressed, ill-spoken, banal nonentities cost me so much.

I re-trained for almost a decade, in the middle of my life, to teach. It is all I had ever really wanted to do with my life. Now I will never be able to be the only thing I ever wanted to be — a Professor of English Literature at a university.

I am now sixty. It's too late for me. Twitter, in collusion with the Biden administration, cost me my hard-won lifelong dream. I've been maligned and censored by Twitter since 2021. Even if the company eventually settles my lawsuit against it, and even though Mr Musk has "let" me back on the platform, that would be, this is, no victory.

Twitter has not sent an advisory to all of the news outlets around the world that depicted me, at Twitter's own direction, as crazy, that they were wrong to do so; there has been no press release stating that they erred, and that I was right, and that they are sorry for wrongly abusing my reputation (and destroying women). No, forever I remain "deplatformed from Twitter for misinformation," even though it is finally being established that sadly I was deplatformed for telling God's truth.

It is unlikely that any university at this point would see past the grotesque imprint on my bio that Twitter, via the White House, CDC and perhaps the FBI, has taken care to embed in my bio and articles about me, around the world. It is unlikely, topo, that I will ever recoup the six figure investments that investors withdrew from my company when Twitter, colluding with the government, was orchestrating the shredding of my reputation. It is unlikely that a 35-year career and legacy online of what had been seen until very recently as a life of significant accomplishment, can ever be re-established.

I try never to complain in public. I try never to show self-pity or weakness, at least not to my enemies. But Twitter's attacks on me are not over, and I am simply sick of the damage these mediocrities have done to me, and continue to try to do.

Just yesterday LinkedIn sent me a notification that a Twitter "Political Staffer" was viewing my bio. A notice of scrutiny by Twitter and their friends in the administration reached my inbox *the day before* Congressional hearings about the censorship they imposed on people such as me.

Intimidate much @Twitter?

I am a brave person — I guess — and I won't be daunted by this obvious act of harassment. But I am also human, and I happen to have a broken shoulder at the moment, and I am simply tired; tired of fighting these monsters.

And yes, it is wearying and threatening and coercive to see that this massive behemoth, with their friends at the highest levels of government, are not done messing with my own, personal, only life.

Yoel Roth is to this very minute, defending the de-platforming of people due to their having "spread COVID misinformation." A nonentity, to this very day defending debunked magical thinking. To which Rep Marjorie Taylor Greene rightly responded: "Mr Roth: who put you in charge of what is true and what is not?"

Rep. Taylor Greene also said to Mr Roth: "You abused the power of Big Tech to censor Americans. I am so glad you are censored now, and that you have lost your job."

I cannot believe that "my own" people, my former tribe on the elite left, are joining forces with the government to violate the First Amendment rights of all Americans and then, worse still, to justify having done so.

I can't believe that people I thought were hostile to America's interests — in this case, the Republicans demanding answers from the hacks and flunkies of Big Tech — are the allies in this hearing's case at least, of truth and the Constitution and freedom of speech.

And I can't believe that the forces who tore my life apart, temporarily half-destroyed my business, ended any hopes of my realizing my one life's best dream, and set a match to my reputation, turn out, now that the curtain has been pulled back, as at the end of The Wizard of Oz - to be such small, small, sad, petty, miserable, mediocre people.

The larger issue is not the damage these smirking, small-minded people did to me. The larger issue is what the experience I underwent at their hands, represents for our culture.

There is a specific kind of damage that Twitter and the Biden administration did, in censoring and smearing the medical doctors — in silencing the signatories of the Great Barrington Declaration. Medical harms, medical damage, limits to medical options and open debate, follow.

But consider my example as an example of something else, that is equally serious.

I am not a medical doctor or a public health official — I am, or I was, an American writer, identified as a feminist leader; a cultural figure. So what happened to me means that any American cultural figure can be taken down. Any American cultural movement can be mis-framed, defamed, broken. Any American writer, musician, artist, sculptor, actor, director, can be taken down. Any American artistic movement can be burned alive. And remember — Twitter is an international company, and wars can be waged, culturally, against us by our adversaries.

So this issue brings us squarely into the cultural climate of 1933, when books were dragged from university libraries to be burned in a pile, in Berlin: or of 1937, when the Nazi party curated and hosted a "Degenerate Art" exhibit in Munich. What happened to me brings us squarely into a climate in which specific American writers, artists, sculptors, musicians, social activists, can be identified as enemies of the state, or identified as culturally or socially untouchable.

"Degeneracy" in 1937 was defined essentially as that of which the Nazi party did not approve.

Today on C-Span, we heard a lot about the decision to violate Americans' rights, based simply on that of which the Biden administration, or Twitter's employees, did not approve.

The larger issue is that once a society crosses this Rubicon, with one cultural figure, this can happen to any cultural figure or any cultural movement. And that if we do not reject (and indeed prosecute and legislate against) this unlawful suppression of views at the behest of the government, then we no longer live in an American culture, in which ideas rise and gain currency on the basis of merit and on the basis of ideas' appeals to others. We will be in a Nazi reality in which petty officials distort and dictate culture itself and reputationally behead those cultural leaders who pose challenges to the power structure.

Berlin, Munich, in this respect, are here again, in their darkest sense; those who decided, based on a party line, on proper and improper art, books, views — are not dead and gone; lost in history; no; here they are again.

But this time they appear in our America, in their bad blue suits, with their hectoring nasal voices; saying "I have no knowledge of this matter"; or "I can't hear the question"; as they occupy, with their damaged consciences, their nauseating excuses, seats in a hearing room on Capitol Hill in the United States of America.

Will we let these cultural functionaries — who operate just like those petty tyrants of the cultures of Berlin and Munich not so long ago — take up space, with impunity, in the heart of our America?

Or will we drag America back into daylight and sunlight again, and force these equivocating wretches to face their own degenerate crimes against freedom of speech and the Constitution?

CHAPTER 26

From High-tech to Citizen Journalist: How They Tried to Silence Me

Steve Kirsch

Entrepreneur & founder of Vaccine
Safety Research Foundation

Steve Kirsch is a high-tech entrepreneur turned investigative journalist. He founded the Vaccine Safety Research Foundation in response to the COVID-19 vaccines. The VSRF's mission is to encourage questions and an open dialogue of transparency on any medical and scientific information, as well as to advance COVID-19 vaccine safety through scientific research, public education, and advocacy, and to support the vaccine injured.

As far as I can see, nobody wants to discuss anything anymore. Certainly while the COVID pandemic and subsequent vaccination campaign was in full swing, nobody wanted to discuss numbers at all - not your mother, father, brother or neighbor, and most certainly not those people who should be looking at numbers.

The thing about good science is that it should be repeatable. If I get a result, then some other scientist should be able to get the same result, right? I'm trying to prove the science with repeatable statistics and I'm asking questions that people don't want to answer. What I'm hoping to do is try to show people that the information they are not getting is not the whole truth and nothing but the truth because it is being censored, because they are being subjected to a propaganda campaign that prevents them from seeing the bigger picture.

I didn't see censorship at the beginning of the pandemic. So, we were just believing the narratives. But once people started speaking out, then they were basically either ignored, censored, de-platformed, or discredited. That has clearly led to a lot of people who were only seeing one side of the narrative. So they were making decisions based on knowing only one set of facts instead of seeing the whole picture.

The mainstream press is supposed to provide objective viewpoints. They're supposed to provide pros and cons. They were just providing pros and failing to seek opinions from anyone on the other side of the government narrative, so that the public could weigh both arguments and make their own decision with regard to the vaccines.

It was a huge mistake to think that you're going to be doing a public service by only airing one side of any argument. They did that because they believed that people were telling the truth and they believed that if they told people the potential downside, it would scare them and they wouldn't take the vaccine. So the press turned into propaganda. And when the press does that, it is extremely dangerous.

My first indication that censorship was at play was when I was banned permanently from Medium. And then I was permanently banned on LinkedIn. I was permanently banned on Twitter. I had two lifetime bans (but have now been reinstated. Thanks Elon.) I was permanently banned from Wikipedia. Those were good hints that I was on to something. Then, as soon as I published my article on TrialSite News with the title "Should you Get Vaccinated?" on May 25th, 2021 within about a week, my entire scientific advisory board of the Vaccine Safety Research Foundation quit and said they never wanted to talk to me again. So that's another form of censorship. In other words, they don't want to hear anything that might challenge their beliefs.

In that TrialSite News article, which has had over one million views, I told the naked truth. Here's an excerpt for those who missed it:

"I always get vaccinated. I have been fully vaccinated with the Moderna COVID vaccine. My three daughters have all been vaccinated.

I recently learned that these vaccines have likely killed over 25,800 Americans (which I confirmed 3 different ways) and disabled at least 1,000,000 more. And we're only halfway to the finish line. We need to PAUSE these vaccines NOW before more people are killed.

The CDC, FDA, and NIH aren't disclosing how many people have been killed or disabled from the COVID vaccines. The mainstream media isn't asking any questions; they are playing along. YouTube, Facebook, Twitter, and others are all censoring content that goes against the "perfectly safe" narrative, so nobody's the wiser."

There were a lot of people who chose to sever all ties with me after I published this article; nearly all of them would be considered "top tier" academics. Challenging the accepted narrative is seen as evil. They said I was risking lives and they didn't want their name associated with me.

So be it. I think it is extremely dangerous for the scientific community to have the attitude that if anyone challenges the narrative that they must be wrong and the correct course of action is to sever all ties and refuse to engage in debate. If I'm wrong, I'll be discredited. If I'm right, I'll be the one saving lives and their views were the ones endangering lives. I wouldn't be spending my time writing this if I wasn't convinced I was right. There are too many things nobody can explain if you buy the hypothesis that the vaccines are safe.

I asked these academics "look if I'm wrong, then how do you explain this....?" None of them would engage. Some of them said, "I heard you are against the vaccine. Never talk to me again." I'm serious. You can't make this stuff up.

On June 6th, 2021 I challenged any doctor on Clubhouse to a debate on the COVID vaccine facts I raised in my May 25th article. The challenge was ignored and to this day, no doctor, nor anybody from the CDC or FDA has taken me up on the million dollar wager I offered to debate. They don't want to discuss it, they don't want to see any evidence.

Nobody's ever seen anything to this level of censorship and deplatforming except perhaps Dr. Andrew Wakefield, when he pointed out the link between vaccines and autism. He was attacked, discredited and fired. People all the time are attacking his credibility; this is what they're going to do to us all, which is why there's such a small pool of people who are prepared to step out and speak up. It's truly tragic because there is a lot of stuff that people are seeing that they're afraid to bring up because they're worried about job loss for sure.

There is a pediatrician at a well-known university who recently reached out to my wife and said, "Hey, your husband's not a whack job. But you can't tell him who I am as I don't want to lose my job." This at least makes me feel that I've been vindicated. And anyway, there's no doubt that I'm right. If nobody wants to listen, then shame on them. I will still do my best and work my hardest to make sure that they know that they're in the wrong.

I have never seen anything like this before in history, but they were trained to do this. They had exercises like Event 201 hosted by Johns Hopkins University to say, " world, we need to prepare for a pandemic." That's actually a good thing; that there is coordination and planning ahead of time, because you don't want to have a disaster and not have done any planning. But the coordinated response should have included treatments such as making sure everybody gets ivermectin and hydroxychloroquine and fluvoxamine and whatever else works. They should have put the coordinated effort into that, as well as the vaccine, had it worked and had it been safe.

I was treated as if I'm an evil person. I'm not evil at all. My sole motivation is to save lives by seeking resolution to key questions. Ostracizing dissenters is bad science in my opinion. I've listened to both sides and I'm convinced that there is an air-tight case to be made here for the counter-narrative because the things I've seen with my own eyes are not consistent with the narrative. Could I be wrong? Sure. Could they be wrong? Absolutely. But my narrative fits the facts and their narrative doesn't. So there you go.

I think the entire academic community should be ashamed of themselves for not speaking out loudly against this vaccine. It shows how inept they are that a computer entrepreneur can clearly see what is happening and they cannot. It is embarrassing for the entire medical community. It's going to come out that I am on the right side of this and they are all wrong. The evidence on the table is so compelling. And the longer academia digs in their heels opposing what I write, the worse they are going to look.

It's also an indictment of the mainstream media. There should be a *New York Times* investigative journalist on this. Do you know how many inbound queries I've gotten (since I know a lot more that I can't disclose publicly): zero.

Ask yourself, if the vaccine is so safe, then why does Facebook keep removing "Vaccine side effects" groups? It's hardly news now in 2023 to understand that Facebook employees were enabling censorship by sitting on their hands while their company silenced innocent vaccine victims. Since when is it OK to censor facts and truth and civil discussion?

Marc Zuckerberg has few comments on this (he has a lot of money tied up in the vaccine and promised Tony Fauci to remove any content that goes against the false NIH narrative). Censoring victims of a dangerous vaccine is not in the public interest.

We are literally silencing free speech.

CHAPTER 27

"On Stupidity"

Dietrich Bonhoeffer's theory
explains much of the COVID-19
Pandemic Response.

John Leake

Historian and co-author of

"The Courage To Face Covid19"

John Leake studied history and philosophy with Roger Scruton at Boston University. He went to Vienna, Austria on a graduate school scholarship and ended up living in the city for over a decade, working as a freelance writer and translator. He is a true crime writer with a lifelong interest in medical history and forensic medicine. He is also Co-author of *"The Courage to Face COVID-19: Preventing Hospitalization and Death While Battling the Biopharmaceutical Complex,"* by John Leake & Peter McCullough, MD, MPH. New York: Skyhorse Publishing, 2022.

In 1943, the Lutheran pastor and member of the German resistance, Dietrich Bonhoeffer, was arrested and incarcerated in Tegel Prison. There he meditated on the question of why the German people—in spite of their vast education, culture, and intellectual achievements—had fallen so far from reason and morality. He concluded that they, as a people, had been afflicted with collective stupidity (German: *Dummheit*).

He was not being flippant or sarcastic, and he made it clear that stupidity is not the opposite of native intellect. On the contrary, the events in Germany between 1933 and 1943 had shown him that perfectly intelligent people were, under the pressure of political power and propaganda, rendered stupid—that is, incapable of critical reasoning. As he put it:

Stupidity is a more dangerous enemy of the good than wickedness. Evil can be protested against, exposed, and, if necessary, it can be prevented by force. Evil always harbors the germ of self-destruction by inducing at least some uneasiness in people. We are defenseless against stupidity. Nothing can be done to oppose it, neither with protests nor with violence. Reasons cannot prevail. Facts that contradict one's prejudice simply don't need to be believed, and when they are inescapable, they can simply be brushed aside as meaningless, isolated cases.

In contrast to evil, the stupid person is completely satisfied with himself. When irritated, he becomes dangerous and may even go on the attack. More caution is therefore required when dealing with the stupid than with the wicked. Never try to convince the stupid with reasons; it's pointless and dangerous.

To understand how to deal with stupidity, we must try to understand its nature. This much is certain: it is not essentially an intellectual, but a human defect. There are people who are intellectually agile who are stupid, while intellectually inept people may be anything but stupid. We discover this to our surprise in certain situations.

One gets the impression that stupidity is often not an innate defect, but one that emerges under certain circumstances in which people are made stupid or allow themselves to be made stupid. We also observe that isolated and solitary people exhibit this defect less frequently than socializing groups of people. Thus, perhaps stupidity is less a psychological than a sociological problem. It is a special manifestation of the influence of historical circumstances on man—a psychological side effect of certain external conditions.

A closer look reveals that the strong exertion of external power, be it political or religious, strikes a large part of the people with stupidity. Yes, it seems as if this is a sociological-psychological law. The power of some requires the stupidity of others. Under this influence, human abilities suddenly wither or fail, robbing people of their inner independence, which they—more or less unconsciously — renounce to adapt their behavior to the prevailing situation.

The fact that stupid people are often stubborn should not hide the fact that they are not independent. When talking to him, one feels that one is not dealing with him personally, but with catchphrases, slogans, etc. that have taken possession of him. He is under a spell; he is blinded; he is abused in his own being.

Having become an instrument without an independent will, the fool will also be capable of all evil, and at the same time, unable to recognize it as evil. Here lies the danger of diabolical abuse. Through this, a people can be ruined forever. But it is also quite clear here that it is not an act of instruction, but only an act of liberation that can overcome stupidity. In doing so, one will have to accept the fact that, in most cases, real inner liberation is only possible after outer liberation has taken place. Until then we will have to refrain from all attempts to convince the stupid. In this state of affairs, we try in vain to know what such people actually think.

Upon reading Bonhoeffer's reflections, some might protest that "stupidity" is a pejorative term that lacks scientific precision. However, it seems to me that the word is, in fact, an accurate characterization of the COVID-19 pandemic response. Consider the unfathomable fit of stupidity required to believe that hydroxychloroquine and ivermectin are *dangerous* while at the same time believing that novel mRNA vaccines—developed at "warp speed"—are perfectly safe. As Bonhoeffer pointed out, such stupidity is *not* an expression of the victim's lack of native intelligence, but of his inability to think when political or religious power is being exerted on his society.

Other writers, such as Carl Jung, have described this phenomenon as **Mass Psychosis** (German: *Massenpsychose*). Mattias Desmet has written in a similar vein about the same phenomenon, which he calls **Mass Formation**. The late Stanford professor, Rene Girard, described a similar process combining the phenomena of **Mimesis** (imitation) and **Scapegoating**. Girard's reflections are consistent with Bonhoeffer's observation: "We also observe that isolated and solitary people exhibit this defect less frequently than socializing groups of people."

It seems to me that all the above authors are using different terms to describe the same thing—namely, that under certain conditions, otherwise intelligent people lose their capacity for rational thinking and evaluation. Most notable to me is Bonhoeffer's observation: "There are people who are intellectually agile who are stupid, while intellectually inept people may be anything but stupid." This reminds me of something we often saw during the pandemic—namely, the spectacle of Ivy League-educated professionals becoming *the most* responsive to crude propaganda about social distancing, masking, the suppression of early treatment, and the fanatical promotion of experimental vaccines. As my co-author, Peter McCullough, often exclaimed, "These people have lost their minds!" What can explain this seemingly paradoxical phenomenon?

A few possibilities come to mind:

1. Educated, affluent professionals live under circumstances of enormous material and personal security and are therefore unaccustomed to thinking about anything that could purportedly cut their lives short. This causes them to feel great fear—an emotion that impairs the normal functioning of their cognitive skills.

2. They have attained great success from their affiliation with people and institutions that are perceived as bearing authority.

This has made them unaccustomed to questioning figures of perceived authority.

3. Likewise, they have attained success by mastering tried and true procedures. When confronted with a novel and stressful situation, they are reluctant to recognize that their longstanding mental habits are of limited utility. For the first time in years, they are called upon *to think* about something they've never encountered before. Threatened by the reality that their authority is being challenged by the situation, they double down on their appeals to authority.

Years from now, when we look back on the COVID-19 pandemic response, we will—like young Germans in the post-war period who reflected on what happened to their country in 1933-45—marvel at the astonishing stupidity that can afflict an intellectually advanced civilization.

Note: Bonhoeffer, Dietrich."Von der Dummheit": *Widerstand und Ergebung. Briefe und Aufzeichnungen aus der Haft.* S. 17–20. Muenchen, Christian Kaiser Verlag, 1951. Translated from the German by John Leake.

CHAPTER 28

My Message to the Ontario College of Physicians and Surgeons

Dr. Mary O'Connor

Family physician

I graduated from the University of Toronto Medical school in 1971. I worked as a solo practitioner in family medicine for 44 years, and in the last 18 years I focused on mental health issues and substance use disorders. I had the most wonderful patients. I advocated for them to the best of my ability.

And then, COVID came; I didn't know the truth for a couple of months. In truth, I was looking forward to a rest during that first 2 week lockdown. Then I began to understand the craziness of it all.

I always tried to go to daily Mass; as I sat in the pew, all of a sudden the questions came... why didn't the priests have to wear masks on the altar, but the parishioners had to wear them in the seats? How is this virus only going in one direction? I felt so confused at times. During lockdown I also had the chance to watch and listen to several American priests who knew and spoke the truth about the non-pandemic. The truth became clearer and clearer.

I began to realize and learn that masks were not needed, and are in fact harmful, but it still took me some weeks to finally take off my mask forever; I was afraid that people would be angry at me, and that I would be responsible for having the Church closed down.

And then the requests for exemptions started ...so many requests. Strange, looking back, that we believed we needed an exemption to prevent an illegal action from being perpetrated against us.

Then on April 30, 2021 Ontario's physician licensing body, the College of Physicians and Surgeons of Ontario (CPSO) issued a statement forbidding physicians from questioning or debating any or all of the official measures imposed in response to Covid 19. The CPSO then went on to threaten us with punishment, investigation and disciplinary action.

This threat was hanging over our heads.

The first exemption requests were for masks, especially for children. I want to say that I am not blaming the parents who did mask their children at first; they didn't know the truth; they were afraid and thought they were doing the right thing.

But it was very distressing. A school principal called me to question an exemption I'd written for one child. This principal totally believed that all 400 children in her school should wear masks..

But I also heard a very uplifting story. A little 4 year old strongly objected when her kindergarten teacher tried to put a mask on her, and asked " Are you trying to kill me"?

And then, more and more requests, hundreds of them, for exemptions from PCR testing, and then from the experimental gene therapy injections.

I was still trying to do my regular patient work

I couldn't keep up with the demand.

I was helped by the most amazing assistant. I give a huge thanks to my helper.

We did not charge for these exemptions.

Every telephone request for an exemption was a long conversation. The people were so grateful to speak to someone who understood and supported their decisions.

I was given the privilege of speaking to so many wonderful people.

All these patients were all being coerced for various reasons; by their workplace, gym, pressure from family members and friends. They were isolated from other family members, not allowed to visit their grandchildren, or visit loved ones in hospitals or Long Term Care. The stories were heartbreaking.

Many of these people had known the truth from day 1. They (as did we all) had valid reasons to never comply with the illegal mandates. Many had never taken any vaccine in their whole life. Others had existing health problems, often cardiac, which would have been exacerbated by the "jab". And others had had "Covid-19", and thus would have had natural immunity.

Many already knew others who had suffered a serious adverse effect from the needle, including death.

And, at first, some exemptions were accepted, but then the College of Physicians and Surgeons quickly changed the criteria, and it was almost impossible to qualify for a "valid" exemption. For example, you would have to prove that you had a life threatening reaction to a first injection. I continued to write exemptions however, stating that exemptions were required for "medical" reasons; the patients were prepared for a refusal, but it gave them a few weeks to sort out their plans for a new life.

Looking back, I wish I had been stronger, and had been able to tell patients...we don't need exemptions; we'll just all say NO.

I became quickly aware of adverse effects in my own patients. One gentleman who, though he knew the truth, was injected so he could visit a family member. He developed, I believe, significant heart problems with pain, shortness of breath, tachycardia, and weakness, which lasted about 6 weeks. However he was afraid to go to hospital, and specific testing wasn't done. Another patient's relative was found dead in bed days after the Pfizer shot. I saw several people with neurological effects, including loss of coherent speech for a few days, paranoia, and facial grimacing.

The College of Physicians and Surgeons of Ontario became aware of my exemption notes, when two employers of patients contacted the College to check the legitimacy of my exemptions.

On October 8, 2021, I received my first letter from the College. They demanded that I give them the names and charts of all the patients for whom I had written exemptions. They started an investigation into my practice. They described my conduct as disgraceful, dis-honourable or unprofessional. They were investigating whether I had engaged in professional misconduct and/or was incompetent. They were concerned "as my behaviour was liable to expose my patients to harm," and that I was putting my patients, and society at large, at risk.

They "recognized" an investigation might be stressful, and offered help from their physician health program. I did not accept their offer.

And, I continued on my path; I did not relinquish my patients' names and charts.

They hired a team of four Investigators to find me and my charts, wherever I might be.

The Investigators did not want to be named, as they did not want to be harassed.

I received written notice that "No one was to obstruct a College investigator or withhold from him or her things that are relevant to the investigation as the investigator exercises his or her powers under section 76(1) and (2) of the Code....under Section 87 of the Health Professions Procedural Code."

They were given authority by the College that they could enter my dwelling any time during working hours.

The chief investigator sent me multiple letters over many months, usually on a Friday afternoon. Eventually, I learned not to let them disturb me. It became a joke, as I waited for the Friday letter.

When I was back in Ottawa, I had to stay with friends, and my hostesses were all nervous that "The Investigator" would show up. We all became a little paranoid for a while. But we firmly decided we would not worry and just call the police, but even that decision was worrying during COVID times.

And, I continued on my path; I did not relinquish my patients' names and charts.

On November 5th, 2021 the inquiry, Complaint and Reports Committee (ICRC) of the College gave me an order, but "WITHOUT NOTICE" to me, in which they forbade me to write more exemptions.

I didn't know about the order, and I continued on my path; I continued to write exemptions.

They wrote, as I saw later, that they were "of the opinion, on reasonable and probable grounds, that the conduct of Dr O'Connor exposes or is likely to expose her patients to harm or injury and urgent intervention is needed. "

They also demanded that I put signs in all office rooms, and on Zoom, and that I say on the telephone that I was not allowed to write exemptions. The College wanted to know each and every location where I was practising. They wanted my permission to contact OHIP to monitor my compliance. And they wanted me to give them a Patient Log every 2 weeks, or whenever they asked. They wanted me to submit to and not interfere with, unannounced inspections of my practice locations.

These people redacted their names on the letters to me.

And so I continued on my path; I continued not to comply.

On November 22, 2021, a private eye, hired by the College, tricked me into giving her an exemption. She wanted to go to the gym. On November 26th, or thereabouts, my lawyer was informed of the order, and passed the instructions on to me. As soon as I learned of the Order, I wrote no more exemptions.

They tried to fool me at least one other time with another "Private Eye," but I had stopped writing exemptions by then.

Due to the threat of surprise visits from the investigators, I had to have a friend act as a guard to open and close the door between patients. My patients were very dismayed by the possibility of this break-in.

On December 8th 2021, what we feared, happened. It happened on a day when I wasn't in the office, and my friend was there by himself, with the door unlocked. The four Investigators entered. My friend heard people rushing up the stairs; they trapped him in the boardroom, and the Chief Investigator pummelled him with questions about the whereabouts of myself and my charts. He was very intimidating. The female Investigator searched all the filing cabinets. The other two stood by the doors of the boardroom, trapping my friend in the room.

My friend was traumatised. He was able to relay some of the conversation on his phone to a colleague. Eventually, he regained his strength, told the Investigators he was leaving and was going to call the police. They followed him out.

And, by the Grace of God, they did not get my charts, as I had relocated them two months before because I had moved.

These Investigators also left a "warrant" for my colleague, demanding that she give them my charts. (She never had access to my charts at all.)

Two of the four left their calling cards with my friend. They released their own names, in spite of their fears!

The Investigator(s) also went to my old neighbourhood to find me, to ask if anyone knew where I moved.

The Chief Investigator then sent a letter to my new post office box, letting me know he knew where I was.

On December 23rd, 2021 at midnight, the College suspended my licence to practise medicine. The ICRC was of the opinion that my behaviour was likely to expose my patients to harm or injury.

They "considered the least restrictive order that was necessary to ensure patient protection," was to suspend my certificate of registration.

On January 7th, 2022, the College took me to Ontario Superior Court. I was co-accused with three other doctors (humbling, with three of my heroes).

It was a ZOOM court, and those on the other side, except for the lawyers, blacked out their faces.

One of the College lawyers actually said out loud that this had nothing to do with vaccine safety. My lawyer said it had everything to do with vaccine safety.

The blacked out faces must have included news reporters Ashleigh Stewart from Global, and Michele Mandel from The Toronto Sun; both wrote defamatory articles about me and my "conspiracy theories." They also mocked other well spoken doctors who were trying to spread the truth, including Dr. Stephen Malthouse and Dr Charles Hoffe.

Looking back on news writing, it was shocking to read about their total lack of knowledge of any truth at the time. But that's how it was for so many then. Even now.

We presented multiple pages to the court about the truth of the Covid situation; the danger of the mandates, and especially the experimental gene therapy injection.

Judge Edward Morgan ruled against my patients, and said I had to hand over their names and charts. And, I continued on my path; I did not relinquish my patients' names and charts.

I was unwilling to violate my Hippocratic Oath or my patients' rights to choose their medical treatment and protect their privacy rights.

And so, I was in Contempt of Court. I knew that could have a possible jail sentence.

Several months went by, and finally the College contacted my lawyer. They told him that they were NOT going to ask for a jail sentence.

A court date for my Contempt charge was set for February 6, 2023. The College cancelled the case on February 4. The College was also bringing me to the Tribunal to discipline me for my "disgraceful" and risky behaviour.

I did attend two pre-hearing conferences with the help of a para-legal. The College lawyer, Ms Widner actually accused me of lying when, in my defence, I said that I had not received the order on November 5, not to write more exemptions.

I did not lie, and I had proof of when I received the notice, which was after I had written that last exemption. The College dropped the Tribunal hearings, and I missed my opportunity to prove my truth.

My case illustrates the danger from the College, the censorship and their propaganda. Had they been successful, it would mean that all patients would have lost their right to privacy, that their most intimate private medical details could be surrendered to the College when they decide there is an emergency. I ask people to speak to their doctors and see if they are willing to protect their information.

I say to the College: to Dr. Nancy Whitmore, the four unnamed (frightened) Investigators, the Private Eyes, the College lawyers: Ms Ruth Ainsworth, Mr Evan Rankin and Mr Peter Wardle, and all the Tribunal members, my Compliance Monitor(s), and to Judge Edward Morgan who ruled against my patients, and to the News reporters, I am not angry at you. I feel great sorrow for you. You are caught in the lie, and on the side of darkness. I hope and pray to Our Good Lord that you will come to know the truth, and see the light, so you will no longer be complicit in the injuries and deaths of so many people.

And, as we say in Ottawa nowadays, "we will hold the line."

CHAPTER 29

Plausibility but Not Science Has Dominated Public Discussions of the COVID Pandemic

Dr. Harvey Risch

Professor Emeritus of Epidemiology, Yale School of
Public Health & Medicine

Dr. Harvey Risch is Professor Emeritus of Epidemiology at the Yale School of Public Health and Yale School of Medicine. Dr. Risch received his MD degree from the University of California San Diego, and PhD, in mathematical modeling of infectious epidemics, from the University of Chicago. Dr. Risch is one of the original contrarians of the pandemic and a major figure. He was among the first to stand publicly and claim that the pandemic management was unscientific and basically a fraud. In May of 2022 Dr Risch published unequivocal evidence for the early and safe use of hydroxychloroquine (the HCQ cocktail) for COVID-19 in the American Journal of Epidemiology titled, "Early Outpatient Treatment of Symptomatic, High-Risk COVID-19 Patients that Should be Ramped-Up Immediately as Key to Pandemic Crisis." Dr. Risch continues to speak out about the false rationales of the pandemic management.

"Attacks on me, quite frankly, are attacks on *science*."
- Anthony Fauci, June 9, 2021 (MSNBC).

Thus, Dr. Fauci proclaims himself "Emperor of Science." *Preposterous.* For one thing, Dr. Fauci has not reported accurately on scientific questions throughout the Covid-19 pandemic. For another, the essential dialectic of science is arguing, questioning, debating. Without debate, science is nothing more than propaganda. Yet, one may ask, how has it been possible to present technical material to the American public, if not to the international public, for more than three years and achieve a general understanding that the matters were "scientific," when in fact they were not. I assert that what has been fed to these publics through the traditional media over the course of the pandemic has largely been plausibility, sometimes called "scientism," but not science, and that both the American and international publics, as well as most doctors, and scientists themselves, cannot tell the difference. However, the difference is fundamental and profound.

Science starts with theories, hypotheses, that have examinable empiric ramifications. Nevertheless, those theories are not science; they *motivate* science. Science occurs when individuals do experiments or make observations that bear upon the implications or ramifications of the theories. Those findings tend to support or refute the theories, which are then modified or updated to adjust to the new observations or discarded if compelling evidence shows that they fail to describe nature. The cycle is then repeated. *Science* is the performance of empirical or observational work to obtain evidence confirming or refuting theories.

In general, theories tend to be plausible statements describing something specific about how nature operates. Plausibility is in the eye of the beholder, since what is plausible to a technically knowledgeable expert may not be plausible to a lay person. For example, we might balk at thinking it plausible that light travels simultaneously as both particles and waves, and that making measurements on the light, what we do as observers, determines whether we see particle behavior or wave behavior, and we can choose to observe either particles or waves, but not both at the same time. But this is how it is; nature is not necessarily plausible.

All the same, plausible theories are easy to believe, and that is the problem. That is what we have been fed for three years of the Covid-19 pandemic. In fact though, we have been fed plausibility instead of science for much longer.

Evidence-Based Medicine

There is perhaps no bigger plausibility sham today than "evidence-based medicine" (EBM). This term was coined by Gordon Guyatt in 1991. As a university epidemiologist at the time, I was insulted by the hubris and ignorance in the use of this term, EBM, as if medical evidence were somehow "unscientific" until proclaimed a new discipline with new rules for evidence.

Responding to criticisms, Sacket et al. (1996) asserted that EBM followed from "Good doctors use both individual clinical expertise and the best available external evidence." This is an anodyne plausibility implication, but both components are wrong or at least misleading. Phrasing it in terms of what individual doctors should do, Sackett was implying that practitioners should use their own clinical observations and experience. However, the general evidential representativeness of one individual's clinical experience is likely to be weak. Just like other forms of evidence, clinical evidence needs to be systematically collected, reviewed and analyzed, to form a synthesis of clinical reasoning.

A bigger failure of evidential reasoning is Sackett's statement to use "the best available external evidence" rather than *all* valid external evidence. Judgements about what constitutes "best" evidence are highly subjective and do not necessarily yield results that are quantitatively the most accurate (Hartling et al., 2013; Bae, 2016). In formulating his now canonical aspects of evidential causal reasoning, Sir Austin Bradford Hill (1965) did not include an aspect of what would constitute "best" evidence, nor did he suggest that studies should be measured or categorized for "quality of study" nor even that some types of study designs might be intrinsically better than others. In the Reference Manual on Scientific Evidence, Margaret Berger (2011) states explicitly, "... many of the most well-respected and prestigious scientific bodies (such as the International Agency for Research on Cancer (IARC), the

Institute of Medicine, the National Research Council, and the National Institute for Environmental Health Sciences) consider all the relevant available scientific evidence, taken as a whole, to determine which conclusion or hypothesis regarding a causal claim is best supported by the body of evidence." This is exactly Hill's approach. That EBM is premised on subjectively cherry picking "best" evidence is a plausible method but not a scientific one.

Over time, the EBM approach to selectively considering "best" evidence seems to have been "dumbed down," first by placing randomized controlled trials (RCTs) at the top of a pyramid of all study designs as the supposed "gold standard" design, and later, as the asserted only type of study that can be trusted to obtain unbiased estimates of effects. All other forms of empirical evidence are "potentially biased" and therefore unreliable. This is a plausibility conceit as I will show below. But it is so plausible that it is routinely taught in modern medical education, so that most doctors only consider RCT evidence and dismiss all other forms of empirical evidence. It is so plausible that this author had an on-air verbal battle over it with a medically uneducated television commentator who provided no evidence other than plausibility (Whelan, 2020): Isn't it "just obvious" that if you randomize subjects, any differences must be caused by the treatment, and no other types of studies can be trusted? Obvious, yes; true, no.

Who benefits from a sole, obsessive focus on RCT evidence? RCTs are very expensive to conduct if they are to be epidemiologically valid and statistically adequate. They can cost millions or tens of millions of dollars, which limits their appeal largely to companies promoting medical products likely to bring in profits substantially larger than those costs. Historically, pharma control and manipulation of RCT evidence in the regulation process provided an enormous boost in the ability to push products through regulatory approval into the marketplace, and the motivation to do this still continues today. This problem was recognized by Congress, which passed the Food and Drug Administration Modernization Act of 1997 (FDAMA) that established in 2000 the ClinicalTrials.gov website for registration of all clinical trials performed under investigational new drug applications to examine the effectiveness of experimental drugs for patients with serious or life-threatening conditions (National Library of Medicine, 2021).

Misrepresentation of evidence under the guise of EBMabounds. One of the worst examples was a paper published in the *New England Journal of Medicine* February 13, 2020, at the beginning of the Covid-19 pandemic, titled, "The Magic of Randomization versus the Myth of Real-World Evidence," by four well-known British medical statisticians having substantial ties to pharma companies (Collins et al., 2020). This paper claims that randomization automatically creates strong studies, and that all nonrandomized studies are evidentiary rubbish. Representing that only highly unaffordable RCT evidence is appropriate for regulatory approvals provides a tool for pharma companies to protect their expensive, highly profitable patent products against competition by effective and inexpensive off-label approved generic medications whose manufacturers would not be able to afford large-scale RCTs.

Randomization

So, what is the flaw of randomization to which I have been alluding, that requires a deeper examination in order to understand the relative validity of RCT studies vs other study designs? The problem lies in the understanding of *confounding*. Confounding is an epidemiological circumstance where a relationship between an exposure and an outcome is not due to the exposure, but to a third variable (the confounder), at least in part. The confounder is somehow associated with the exposure but is not a result of the exposure. In such case, the apparent exposure-outcome relationship is really due to the confounder-outcome relationship. For example, a study of alcohol consumption and cancer risk could be potentially confounded by smoking history which correlates with alcohol use (and isn't caused by alcohol use) but is really driving the increased cancer risk. A simple analysis of alcohol and cancer risk, ignoring smoking, would show a relationship. However, once the effect of smoking was controlled or adjusted, the alcohol relationship with cancer risk would decline or disappear.

The purpose of randomization, of balancing everything between the treatment and control groups, is to remove potential confounding. Is there any other way to remove potential confounding? Yes: measure the factors in question and adjust or control for them in statistical analyses. It is thus apparent that randomization has exactly one possible benefit not available to non-randomized studies: the control of *un*measured confounders. If biological, medical, or epidemiological relationships are incompletely understood about an outcome of interest, then not all relevant factors may be measured, and some of those unmeasured factors could still confound an association of interest.

Thus, randomization, *in theory*, removes potential confounding by unmeasured factors as an explanation for an observed association. That is the plausibility argument. The question, though, concerns how well randomization works in reality, and what exactly needs to be balanced by the randomization. Clinical trials apply randomization to all participating subjects to determine treatment group assignments. If the study outcome event individuals comprise a subset of the total study, then those outcome people need to be balanced in their potential confounders as well. For example, if all of the deaths in the treatment group are males and all in the placebo group are females, then gender likely confounds the effect of treatment. The problem is, RCT studies essentially never explicitly demonstrate adequate randomization of their outcome subjects, and what they purport to show of randomization for their total treatment groups is almost always scientifically irrelevant. This problem likely arises because the individuals carrying out RCT studies, and the reviewers and journal editors who consider their papers, do not sufficiently understand epidemiologic principles.

In most RCT publications, the investigators provide a perfunctory initial descriptive table of the treatment and placebo groups (as columns), vs various measured factors (as rows). For example, the percent distributions of treatment and placebo subjects by gender, age group, race/ethnicity. The third column in these tables is usually the p-value statistic for the frequency difference between the treatment and placebo subjects on that measured factor. Loosely speaking, this statistic estimates a probability that a frequency difference between treatment and placebo subjects this large could have occurred by chance. Given that the subjects were assigned their treatment groups entirely by chance, statistical examination of the randomization chance process is tautological and irrelevant.

What is needed in the third column of the RCT descriptive table is not p-value, but a measure of the magnitude of confounding of the particular row factor. *Confounding is not measured by how it occurred, but by how bad it is.* For example, if with adjustment for gender, treatment cuts mortality by 25% (relative risk = 0.75), but without adjustment cuts it by 50%, then the magnitude of confounding by gender would be (0.75 − 0.50)/0.75 = 33%. Epidemiologists generally consider more than a 10% change with such adjustment to imply that confounding is present and needs to be controlled.

The potential fatal flaw of RCT studies, what can make them no better than nonrandomized studies and sometimes worse, is that randomization only works when large numbers of subjects have been randomized (Deaton and Cartwright, 2018), and this applies specifically to the outcome subjects, not just to the total study. Consider: flip a coin ten times. It might come up at least seven heads and three tails, or vice versa, easily by chance (34%). However, the magnitude of this difference, $7/3 = 2.33$, is potentially quite large in terms of possible confounding. On the other hand, occurrence of the same 2.33 magnitude from 70 or more heads out of 100 flips would be rare, p=.000078. For randomization to work, the study needs sizeable numbers of outcome events in both the treatment and placebo groups, say 50 or more in each group. This is the unspoken potential major flaw of RCT studies that makes their plausibility argument useless, because RCT studies are generally designed to have enough statistical power to find statistical significance of their primary result if the treatment works as predicted, but not designed to have enough outcome subjects to reduce potential confounding to less than 10% say.

An important example of this issue can be seen in the first published efficacy RCT result for the Pfizer BNT162b2 mRNA Covid-19 vaccine (Polack et al., 2020). This study was considered large enough (43,548 randomized participants) and important enough (Covid-19) that because of its assumed RCT plausibility it secured publication in the "prestigious" *New England Journal of Medicine*. The primary outcome of the study was the occurrence of Covid-19 with onset at least seven days after the second dose of the vaccine or placebo injection. However, while it observed 162 cases among the placebo subjects, enough for good randomization, it only found eight cases among the vaccine subjects, nowhere near enough for randomization to have done anything to control confounding. From general epidemiologic experience, an estimated relative risk this large (approximately $162/8 = 20$) would be unlikely entirely to be due to confounding, but the accuracy of the relative risk or its implied effectiveness ($(20 - 1)/20 = 95\%$) is in doubt. That this vaccine in use was observed not to be this effective in reducing infection risk is not surprising given the weakness of the study result because of inadequate sample size to assure that randomization worked for the outcome subjects in both the treatment and placebo groups.

Empirical Evidence

You might think that these arguments concerning randomized vs nonrandomized trials are very plausible, but what about empirical evidence to support them? For that, a very thorough analysis was carried out by the Cochrane Library Database of Systematic Reviews (Anglemyer et al., 2014). This study comprehensively searched seven electronic publication databases from January 1990 through December 2013, to identify all systematic review papers that compared "quantitative effect size estimates measuring efficacy or effectiveness of interventions tested in [randomized] trials with those tested in observational studies." In effect a meta-analysis of meta-analyses, the analysis included many thousands of individual study comparisons as summarized across 14 review papers. The bottom line: an average of only 8% difference (95% confidence limits, −4% to 22%, not statistically significant) between the RCTs and their corresponding nonrandomized trials results.

In summary, this body of knowledge—the empirical as well as that based upon epidemiologic principles—demonstrates that, contra so-called "plausibility," randomized trials have no automatic ranking as a gold-standard of medical evidence or as the only acceptable form of medical evidence, and that every study needs to be critically and objectively addressed for its own strengths and weaknesses, and for how much those strengths and weaknesses matter to the conclusions drawn.

Other Plausibilities

During the Covid-19 pandemic, numerous other assertions of scientific evidence have been used to justify public health policies, including for the very declaration of the pandemic emergency itself. Underlying many of these has been the fallacious but plausible principle that the goal of public health pandemic management is to minimize the number of people infected by the SARS-CoV-2 virus. That policy may seem obvious, but it is wrong as a blanket policy. What need to be minimized are the harmful consequences of the pandemic. If infection leads to unpleasant or annoying symptoms for most people but no serious or long-term issues—as is generally the case with SARS-CoV-2, particularly in the Omicron era—then there would be no tangible benefit of general public-health limitations infringing upon natural or economic rights and causing harms in themselves. Western societies, including the U.S., take annual respiratory infection waves in stride without declared pandemic emergencies, even though they produce millions of infected individuals each year, because the consequences of infection are considered generally medically minor, even allowing for some tens of thousands of deaths annually. It was established in the first few months of the Covid-19 pandemic that the infection mortality risk varied by more than 1000-fold across the age span, and that people without chronic health conditions such as diabetes, obesity, heart disease, kidney disease, cancer history etc., were at negligible risk of mortality and very low risk of hospitalization. At that point, it was straightforward to define categories of high-risk individuals who on average would benefit from public health interventions, vs low-risk individuals who would successfully weather the infection without appreciable or long-term issues. Thus, an obsessive, one-size-fits-all pandemic management scheme that did not distinguish risk categories was unreasonable and oppressive from the outset.

Accordingly, measures promoted by plausibility to reduce infection transmission, even had they been effective for that purpose, have not served good pandemic management. These measures however were never justified by scientific evidence in the first place. The Six-Foot Social Distancing Rule was an arbitrary concoction of the CDC (Dangor, 2021). Claims of benefit for wearing of face masks have rarely distinguished potential benefit to the wearer—for whom such wearing would be a personal choice whether to accept more theoretical risk—vs benefit to bystanders, so-called "source control," wherein public health considerations might properly apply. Studies of mask-based source control for respiratory viruses, where the studies are without fatal flaws, show no appreciable benefit in reducing infection transmission (Alexander, 2021; Alexander, 2022; Burns, 2022).

General population lockdowns have never been used in western countries and have no evidence of effect for doing anything other than postponing the inevitable (Meunier, 2020), as Australia population data make clear (Worldometer, 2022). In the definitive discussion of public health measures for control of pandemic influenza (Inglesby et al., 2006), the authors state, "There are no historical observations or scientific studies that support the confinement by quarantine of groups of possibly infected people for extended periods in order to slow the spread of influenza. A World Health Organization (WHO) Writing Group, after reviewing the literature and considering contemporary international experience, concluded that 'forced isolation and quarantine are ineffective and impractical.' ... The negative consequences of large-scale quarantine are so extreme ... that this mitigation measure should be eliminated from serious consideration."

On travel restrictions, Inglesby et al. (2006) note, "Travel restrictions, such as closing airports and screening travelers at borders, have historically been ineffective." On school closures (Inglesby et al., 2006): "In previous influenza epidemics, the impact of school closings on illness rates has been mixed. A study from Israel reported a decrease in respiratory infections after a 2-week teacher strike, but the decrease was only evident for a single day. On the other hand, when schools closed for a winter holiday during the 1918 pandemic in Chicago, 'more influenza cases developed among pupils ... than when schools were in session.'"

This discussion makes clear that these actions supposedly interfering with virus transmission on the basis of plausibility arguments for their effectiveness have been both misguided for managing the pandemic, and unsubstantiated by scientific evidence of effectiveness in reducing spread. Their large-scale promotion has demonstrated the failure of public-health policies in the Covid-19 era.

Plausibility vs Bad Science

An argument could be entertained that various public-health policies as well as information made available to the general public have not been supported by plausibility but instead by bad or fatally flawed science, posing as real science. For example, in its in-house, non-peer-reviewed journal, *Morbidity and Mortality Weekly Reports*, CDC has published a number of analyses of vaccine effectiveness. These reports described cross-sectional studies but analyzed them as if they were case-control studies, systematically using estimated odds ratio parameters instead of relative risks to calculate vaccine effectiveness. When study outcomes are infrequent, say fewer than 10% of study subjects, then odds ratios can approximate relative risks, but otherwise, odds ratios tend to be overestimates. However, in cross-sectional studies, relative risks can be directly calculated and can be adjusted for potential confounders.

A representative example is a study of the effectiveness of third dose Covid-19 vaccines (Tenforde et al., 2022). This study reported a vaccine effectiveness of 82% among patients without immunocompromising conditions. However, the fraction of case patients among the vaccinated was 31% and among the unvaccinated was 70%, neither of which is sufficiently infrequent to allow use of the odds ratio approximation to calculate vaccine effectiveness. By the numbers in the study report Table 3, I calculate a true vaccine effectiveness of 57% which is substantially different and much worse than the 82% presented in the paper.

In a different context, after I published a summary review article on the use of hydroxychloroquine (HCQ) for early outpatient Covid-19 treatment (Risch, 2020), several clinical trials papers were published in attempt to show that HCQ is ineffective. The first of these so-called "refutations" were conducted in hospitalized patients, whose disease is almost entirely different in pathophysiology and treatment than early outpatient illness (Park et al., 2020). The important outcomes that I had addressed in my review, risks of hospitalization and mortality, were distracted in these works by focus on subjective and lesser outcomes such as duration of viral test positivity, or length of hospital stay.

Subsequently, RCTs of outpatient HCQ use began to be published. A typical one is that by Skipper et al. (2020). The primary endpoint of this trial was change in overall self-reported symptom severity over 14 days. This subjective endpoint was of little pandemic importance, especially given that the subjects in studies by this research group were moderately able to tell whether they were in the HCQ or placebo arms of the trial (Rajasingham et al., 2021). From their statistical analyses, the authors appropriately concluded that "Hydroxychloroquine did not substantially reduce symptom severity in outpatients with early, mild COVID-19." However, the general media reported this study as showing that "hydroxychloroquine doesn't work." For example, Jen Christensen (2020) in *CNN Health* stated about this study, "The antimalarial drug hydroxychloroquine did not benefit non-hospitalized patients with mild Covid-19 symptoms who were treated early in their infection, according to a study published Thursday in the medical journal Annals of Internal Medicine." But in fact, the Skipper study did report on the two outcomes of importance, risks of hospitalization and mortality: with placebo, 10 hospitalizations and 1 death; with HCQ, 4 hospitalizations and 1 death. These numbers show a 60% reduced risk of hospitalization which, though not statistically significant (p=0.11), is entirely consistent with all other studies of hospitalization risk for HCQ use in outpatients (Risch, 2021). Nevertheless, these small numbers of outcome events are not nearly enough for randomization to have balanced any factors, and the study is essentially useless on this basis. But it was still misinterpreted in the lay literature as showing that HCQ provides no benefit in outpatient use.

Conclusions

Many other instances of plausible scientific claptrap or bad science have occurred during the Covid-19 pandemic. As was seen with the retracted Surgisphere papers, medical journals routinely and uncritically publish this nonsense as long as conclusions align with government policies. This body of fake knowledge has been promulgated at the highest levels, by NSC, FDA, CDC, NIH, WHO, Wellcome Trust, AMA, medical specialty boards, state and local public health agencies and licensing boards, multinational pharma companies and other organizations around the world that have violated their responsibilities to the public or have purposely chosen not to understand the fake science.

Massive censorship by the traditional media and much of social media has blocked most public discussion of this bad and fake science. Censorship is the tool of the undefendable, since valid science inherently defends itself. Until the public begins to understand the difference between plausibility and science and how large the effort has been to mass-produce science "product" that looks like science but is not, the process will continue and leaders seeking authoritarian power will continue to rely on it for fake justification.

Over the last 3 years, technical matters about the Covid-19 pandemic have been presented to the American public as if they were "scientific." Many of these messages have been plausible and easy to believe, but in fact were not scientific, or reflected bad or fatally flawed science posing as real science. Examination of these matters shows that plausibility is not a substitute for science, and that individuals including scientists themselves may have a hard time telling the difference.

(For complete essay and references visit https://brownstone.org/articles/ plausibility-but-not-science-has-dominated-public-discussions-of-the- covid-pandemic/)

CHAPTER 30

Fact Checkers are
Narrative Enforcers,
Consensus is
not Science and
Propaganda is a Hell
of a Drug

Dr. Sam Dubé

Mathematician, physician, strength coach, and
broadcaster

Dr. Sam Dubé is a mathematician, retired award-winning university faculty, educator, academic physician, master strength coach, and broadcaster. He was one of the first Canadian physicians to attempt to expose the truth during the pandemic of fear, and continues to do so on his Rumble channel "The Fifth Doctor", and abroad.

On Becoming "The Fifth Doctor" and Helping Expose the Truth

At the end of January of 2020, in seeking information on the internet concerning the "flu-like virus" alleged by the mainstream media to have emerged from China a couple of months prior, I came across a scientific paper that made my internal "red alert" klaxon go off. I was previously wary of any news coming from the MSM (MainStream Media), in particular concerning China, and so was already at a stage of "amber alert," which motivated my search. The research article from India stated that there were four subdomains on the spike protein that had essentially a close-to-zero chance of having evolved naturally. The authors concluded that the virus had to be the product of genetic engineering. In other words, gain-of-function research. This was a game-changer for me, and I shuddered internally at the implications, both past and future.

Three days later, the paper had disappeared, with nothing but a committed yet cryptic message from the Indian team promising to someday publish their findings. Rumours proliferated that the Chinese had exerted pressure to have the work withdrawn.

On March 11, 2020, the World Health Organization declared a "pandemic," and our world would never be the same again.

***

Years ago I had found my niche, putting my education and interests to good use. As an academic physician, albeit one trained in family and sports medicine with an avid interest in alternative and complementary therapies and human potential in general, I worked as a consultant in the health and wellness industry. Scientific writing, editing, idea generation, and presenting formed the basis of my diverse contract work. My background in mathematics and physics, as a retired university faculty member with a love of teaching, had me freelance tutoring, which included large in-person groups of students. I was also doing a fair amount of athletic coaching and training of trainers, mainly in strength sports, which had been a long-time passion of mine. Two decades earlier, this passion had led me to co-host The Canadian Strength Athletes' series on TSN (The Sports Network) and other related shows, which motivated me to extend my media work to other fields.

On the evening of March 12, 2020, I fell ill. I had been feeling tired and run-down all day. Three days prior, I had spent several hours sitting next to a student who had insisted, despite his flu-like symptoms, to proceed with our lesson due to an upcoming final exam. He had just returned from March break after spending a couple of weeks with his parents on the west coasts of Canada and the U.S. His parents had tested positive for COVID and were symptomatic. I was hit with a high fever, a dry unproductive cough and some of the worst body aches I'd ever experienced. Despite the discomfort, I wasn't too concerned, and took 1-2 grams of vitamin C every hour until I went to bed. The next day, the fever had broken and the cough subsided. Apart from some fatigue, mild shortness of breath on exertion, and a low nocturnal fever for the next few days, I was fine. I stayed home for a day and worked online. I took a couple of days off working out. On the fifth day, I hit repetitions in my weightlifting workout that I had not achieved for years. I didn't give my illness much second thought.

***

Here in Canada, the public health response was similar to that of the U.S.: "two weeks to flatten the curve" of unending lockdowns, social distancing and inconsistent information about masking. Official case diagnoses were made using the amplification PCR technique with wildly exaggerated cycle thresholds. This, despite the fact that its Nobel Prize-winning inventor, Dr. Kary Mullis, had said emphatically that it could never be used as a diagnostic tool. Apparent sky-rocketing COVID death numbers were compounded by the conflation of dying FROM COVID or dying WITH a positive COVID test. This obfuscation of data was employed again after the rollout of the vaccines, when one was not considered "fully vaccinated" until two weeks AFTER one's last injection. This artificially and drastically diminished the number of people reported to have suffered adverse events or death after being vaccinated, as any such event that occurred in the two-week window was recorded as unvaccinated.

In addition, those questioning the official zoological explanation of viral origin were ridiculed in spite of the dearth of evidence to support this narrative, and in contrast to actual facts. And it got rapidly worse – individuals speaking out against the measures or attempting to report success with known medications and treatments were censored, then vilified, even persecuted and prosecuted. Some even disappeared. There was no official emphasis on lifestyle modification such as weight loss, exercise, nutrition and vitamin D consumption. The concept of natural immunity was suppressed and dismissed. Published data were generally not age-stratified, which would have shown a disproportionate risk to the elderly, and in October of 2020 the Great Barrington Declaration, its authors and supporters were condemned. The Declaration suggested targeted protection for those most at risk - notably the elderly and those with severe health challenges.

People were told to stay home and not present to hospital unless very ill. Government overreach was rampant. It seemed to me as if a pandemic was being manufactured, in lockstep worldwide. Political science trumped science. And scientism became the new religion. Was it more a pandemic of fear than a pathogen?

During the next several months of 2020, like many of you, I was witness to these things. In the National Capital Region of Canada where I lived, few people questioned the government and public health narrative, promoted by MSM. It was difficult to find like-minded people, those who were aware of what was happening. It was only going to get worse.

Due to lockdowns, I had adapted much of my teaching and coaching work, moving it online; for me, it was not ideal. Most of my consulting work was paused as business shrunk for many of my clients. I decided to increase my freelance online interviewing in an effort to educate the public and to bring people together. This included a separate interview series featuring new Canadian authors and Toronto-area business owners, some of the world's greatest dating experts, as well as a web TV show on dating that got picked up by a New York City lifestyle and news site. In exchange for doing these features for a small publishing company and its YouTube-based channel, they allowed me to use their channel to post my own interviews.

Unfortunately, it became apparent that YouTube had algorithms to "discourage" the use of certain terms in the audio of the interviews, as well as certain words featured in the titles and descriptions. Words such as "COVID," "virus," and (later) "vaccine," relegated these interviews very low on searches and recommendations. It became clear that Big Brother was watching.

Keeping an ear to the medical world, I had also been hearing of off-label treatments being used successfully for COVID; notably corticosteroids, hydroxychloroquine and ivermectin. But there appeared to be a concerted effort by public health and MSM to limit the good news of these medications as treatments for COVID. This censorship was expanded to outright falsehoods, alleging adverse effects from hydroxychloroquine and ivermectin and attacking any doctor who dared to endorse their use. Later, this evolved into studies clearly designed to fail, as it became clear the depth of pharma corruption, extending to researchers and medical journals. Whistleblowers were being fired or otherwise silenced. But there was the promise of a vaccine that would save us all.

***

In November of 2020, I heard the following words, in a town hall broadcast from Edmonton, Alberta. "This is the greatest hoax perpetrated on an unsuspecting public."

The voice was a familiar one from my medical school days, distinctive with its deep tone, confidence, defiance, and cultured British accent. It was Dr. Roger Hodkinson, a venerated and senior Canadian pathologist, who had been very active in smoking cessation campaigns and in confronting the tobacco industry. I urge you to seek out the full broadcast, which is still on Bitchute under the title "Listen to Dr Roger Hodkinson lay out some much needed rational sanity." Remember, this was very early during the "pandemic." It was almost funny watching the fact checkers (a.k.a. narrative enforcers) futile attempts to discredit his identity, then his credentials. Roger's words not only confirmed what I had been seeing, but affirmed and validated my feelings and my desire to do more. He was truly inspiring.

I immediately got in touch with Roger and we've been friends ever since. He told me that he had waited over five hours to speak on that call during the town hall meeting, but that he HAD to do it. I interviewed Roger for the YouTube channel where I did most of my freelancing. It was the first of a series of interviews with him.

The owner of the channel and I agreed that the public health narrative was propagating true misinformation, generating confusion and harm. With Roger's interviews it became clear the extent of YouTube's suppression of free speech. They were all eventually deleted. But we were undaunted, and at that point started posting simultaneously on Bitchute, a free speech platform which had a far smaller audience.

On December 8th, 2020, I watched Dr. Pierre Kory testify before a U.S. Senate Committee formed by Senator Ron Johnson, the Wisconsin Republican Senator who has become a beacon of hope for so many over the last years. Dr. Kory was a frontline physician treating patients in the ICU, an expert from a team of experts in critical care led by Dr. Paul Marik. Some months before, Dr. Kory had addressed another Senate Committee organized by Senator Johnson on the beneficial use of corticosteroids in the treatment of COVID. This time, he was going up to bat for ivermectin. Dr. Kory was moved to tears when pleading with the committee to look at the highly favourable data using ivermectin to treat COVID. They were saving lives with this well-known and eminently safe repurposed medication.

I'll never forget what Joyce, Dr. Kory's assistant said when I called his office: "Dr. Dubé, apart from Senator Johnson you're the only person in the world that wants to speak to us right now. Dr. Kory graciously accepts your kind offer of an interview." I was dumbfounded. How could this be? Was I the only one that saw the importance of his team's results? Pierre and I spoke over the phone and we hit it off. I understood the need not to rock the boat too much in order to get some official recognition for their work, with the goal of saving lives. At the time, neither of us knew really how deep the corruption went. On December

16th, 2020 we recorded an interview. We were careful with our words and statements. The "vaccines" were just starting to roll out, accompanied by much fanfare and many promises. Despite our precautions, something odd happened. The video rapidly acquired over five thousand views – and then never budged further. In searches using its EXACT title, the video would show up on the second or third page of the results. It had been shadowbanned and I was angry. The content was SO important. Who would do this? Who would purposely sabotage people's chance at recovery, at life? How deep did this go? Such was often the fate of efforts to inform that went counter to the narrative. I've seen it happen time and again, even while parents tearfully recounted the death of their child following the COVID vaccine.

***

Many more people saw my interviews with Roger and Pierre than I had anticipated. I started getting requests from people to be interviewed. My open mind, scientific and medical background meant I was well-placed to ask relevant questions that doctors and researchers were keen to answer, and for those answers to be understood by as many people as possible. My long-format interviews gave subjects the time to establish a rapport and for the really important content to surface. My focus was accurate information and human stories. Through this, I hoped to bring people closer together during this time of social, physical, and ideological isolation.

In 2021 I expanded my online interviewing. I did two long interviews with one of the top experts on vitamin C in the world, Patrick Holford of the U.K. I recall it vividly because we had to omit the words "virus," "COVID," and others in an effort to not trigger the algorithms, get shadow-banned or deleted with punitive strikes. There were a few challenges along the way. I wanted only to focus on interviews that exposed what I believed to be the truth, but I also wanted to spread the word. YouTube reached a MUCH larger audience, but what good would that be if you were constantly walking on eggshells, censored, shadowbanned, or deleted? I was feeling constrained.

In mid-June of 2021 I had the opportunity to interview mainstream news broadcaster Ivory Hecker, the Fox News whistleblower who exposed the censorship and persecution she suffered at the hands of her bosses when she tried to expose the success of alternative treatments to COVID. She blew the whistle on live TV while reporting for Fox News' Houston affiliate on a story about air conditioning. It was priceless and she inspired others to do the same. Ivory was the first recipient of my "Ovaries of Steel" award.

Ivory inspired me to raise the bar. I established my own channel on Rumble, called The Fifth Doctor. I planned another large long-format interview with four Canadian doctors being persecuted by their provincial governing bodies, and a lawyer from the Justice Centre for Constitutional Freedoms.

On July 1st, 2021, I hosted a panel interview with Drs. Roger Hodkinson, Francis Christian, Chris Milburn and Charles Hoffe, along with John Carpay, attorney. Each physician told their story, questioning the public health response and the safety and efficacy of the experimental gene therapy injections. They described how they stood up for their patients. John Carpay provided legal commentary. Dr. Hoffe described how he had tested COVID-vaccinated patients coming into Emergency using a d-dimer test, a test of blood coagulation that might not show up on other tests. Although a relatively small sample size, he found that 62 percent of vaccinated patients had high d-dimers. This was very big news; it all went viral. On YouTube, the video started off slow, but accelerated, hitting thirteen thousand views within a couple of days. It then disappeared, although it did appear on other platforms, having been downloaded and shared. However, YouTube had *the* big audience. When it was deleted, my YouTube host sent a strongly-worded letter, alleging violation of free speech and the Canadian Charter of Rights and Freedoms. Three days later, the video returned. It rose rapidly to three hundred thousand views. Then strangely, it dropped spontaneously to eighty thousand views, only to ascend even more rapidly than the first time to two hundred and eighty thousand views, at which point it disappeared for good.

The video was now "out there." Conservatively speaking, this video entitled *"Exposed: The Persecution of Canadian Physicians by Organized Medicine,"* was viewed at least two million times, and on multiple platforms, particularly in the alternative media. An equally successful sequel with a new set of persecuted physicians followed. The world awakened to what was happening in Canada thanks to the brave physicians who were speaking out against the narrative. Similar stories of censorship and persecution flooded in from around the world.

Those interviews seem like a lifetime ago, and so much has happened since. Death, disability, destruction, despair and hate. But so many good things too; connections, people coming together to fight for a common cause, our God-given rights and freedoms.

***

Something happened in Canada that changed the world. A beacon of tremendous hope, and a driver of ongoing positive change: The Canadian Freedom Convoy.

Technically, it was a legal protest in support of health freedom and against vaccine mandates, but really it was a massive celebration, an incredibly festive gathering of people of diverse backgrounds, ages, religions, and ethnicities. I was there. Most of the people I spoke to were unvaccinated. For them, the convoy was a demonstration against injections that they believed to be neither safe nor effective, or that they knew to be harmful, even deadly.

The spirit of joy, hope, humanity and freedom was palpable. It was the greatest expression of Canadian patriotism I had ever seen. It began in Western Canada and picked up steam and trucks across the country, before converging on Ottawa. In the dead of winter in one of the coldest capital cities on the planet, the streets of downtown Ottawa were immaculate, the homeless fed and cared for. Alternative media were streaming live in an effort to show reality on the ground. Some mainstream media outlets from other parts of the world, in particular the U.S. and Europe, reported objectively. But convoy coverage revealed the total capture of Canadian mainstream media. MSM vilified the convoy as a "small fringe minority" in the words of Prime Minister Justin Trudeau, portraying them as malcontents with unacceptable and unscientific views, consisting largely of misogynists and white supremacists.

When the Liberal government crushed the protest, ruthlessly invoking the Emergencies Act, it was disheartening and demoralising for so many of us. Those were very dark days. But the Canadian Freedom Convoy inspired similar protests worldwide, including the Dutch farmers and the massive American Trucker Convoy. It continues to inspire us to this day.

Much has changed since March of 2020. We've seen a surge of vaccine-associated injury and death reports worldwide with significant research, observation, and data analysis backing this up. We've seen documented evidence of the U.S. Department of Defence and Department of Health and Human Services involvement in the creation of the vaccines. We know that there was no scientific justification for travel mandates restricting the movement of the unvaccinated in Canada. We've seen major resignations in public health and political spheres, and many whistleblowers have come forward. We've heard public health and government officials backtrack on past statements. We've even heard calls for a "COVID amnesty," justifying measures that violated legal rights and freedoms, and isolated, stigmatised, persecuted and prosecuted dissenters under the false defence of "we didn't know!" People DID know. They were simply ostracised, censored, or crushed. We now know that regulatory bodies knew of vaccine harms and authorized them anyway. And we've seen both excess and sudden death reports surging.

In Canada we are also seeing the passage of legislation focused on censorship and securing the public health narrative. We're seeing people vehemently declaring an illness or injury is due to ABV ("All But the Vaccine"). Mainstream media seems completely disinterested in reporting or investigating potential causes of unknown illness or death. We're seeing a major push to convert to Central Bank Digital Currencies (CBDCs) as well as Digital Identification. We're seeing efforts to control and confine people under the guise of dubious and scientifically unsound arguments, using these conversions to facilitate them. We're hearing about plans to inject livestock and even crops with the mRNA technology, and mRNA vaccine plants are being built, despite the safety data. MSM continues to push a narrative that now includes climate change and the sexualisation of children.

A few final thoughts to bookend this essay. Be aware of the use of language to change thoughts and perceptions. This is a very old technique, characteristic of totalitarian regimes, as are censorship and the persecution of those speaking out against a false narrative. Thus "misinformation" in an official context just means "not government approved information."

Consensus is not science, nor is it a single person or organisation. Hence the name of my podcast, The Fifth Doctor on Rumble, which gives a nod to the "four out of five" doctors who, historically, have made some very harmful recommendations. Science is a dynamic process of inquiry and experiment and is never settled.

Be vigilant.

Be the best of humanity.

Be free.

CHAPTER 31

A Primer for the Propagandized

Margaret Anna Alice

Writer who blogs about propaganda, mass control, psychology, politics, and health with a focus on COVID

Margaret Anna Alice writes about propaganda, mass control, psychology, politics, and health with a focus on COVID at her Substack, Margaret Anna Alice Through the Looking Glass. She is the author of the fairy tale The Vapor, the Hot Hat, & the Witches' Potion and has presented her research to the Corona Investigative Committee. Described as "COVID's Best Chronicler" by Dr. Meryl Nass and "my favourite writer anywhere" by Dr. Mike Yeadon, Margaret Anna aims to unmask totalitarianism and awaken the sleeping before tyranny triumphs.

Fear Is the Mind-Killer

"Totalitarianism, if not fought against, could triumph anywhere."
—George Orwell

The noose is dangling gently around our necks. Every day, they cinch it tighter. By the time we realize it's strangling us, it will be too late.

Those who gradually and gleefully sacrifice their freedoms, their autonomy, their individuality, their livelihoods, and their relationships on the altar of the "common good" have forgotten this is the pattern followed by every totalitarian regime in history.

Everyone wonders how ordinary Germans could have been manipulated to participate or stand dumbstruck while their government was transformed into a genocidal juggernaut. This is how. Read Sebastian Haffner's *Defying Hitler* memoir to see how this **can** happen anywhere—including here.

Everyone wonders how Russians could have permitted and even zealously reported fellow citizens for imprisonment and execution under

Article 58, the penal code invented to incarcerate anyone who expressed the slightest whisper of noncompliance under Stalin's homicidal state. This is how. Read Aleksandr Solzhenitsyn's meticulously documented *The Gulag Archipelago* to witness this progression of authoritarian lunacy.

Everyone wonders how Hutus could have suddenly started axing their Tutsi neighbors to death after being inundated with waves of anti-Tutsi propaganda from Radio Télévision Libre des Mille Collines. Read Philip Gourevitch's *We Wish to Inform You That Tomorrow We Will Be Killed with Our Families: Stories from Rwanda*.

The list goes on. And on. And on. From Machiavelli's *The Prince* to Étienne de La Boétie's *The Politics of Obedience: The Discourse of Voluntary Servitude* to Edward Herman's and Noam Chomsky's *Manufacturing Consent* (and accompanying documentary) to BBC's *The Century of the Self*, mechanisms of mass control have been chronicled for millennia.

George Orwell writes: "As far as the mass of the people go, the extraordinary swings of opinion which occur nowadays, the emotions which can be turned on and off like a tap, are the result of newspaper and radio hypnosis."

Can you imagine what master propagandist Edward Bernays would have done with access to today's mainstream media conglomerate combined with the global surveillance infrastructure of Big Tech? And you really think that's not happening now—with another century of psychological, neurological, and technological research under their belts?

The present ability to curate reality and coerce obedience is unprecedented, far beyond what Orwell envisioned in *1984*, Bradbury in *Fahrenheit 451*, Huxley in *Brave New World*, and Burgess in *A Clockwork Orange*. A textbook example of Problem Reaction Solution, the current tsunami of worldwide hysteria is the latest and potentially most threatening example of mass control in history.

The recipe is simple. Take a naturally occurring phenomenon, say a seasonal virus, and exaggerate its threat far beyond every imagining—despite exhaustive evidence to the contrary. Suppress, silence, ostracize, and demonize every individual who dares present facts that expose the false mono-narrative.

Whip up a witches' brew of anger, envy, and, most importantly, fear, escalating emotions to a boil so as to short-circuit our faculties of reason and logic.

Isolate us from one another, supplant real-world interactions with virtual feuds, label nonconformists as a threat to the group, and pump the public with a disinformation campaign designed to confuse and atomize. In essence, foster a cultlike mentality that shuts down thought to guarantee assent.

Cultivate and wield our cognitive biases—especially ingroup bias, conformity bias, and authority bias—against us in a comprehensive divide-and-conquer policy that keeps us too busy squabbling amongst ourselves to recognize and unite against those corralling us into a *Matrix*-like collective delusion that enables the powerful to extract our resources for their own gain.

This ideological mass psychosis is religion—not science. If this were about science, the Media–Pharmaceutical–Big-Tech complex would not be memory-holing every dissenting voice, vilifying every thought criminal, and censoring every legitimate inquiry in quest of the truth.

This apocryphal Mark Twain quote applies: "It's easier to fool people than to convince them that they have been fooled."

Twain also (actually) said: "In religion and politics people's beliefs and convictions are in almost every case gotten at second-hand, and without examination, from authorities who have not themselves examined the questions at issue but have taken them at second-hand from other non-examiners, whose opinions about them were not worth a brass farthing."

The next time you're watching the news, reading a social media post, listening to a friend repeat a scripted talking point, pay attention. Learn to identify the earmarks of propaganda, the clickbait used to trigger your emotions, the mechanisms employed to engineer your cognitive biases.

Don't let your pride prevent you from seeing—and admitting—the Emperor is naked. We are losing our last sliver of opportunity to resist authoritarianism.

This is not a partisan issue. Those who wish to control us have made it such because disunited lemmings are easier to steer than independent, critical thinkers.

This is a human issue. This is about crushing the middle class— the backbone of a democratic republic—and transferring trillions from the middle and lower classes to the ruling plutocracy. This is about demolishing the foundations of a free society and building it back—not better, but better-controlled.

Dare to question. Dare to disbelieve. Dare to defy ideology in favor of science while you still can.

CHAPTER 32

The COVID Regime and Its Dissidents

Dr. Michael Rectenwald

Author and Distinguished Fellow at Hillsdale College

Dr. Michael Rectenwald is the author of twelve books, including *The Great Reset and the Struggle for Liberty: Unraveling the Global Agenda* (2023), *Thought Criminal* (a novel, 2020); *Beyond Woke* (2020); *Google Archipelago: The Digital Gulag and the Simulation of Freedom* (2019); *Springtime for Snowflakes: "Social Justice" and Its Postmodern Parentage* (an academic's memoir, 2018); *Nineteenth-Century British Secularism: Science, Religion and Literature* (2016); *Academic Writing, Real World Topics* (2015); *Global Secularisms in a Post-Secular Age* (2015), and others. Michael is a Distinguished Fellow at Hillsdale College. He was a Professor of Liberal Studies and Global Liberal Studies at NYU from 2008 to 2019. A former Marxist, Professor Rectenwald is a champion of liberty and opposes all forms of totalitarianism and political authoritarianism, including socialism-communism, "social justice," fascism, political correctness, and "woke" ideology.

I remember when news of covid-19 first reached me. I was living with my eldest son, John-Michael, in the guesthouse of an old flame from my early 20s. It was a rainy, cold March in L.A. and we shivered in my old flame's "guesthouse," which was really a refurbished garage with a broken heater. As the news of the imminent crisis became more insistent, I told John-Michael that the real enemy was not the virus itself but the state and what it would do to us. I was already a libertarian by then, having been through one of the first academic cancel culture ordeals (at New York University), where the "woke" mob among my colleagues tried to ruin my life. John-Michael said then that the state would save us from the virus, a belief that he now completely disavows.

I told him, no, the state, not the virus, will ravage us. I already had the sense that the real enemy we would face would be a mind virus. What really terrified me was not covid; it was the potential that the public would become a reactionary mob, just like the one that had attacked me at NYU, only much, much bigger. The state would enlist large swaths of the population to do its bidding. Millions would become state agents, sentinels of surveillance, and enforcers of a new totalitarian regime.

When John-Michael and I went to a grocery store one day before the crisis was deemed a "pandemic," I pretended to shrink away from a woman in the cashier's line, while mockingly repeating the phrase "social distancing." I thought she would appreciate the humor. Instead, she shrunk away from us, as if we were mortal enemies of humankind.

One afternoon, we decided to play tennis. As we attempted to enter the courts, a squadron of police officers rushed us, one of them warning us through a bullhorn that the courts were closed and that playing tennis was not permitted. The covid police state was already in full force. I would later read about surfers being hauled off the beach and arrested. It was as if sunshine had ceased to be a disinfectant and the whole world had gone completely mad.

I soon left John-Michael in L.A. and returned to Pittsburgh. Tired of fighting the propaganda and censorship with counter arguments deemed "conspiracy theories," I decided to write a novel. In the early days of the covid regime, fiction seemed to be the best avenue for showing how almost all the members of society could succumb to a collectivist ideology, become victims of non-stop propaganda, and thus lose their individuality and self-determination—while dissent was simultaneously censored and criminalized.

Thought Criminal is about an AI researcher who discovers that the state, while claiming to treat a virus, is intentionally administering the virus with "the treatment."[1] The truth is the exact inverse of what the state declares. Only the virus is a mind virus; it is a cloud of nanobots that attach themselves to the neurons of the neo-cortexes of their hosts, such that their brains become connected to a central database and processing system called Collective Mind. Thus, the thoughts of the "infected" are no longer wholly their own; they are supplied by Collective Mind. The AI researcher finds a group of other "thought deviationists," those who know about the true nature of the virus and who communicate on an encrypted network. Not only do they attempt to elude the mind virus; they are also struggling to maintain their sanity and freedom. They know about the "virus" and take a drug called Eraserall in order to stay "virus-free"—that is, disconnected from Collective Mind and thus able to have their own thoughts and individuality. Along with the other thought deviationists, the AI researcher is under the constant fear of future arrest, the treachery of friends, and the loss of his identity. I won't issue a spoiler here. The novel has been called "the 1984 of the covid era."

***

The covid regime, as I have noted elsewhere,[2] uncannily resembled the "post-totalitarianism" of the Soviet bloc, as elaborated by the Czechoslovakian dissident, Václav Havel. By post-totalitarianism, Havel did not mean a state or condition after totalitarianism. He meant a new form of bureaucratic rule, a totalizing system under which power does not simply originate from a singular dictator and flow downward.

1   Michael Rectenwald, *Thought Criminal*. Nashville, TN: New English Review Press, 2020.

2   Michael Rectenwald, "Living in the Age of Covid: 'The Power of the Powerless.'" Mises Institute, August 17, 2021. https://mises.org/wire/living-age-covid-power-powerless.

Rather, the totalitarian regime involves the entire society; it conscripts the population into its very structure. "In the post-totalitarian system," Havel wrote, "this line [of power] runs de facto through each person, for everyone in his or her own way is both a victim and a supporter of the system." Everyone is forced to "live within the lie," and all subjects become "agents of its automatism"—automatic receivers, messengers, and executors of the post-totalitarian logic.[3]

Havel provides an example of one such subject: a typical greengrocer. The greengrocer routinely puts a sign in his storefront window that reads, "Workers of the World Unite!" He does so, not necessarily because he believes in the semantic content of the slogan, although he may. But he puts the sign in his window because he would become conspicuous by the sign's absence if he did not. By posting the sign, he consciously or unconsciously seeks to stay out of the crosshairs of severe repression. Surely, the mask and the vaccine passport served the same function.

The greengrocer's sign is ideological because its semantic content is "noble," while its semiotic function works in an opposite direction. It is debasing; it helps him to conceal from himself the low foundations of his obedience: fear. Its function is to ensure conformity to a system that has nothing to do with the welfare of "the workers." (Under communism, it is the Marxist true believers who live in "false consciousness.") The sign is only a sign of compliance and complicity and not a statement of belief.

And the sign feeds into a wider "panorama" of compliance and complicity while compelling others to do the same. The greengrocer's plastering of the sign is a piece within a system that enrolls its subjects in its own administration, subjects who, by their participation, ensure

---

3   Václav Havel, "The Power of the Powerless," in Václav Havel et al., The Power of the Powerless: Citizens against the State in Central-Eastern Europe, ed. John Keane (Abingdon, UK: Routledge, 2015), p. 37 and passim.

the participation of others and who together help to constitute post-totalitarianism at large:

> *Part of the essence of the post-totalitarian system is that it draws everyone into its sphere of power ... so they may become agents of the system's general automatism and servants of its self-determined goals....* More than this: so they may create through their involvement a general norm and, thus, *bring pressure to bear on their fellow citizens.* And further: *so they may learn to be comfortable with their involvement, to identify with it as though it were something natural and inevitable and, ultimately, so they may—with no external urging—come to treat any non-involvement as an abnormality, as arrogance, as an attack on themselves, as a form of dropping out of society. By pulling everyone into its power structure, the post-totalitarian system makes everyone instruments of a mutual totality, the auto-totality of society.*[4]

Not everyone can live the lie of ideological conformity under post-totalitarianism, however. Havel points to those who begin to "live within the truth." They no longer feign belief and thus cease to be complicit with the system. But those who do so are promptly cancelled:

> Let us now imagine that one day something in our greengrocer snaps and he stops putting up the slogans merely to ingratiate himself... The bill is not long in coming. He will be relieved of his post as manager of the shop and transferred to the warehouse. His pay will be reduced. His hopes for a holiday in Bulgaria will evaporate. His children's access to higher education will be threatened. His superiors will harass him and his fellow workers will wonder about him. *Most of those who apply these sanctions, however, will not do so*

---

4   Havel, "The Power of the Powerless," pp. 36–37, emphasis mine.

from any authentic inner conviction but simply under pressure from conditions, the same conditions that once pressured the greengrocer to display the official slogans.[5]

Thus, the non-compliant is marked by his lack of signalling. He is isolated and demonised. He becomes a pariah and is exiled from the community. He loses his status and faces hardship, or worse. Sound familiar?

***

While the "pandemic" has passed, the covid crisis is not over. The damage to our social, political, economic, and scientific institutions, and to billions of people, has been immeasurable and is still being felt. Not only that, but there remains the justifiable suspicion that it could happen again, that the ruling elite could very well declare other emergencies, including a climate emergency, replete with lockdowns or partial lockdowns. As Klaus Schwab, the founder and chair of the World Economic Forum declared at the 2022 annual meeting of that organization: "We have to reinforce our resilience against *a new virus,* possibly, *or other risks which we have on the global agenda.* The future is not just happening," Schwab declared in the same speech, "*the future is built by us, by a powerful community, as you here in this room.*"[6]

I am not hereby saying that the entire covid crisis was planned by ruling "elites." But I am saying that it wouldn't have unfolded much

5   Havel, "The Power of the Powerless," p. 39, emphasis mine.

6   "Welcoming Remarks and Special Address, World Economic Forum Annual Meeting 2022, Davos," World Economic Forum, May 23, 2022, https://www.weforum.org/events/world-economic-forum-annual-meeting-2022, emphasis mine.

differently if it had been. At the very least, they had already planned the responses to a coronavirus pandemic.[7] Likewise, we should be prepared for the declaration of other emergencies and the pre-planned responses to them by governments, international governmental agencies, NGOs, national and international health agencies, universities, the media, corporations, and the public at large.

The question now is whether the fallout from the covid crisis has produced enough dissidents who will no longer comply when a new emergency is declared. Will enough people recognize the by-now familiar pattern? Will non-compliance be exerted to a necessary extent such that the regime cannot crush us again? What can we do, besides hope and pray? We can and must continue telling the counternarratives, so that the power of the powerless poses a threat and becomes paramount, thus forewarning the regime before they dare strike again.

---

7   JHCHS website, "The Event 201 Scenario: A Pandemic Tabletop Exercise," Johns Hopkins Center for Health Security, October 18, 2019, https://www.centerforhealthsecurity.org/event201/scenario.html.

CHAPTER 33

Confronting the
COVID Global
Predators. How it
Overturned Our View
of the World—and of
Human Life Itself

Dr. Peter & Ginger Breggin

Psychiatrist

Peter Breggin MD and Ginger Ross Breggin have been married and working together for almost 40 years. Peter graduated Harvard College, took part of his psychiatric residency at Harvard where he was a Teaching Fellow at Harvard Medical School, and became a full-time Consultant at the National Institutes of Mental Health (NIMH). Peter is known as "The Conscience of Psychiatry" for his many decades of successful reform work in mental health, including stopping the returning of lobotomy and transhumanistic experiments in the 1970s and stopping a giant eugenical program by the federal government working with his wife Ginger in the 1990s. He has published more than 20 medical and popular books, several coedited or coauthored by Ginger, including the huge bestseller Talking Back to Prozac. He has written more than 70 peer-reviewed publications and testified in court more than 100 times with many cases related to drug company and medical malfeasance. The couple has now turned their attention to the misuse of science and the suppression of freedoms surrounding COVID-19 and its origins by those they identify as "global predators."

Peter and Ginger have written the bestselling book, *"COVID-19 and the Global Predators: We are the Prey"* with introductions by top COVID-19 scientists and physicians, Peter A. McCullough MD, MPH; Elizabeth Lee Vliet MD; and Vladimir "Zev" Zelenko. The book is available everywhere.

From the beginning in February and March 2020, it seemed that COVID-19 "science" was being distorted and used to enforce the government narrative about the need for draconian political measures. Troubled by what we saw, we began to weigh whether or not to become more fully engaged in research and perhaps activism surrounding COVID-19.

I anticipated that I might be unusually well-prepared for the task of examining COVID-19 policies. As a physician, psychiatrist, medical-expert, and scientist, I have written more than twenty popular books and medical textbooks, many of them examining what I called the Psychopharmaceutical Complex, which we now see as the tip of the globalist empires. I had already written more than 70 peer-reviewed scientific reports as well as chapters in medical and scientific books dealing with everything from the fraudulent approval process for vaccines and the suppression of vaccine harms[1] to how the FDA works behind the scenes to help drug companies hide their more serious adverse effects, such as violence and suicide from Prozac (fluoxetine) and other antidepressants.[2] But I remained unprepared for the kind of disclosures of evil that would explode out of our research into COVID-19.

My background was also unique in having been approved as a scientific and medical expert more than 100 times in court in the U.S. and Canada, often testifying about medical malpractice, negligence by medical institutions, drug company malfeasance, and the failures of federal agencies including the FDA and NIH. Some of my successful cases involved applying the Nuremberg Code and other principles of medical ethics to human experimentation.[3] I was far more sophisticated about issues surrounding consent, coercion, fraud and dereliction in medicine, the pharmaceutical industry, and science than the vast

---

1   Breggin, Peter. (2021). Moving past the vaccine/autism controversy - to examine poten-
    tial vaccine neurological harms. *International Journal of Risk & Safety in Medicine, 32,*
    25-29.

2   Breggin, Peter, and Breggin, Ginger. (1994). *Talking Back to Prozac.* New York: St.
    Martin's Press.

3   Breggin.com | Article Detail for a review of some of my reform work.

majority of my colleagues. *But I was not nearly prepared for what we would quickly discover—a conspiracy to hide a widespread global plan— more than a decade in the works—to impose a kind of martial law on the world with the next pandemic in order to increase the power and the wealth of those at the top of human pyramid.*

The Origin of SARS-CoV-2

In mid-March 2020, Anthony Fauci, the government czar of COVID-19, as well as legions of supposedly reputable scientists, science writers, and high-ranking officials in medicine and science were rejecting the possibility that a SARS-CoV virus could have been made in a virology lab, specifically including the Wuhan Institute of Virology in China. Often they denied that such a virus could be made in any lab and certainly not by the Chinese. They argued with certainty that SARS-CoV-2 had originated in animals in nature and then been accidentally transferred from an animal to a human. This alleged risk of animal to human transmission, they argued, required constant preparation by creating new pathogens and then making vaccines for them. The flaw in this thinking? It is far more likely that humanity will continue to be struck down by pandemics originating out of the innumerable labs around the world rather than out of nature.

Blowing up the COVID Narrative as a Huge Conspiratorial Lie

Amid that avalanche of misinformation and lies, Ginger unearthed a scientific article that blew apart the entire unified political and scientific consensus that SARS-CoV-2 could not and did not come out of a lab. Although published six years earlier in a prestigious British journal, *Nature Medicine*, censorship had become so thorough that no one was talking or writing about this political and scientific bombshell.

The title of the article is "A SARS-like Cluster Of Circulating Bat Coronaviruses Shows Potential For Human Emergence."[4] The lab study describes how U.S. and Chinese scientists were collaborating in making SARS-CoV viruses in labs in the U.S. and in China—and had been doing so for years with a team led by Ralph Baric, the nation's most respected virologist and Anthony Fauci's favorite gain-of-function researcher.

The subject of the article was gain-of-function research—successfully turning harmless bat viruses from Chinese caves into toxic pandemic viruses that cause the deadly and infamous SARS or Severe Acute Respiratory Syndrome. In addition, the virus was a CoV—a coronavirus. From this comes the abbreviation SARS-CoV.

There had been a limited but more deadly outbreak of a SARS-CoV in 2003-2004—and hence the "2" in SARS-CoV-2. In fact, many SARS-CoV pathogens have been invented or re-engineered in laboratories around the world ever since the original pandemic. There were more than six accidental releases from labs, resulting in several deaths. As we document in our book, *COVID-19 and the Global Predators: We Are the Prey*, even the original pandemic SARS-CoV from 2003-2004 remains of unknown origin—nature or a lab.

In the 2015 report, American and Chinese researchers collaborated to document that their new variant of SARS-CoV killed mice, especially those who were old or immune compromised, and left the young mice

---

4   Vineet D Menachery, Boyd L Yount Jr, Kari Debbink1, Sudhakar Agnihothram, Lisa E Gralinski, Jessica A Plante, Rachel L Graham, Trevor Scobey, Xing-Yi Ge, Eric F Donaldson, Scott H Randell, Antonio Lanzavecchia, Wayne A Marasco, Zhengli-Li Shi & Ralph S Baric. A SARS-like cluster of circulating bat coronaviruses shows potential for human emergence. Nature Medicine, 21 (12), 1508-1514. December 2015. With follow-up letter included: https://www.nature.com/articles/nm.3985. This version was updated in the acknowledgement with an additional funding source, "USAID-EPT-PREDICT funding from EcoHealth Alliance (Z.-L.S.)," indicating that US EcoHealth Alliance funding went directly to Zhengli-Li Shi.

unaffected—very much like SARS-CoV-2 would later behave. It attacked human lung tissue in a petri dish and in the lungs of Frankenstein mice bred with genetic human respiratory epithelium.

The researchers lamented the continued failures, including their own, to make safe and effective vaccines for any SARS-CoVs. In their labs, a number of mice infected purposely with their new SARS-CoV died after being vaccinated. Although no genetic vaccines were involved, these warning signs made us concerned about the rush to make and distribute new SARS-CoV experimental vaccines. No safe and effective coronavirus vaccine had ever been made, despite decades of trying—and the ghastly truth is that none has been made to this day.

The 2015 research study confirms the high probability of SARS-CoV-2 coming from one of several labs in Wuhan because the outbreak began nearby them and because Wuhan Institute researchers were already conducting gain-of-function research turning harmless bat viruses into virulent ones that could infect people and cause SARS.

To top it off, we quickly found a second article published a year later in 2016 by the same lead U.S. researchers.[5] In the acknowledgements, the Americans thanked one of the original two Wuhan researchers for providing them some of the elements of the spike protein that made the SARS-CoV deadly to mice and human lung tissue. Their benefactor was Shi Zhengli, the famed coronavirus bat women adored by the American scientific press.

---

5   Vineet D Menachery, Boyd L Yount Jr, Amy C Sims, Kari Debbink, Sudhakar S Agni-hothram, Lisa E Gralinski, Rachel L Graham, Trevor Scobey , Jessica A Plante, Scott R Royal, Jesica Swanstrom, Timothy P Sheahan, Raymond J Pickles, Davide Corti, Scott H Randell, Antonio Lanzavecchia, Wayne A Marasco, Ralph S Baric. (2016). SARS-like Wav -CoV poised for human emergence. Proc Natl Acad. Sci US A 113, 3048-53 (2016). https://pubmed.ncbi.nlm.nih.gov/26976607/ Also obtainable at https://www.pnas.org/content/pnas/113/11/3048.full.pdf

Shock and Awe of The Disclosures

There were so many shocking revelations packed into that one 2015 scientific report and the 2016 follow up. It was stupefying that Anthony Fauci's National Institute of Allergy and Infectious Diseases (NIAID) was utterly denying the possibility of something Fauci himself was already funding—the 2015 "gain-of-function" lab research creating SARS-CoV viruses in American and Chinese labs. Again and again, Fauci denied the Wuhan lab origin of the pandemic virus and even today he and others waffle about it.

In addition, the article had a total of 15 authors including representatives from the Food and Drug Administration (FDA), Harvard Medical School, and a Swiss university, as well as from several departments at the University of North Carolina and the Wuhan Institute of Virology in China. How could so many other well-informed researchers act as if they knew nothing about SARS-CoVs being manipulated and rebuilt in U.S. or China labs—let alone *in a stunning globalist collaboration between the U.S. and China*?

How could this research have continued to escape attention? The studies had to be known by hundreds and perhaps thousands of professionals working in the field who would have to choose to outright lie or to bite their tongues into silence about an issue of worldwide importance and controversy with real life and death consequences. Keeping silent about this SARS-CoV lab research further required silence from others on the periphery as well—scientists, science reporters, media and others who could easily have found and publicly described the 2015 and 2016 reports. Some of them could have discovered the four documented leaks of manmade SARS-CoVs from Chinese labs as far back as 2003-2004, as well as leaks from labs in Singapore and Taiwan.[6]

---

6   Breggin, Peter, and Breggin, Ginger. (2021). *COVID-19 and the Global Predators: We Are the Prey*. Ithaca, NY: Lake Edge Press. See Chapter 3.

How could we become the first to discover and to publicize this important article amid all the "scientific" pronouncements about the supposed certainty that SARS-Co-V-2 had to come from nature and not a lab? How could the collaboration between the U.S. and the Chinese have been missed? How could the likelihood of it originating from a world renown Chinese lab be so easily dismissed when it was near to the point of origin of the pandemic? Who could have wielded the power to cover up all this and many similar revelations, keeping them to this very day a secret from the general public and the media?

Was it possible that a worldwide collusion existed involving virtually the entire medical and scientific establishment that could suppress an enormous amount of laboratory research on SARS-CoV viruses, as well as leaks from six labs, to make sure no blame would fall on China or the U.S. for making the new pandemic agent in their labs?

We had never imagined something like this seemingly enormous conspiracy. And it reached out far beyond the medical, scientific and pharmaceutical establishments into spheres we had never, until then, begun to investigate, from the Deep State to the military-industrial complex and on to world banking. We never foresaw that our own book would make the deepest dives ever into exposing the global predators who had been organizing for a decade precisely how they would use the coming pandemic to vastly increase their wealth and power—and to take their greatest steps toward empowering their own global empires.

Going Public and Blowing the Whistle

Based on the 2015 research article about the U.S./Chinese collaboration in making pandemic SARS-CoV viruses, in mid-April 2020 we authored a report and I presented a YouTube video. The column and the video was the first alert to the world of Fauci-funded collaborative "gain-of-function" research with the Chinese Communist Party. We immediately sent the column and the video to the media and other interested individuals.

Fortunately, we knew someone close to the Trump family who sent the video and the report to their inner circle. Two days later, President Trump announced he was cancelling Anthony Fauci's funding of the joint U.S. and Chinese gain-of-function research. The President stopped a treasonous joint effort with the Chinese Communists making viruses that could be used as biological weapons.[7]

Since the publication of our book, it has become more apparent that the gain-of-function research was always aimed at making biological weapons with the Department of Defense playing a major and guiding role in Operation WARP Speed, in effect, first making weapons (manmade deadly SARS-CoVs) and then making experimental mRNA and DNA vaccines against them.[8]

To whose benefit would the Department of Defense and other federal agencies be working? These so-called public-private collaborations benefit those who are seeking more government power over the people through the erosion of democratic republics along with those seeking to drain more wealth from the poorer nations and people into the already bloated coffers of the elite.

The Communists Spread the Virus

It soon became apparent that the Chinese were spreading SARS-CoV-2 around the world by continuing to fly potentially infected people from China by the hundreds of thousands, with more than half-a-million going by direct flights to the U.S. China used the virus as a biological

7 Breggin, Peter, and Breggin, Ginger. (2021). *COVID-19 and the Global Predators: We Are the Prey*. Ithaca, NY: Lake Edge Press. See Chapter 1.

8 Kennedy, Robert F., Jr. (2021). *The Real Anthony Fauci*. New York: Skyhorse Publishing. See the final subheading in the book, "COVID-19: A Military Project" (p. 433).

weapon against Western civilization and especially the U.S. Many researchers and concerned citizens began reporting on this—but wholly outside the major media which remained under the control of the globalists who were keeping the world in the dark about their intentions and actions.

The organized denial was so effective that, without being challenged, more than two dozen researchers published a letter in the world's oldest medical journal, *Lancet*, in effect swearing that the Chinese had nothing to do with the origin of SARS-Co-2. Later it was revealed that 26 out of 27 signers had financial connections to the Chinese and their labs and that the organizer of the letter, Peter Daszak of the EcoHealth Alliance, was Fauci's main conduit of money to Chinese researchers and the Wuhan Institute.[9]

To this day, SARS-CoV viruses are *defined* by popular sources as zoonotic, meaning jumping from animals to humans.[10] Meanwhile, the truth is that not one SARS-CoV has been proven to originate in nature. That is, none of the circulating coronaviruses cause the Severe Acute Respiratory Syndrome (SARS). SARS is very likely a product of human engineering.

There are many different kinds of circulating coronaviruses and some of them cause the common cold; but there are no coronaviruses in nature that are known to cause the potentially lethal disease. Meanwhile, many dangerous SARS-CoV are housed around the world as a result of experiments in labs. It is worth repeating that the Chinese Communists

---

9   https://www.dailymail.co.uk/news/article-9980015/26-Lancet-scientists-trashed-theo-ry-Covid-leaked-Chinese-lab-links-Wuhan.; html https://www.washingtontimes.com/news/2022/jan/6/the-lancet-chides-wuhan-defender-daszak/

10   https://duckduckgo.com/?q=SARS&ia=web;

had four SARS-CoV leaks from their own labs in 2003-2004 while experimenting with making variations of SARS-CoV.[11]

The further we research, the more we realize that COVID-19 was and remains like a wormhole from our old more naïve reality into a world of global predation whose existence had been unknown to us and which no one had analyzed as a whole in great detail. We found a world of vying global empires whose common goal is, to this day, to make the world increasingly vulnerable to their predations by destroying its leading republic, the United States of America, paving their way to a takeover of the world.

Discovering the Master Plan

The final enlightenment of this naïve "canary" was our discovery of the master plan that had been gathering steam over a ten year period, following Bill Gates' announcement that 2010 was the start of the Decade of Vaccines. In 2017, Gates created a new foundation around which he organized preparations for the coming pandemic—the Coalition for Epidemic Preparedness Innovations (CEPI).

The COVID-19 global plan that unfolded was a nearly exact fulfillment of the decade of planning. For example, of the hundreds of companies vying to make experimental vaccines, Gates and his cohort specifically backed Moderna and Pfizer years ahead of time and like clockwork Moderna and Pfizer became the two companies that would be given billions of dollars by the government, often in advance, to flood the United States with ineffective, deadly and wholly experimental "vaccines."

Our first inkling of the master plan came with our discovery of a PowerPoint presentation from 2017 buried inside the WHO archives in

11   Breggin, P. and Breggin, G. (2021). *COVID-19 and the Global Predators: We Are the Prey*. Ithaca, NY: Lake Edge *Press*. See Chapter 4: Was SARS-CoV-2 "Made in China"?

which Gates' CEPI described a formal mutual agreement with the World
Health Organization (a memorandum of understanding). The agreement
divided up control over industry, finance, and banking (under Gates and
CEPI) and medicine and science (under WHO) in order to completely
dominate and control the coming pandemic. Gates even guaranteed
that the vaccine manufacturers would be paid back for all their direct
and indirect expenses and that any "excess" profits would go back to his
CEPI.[12]

Then we found the original plan itself, upon which the PowerPoint
was based. It is the *Preliminary CEPI Business Plan*, a glossy business
proposal giving the details of an open collusion between the banks,
the drug companies, the UN, WHO, federal agencies, and specific
individuals including Anthony Fauci and Rick Bright and other Deep
State luminaries. This is the model for what is now called the Great
Reset—setting up the elite to continue to grow wealthier and more
powerful through "partnerships" (really, collusions) among the most
powerful and wealthiest individuals, agencies, and institutions in the
world.

*These collusions are essentially conspiracies to bypass or ignore the
normal political and governmental processes, especially any checks and
balances on their own power.* The globalists do not want to be supervised
or constrained by government executives, agencies, legislatures, or
courts. In general, they want to make the sovereign state irrelevant,
except as it can be used to their own ends as it was during COVID-19.
The goal of the globalists is to make sure that their investments will be
as risk free as possible while vastly increasing their wealth and power.

---

12   Breggin and Breggin, Op. Cit., 2021, See Chapter 15: Bill Gates Master Plan Found:
       mplements Operation Warp Speed in 2915-2017. Our latest findings regarding these
       global predatory arrangements are documented on @ Breggin.com | News Flash Topics.

Confirmation of Our Findings

As Robert F. Kennedy, Jr. was about to publish his groundbreaking book, *The Real Anthony Fauci,* he generously endorsed our own book, stating:

> No other book so comprehensively covers the details of COVID-19 criminal conduct as well as its origins in a network of global predators seeking wealth and power at the expense of human freedom and prosperity, under cover of false public health policies.

In addition, three of the top COVID treating physicians and scientists in the world wrote appreciative Introductions to our book: Peter A. McCullough, MD, PhD; Vladimir "Zev" Zelenko, MD; and Elizabeth Lee Vliet, MD. Others, including Paul Alexander, Ph.D., former COVID consultant to the Trump administration, have also endorsed our book.

This canary (PRB), on numerous occasions, has felt nearly asphyxiated by these incredible research findings on the breadth and depth of conspiratorial planning and actions behind COVID-19. Completing our book, *COVID-19 and the Global Predators: We Are the Prey,* I felt very much as if I had survived numerous face-to-face spiritual and even physical encounters with global evil.

CHAPTER 34

There Was No Pandemic

Professor Denis Rancourt

Scientist

Denis Rancourt holds B.Sc. and M.Sc. degrees in physics, and a Ph.D. in physics from the University of Toronto. He was a Natural Sciences and Engineering Research Council (NSERC) of Canada international post-doctoral candidate in national scientific laboratories in France and in The Netherlands. He then became a national NSERC University Research Fellow (NSERC-URF), in Canada, and a lead researcher and professor at the University of Ottawa for 23 years, where he attained the highest academic rank of tenured Full Professor. He is an interdisciplinary research scientist, and has published over 100 articles in peer reviewed science journals, in many different areas of science. He is presently co-director and researcher at the non-profit "CORRELATION Research in the Public Interest" (correlation-canada.org).

This is radical.

The essay is based on my May 17, 2023 testimony for the National Citizens Inquiry (NCI) in Ottawa, Canada, my 894-page book of exhibits in support of that testimony, and our continued research.

I am an accomplished interdisciplinary scientist and physicist, and a former tenured Full Professor of physics and lead scientist, originally at the University of Ottawa.

I have written over 30 scientific reports relevant to COVID, starting April 18, 2020 for the Ontario Civil Liberties Association (ocla.ca/covid), and recently for a new non-profit corporation (correlation-canada.org/research). Presently, all my work and interviews about COVID are documented on my website created to circumvent the barrage of censorship (denisrancourt.ca).

In addition to critical reviews of published science, the main data that my collaborators and I analyse is all-cause mortality.

All-cause mortality by time (day, week, month, year, period), by jurisdiction (country, state, province, county), and by individual characteristics of the deceased (age, sex, race, living accomodations) is the most reliable data for detecting and epidemiologically characterizing events causing death, and for gauging the population-level impact of any surge or collapse in deaths from any cause.

Such data is not susceptible to reporting bias or to any bias in attributing causes of death. We have used it to detect and characterize seasonality, heat waves, earthquakes, economic collapses, wars, population aging, long-term societal development, and societal assaults such as those occurring in the COVID period, in many countries around the world, and over recent history, 1900-present.

Interestingly, none of the post-second-world-war Centers-for-Disease-Control-and-Prevention-promoted (CDC-promoted) viral respiratory disease pandemics (1957-58, "H2N2"; 1968, "H3N2"; 2009, "H1N1 again") can be detected in the all-cause mortality of any country. Unlike all the other causes of death that are known to affect mortality, these so-called pandemics did not cause any detectable increase in mortality, anywhere.

The large 1918 mortality event, which was recruited to be a textbook viral respiratory disease pandemic ("H1N1"), occurred prior to the inventions of antibiotics and the electron microscope, under horrific post-war public-sanitation and economic-stress conditions. The 1918 deaths have been proven by histopathology of preserved lung tissue to have been caused by bacterial pneumonia. This is shown in several independent and non-contested published studies.

My first report analysing all-cause mortality was published on June 2, 2020, at censorship-prone Research Gate, and was entitled "All-cause mortality during COVID-19 - No plague and a likely signature of mass homicide by government response". It showed that hot spots of sudden surges in all-cause mortality occurred only in specific locations in the Northern-hemisphere Western World, which were synchronous with the March 11, 2020 declaration of a pandemic. Such synchronicity is impossible within the presumed framework of a spreading viral respiratory disease, with or without airplanes, because the calculated time from seeding to mortality surge is highly dependent on local societal circumstances, by several months to years. I attributed the excess deaths to aggressive measures and hospital treatment protocols known to have been applied suddenly at that time in those localities.

The work was pursued in greater depth with collaborators for several years and continues. We have shown repeatedly that excess mortality most often refused to cross national borders and inter-state lines. The invisible virus targets the poor and disabled and carries a passport. It also never kills until governments impose socio-economic and care-structure transformations on vulnerable groups within the domestic population.

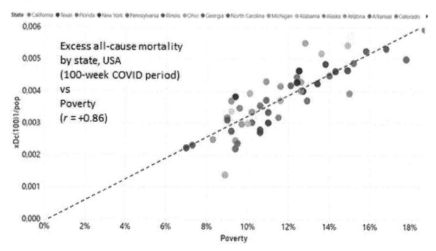

Denis Rancourt et al., 2022

Here are my conclusions, from our detailed studies of all-cause mortality in the COVID period, in combination with socio-economic and vaccine-rollout data:

1. If there had been no pandemic propaganda or coercion, and governments and the medical establishment had simply gone on with business as usual, then there would not have been any excess mortality

2. There was no pandemic causing excess mortality

3. Measures caused excess mortality

4. COVID-19 vaccination caused excess mortality

Regarding the vaccines, we quantified many instances in which a rapid rollout of a dose in the imposed vaccine schedule was synchronous with an otherwise unexpected peak in all-cause mortality, at times in the seasonal cycle and of magnitudes that have not previously been seen in the historic record of mortality.

In this way, we showed that the vaccination campaign in India caused the deaths of 3.7 million fragile residents. In Western countries, we quantified the average all-ages rate of death to be 1 death for every 2000 injections, to increase exponentially with age (doubling every additional 5 years of age), and to be as large as 1 death for every 100 injections for those 80 years and older. We estimated that the vaccines had killed 13 million worldwide.

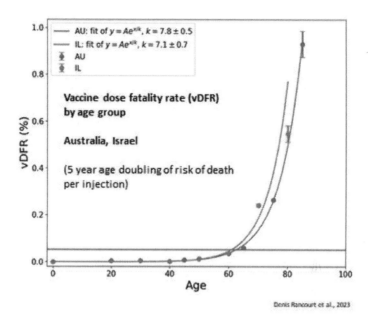

Denis Rancourt et al., 2023

If one accepts my above-numbered conclusions, and the analyses that we have performed, then there are several implications about how one perceives reality regarding what actually did and did not occur.

First, whereas epidemics of fatal infections are very real in care homes, in hospitals, and with degenerate living conditions, the viral respiratory pandemic risk promoted by the USA-led "pandemic response" industry is not a thing. It is most likely fabricated and maintained for ulterior motives, other than saving humanity.

Second, in addition to natural events (heat waves, earthquakes, extended large-scale droughts), significant events that negatively affect mortality are large assaults against domestic populations, affecting vulnerable residents, such as:

- sudden devastating economic deterioration (the Great Depression, the dust bowl, the dissolution of the Soviet Union),
- war (including social-class restructuring),

- imperial or economic occupation and exploitation (including large-scale exploitative land use), and
- the well-documented measures and destruction applied during the COVID period.

Otherwise, in a stable society, mortality is extremely robust and is not subject to large rapid changes. There is no empirical evidence that large changes in mortality can be induced by sudden appearances of new pathogens. In the contemporary era of the dominant human species, humanity is its worst enemy, not nature.

Third, coercive measures imposed to reduce the risk of transmission (such as distancing, direction arrows, lockdown, isolation, quarantine, Plexiglas barriers, face shields and face masks, elbow bumps, etc.) are palpably unscientific; and the underlying concern itself regarding "spread" was not ever warranted and is irrational, since there is no evidence in reliable mortality data that there ever was a particularly virulent pathogen.

In fact, the very notion of "spread" during the COVID period is rigorously disproved by the temporal and spatial variations of excess all-cause mortality, everywhere that it is sufficiently quantified, worldwide. For example, the presumed virus that killed 1.3 million poor and disabled residents of the USA did not cross the more-than-thousand-kilometer land border with Canada, despite continuous and intense economic exchanges. Likewise, the presumed virus that caused synchronous mortality hotspots in March-April-May 2020 (such as in New York, Madrid region, London, Stockholm, and northern Italy) did not spread beyond those hotspots.

Interestingly, in this regard, the historical seasonal variations (12 month period) in all-cause mortality, known for more than 100 years, are inverted in the northern and southern global hemispheres, and show no evidence of "spread" whatsoever. Instead, these patterns, in a given hemisphere, show synchronous increases and decreases of mortality across the entire hemisphere. Would the "spreading" causal agent(s) always take exactly 6 months to cross into the other hemisphere, where it again causes mortality changes that are synchronous across the hemisphere? Many epidemiologists have long-ago concluded that person-to-person "contact" spreading of respiratory diseases cannot explain and is disproved by the seasonal patterns of all-cause mortality. Why the CDC *et al.* are not systematically ridiculed in this regard is beyond this scientist's comprehension.

Instead, outside of extremely poor living conditions, we should look to the body of work produced by Professor Sheldon Cohen and co-authors (USA) who established that two dominant factors control whether intentionally challenged college students become infected and the severity of the respiratory illness when they are infected:

- degree of experienced psychological stress
- degree of social isolation

The negative impact of experienced psychological stress on the immune system is a large current and established area of scientific study, dutifully ignored by vaccine interests, and we now know that the said impact is dramatically larger in elderly individuals, where nutrition (gut biome ecology) is an important co-factor.

Of course, I do not mean that causal agents do not exist, such as bacteria, which can cause pneumonia; nor that there are not dangerous environmental concentrations of such causal agents in proximity to fragile individuals, such as in hospitals and on clinicians' hands, notoriously.

Fourth, since our conclusion is that there is no evidence that there was any particularly virulent pathogen causing excess mortality, the debate about gain-of-function research and an escaped bioweapon is irrelevant.

I do not mean that the Department of Defence (DoD) does not fund gain-of-function and bioweapon research (abroad, in particular), I do not mean that there are not many US patents for genetically modified microbial organisms having potential military applications, and I do not mean that there have not previously been impactful escapes or releases of bioweapon vectors and pathogens. For example, the Lyme disease controversy in the USA may be an example of a bioweapon leak (see Kris Newby's 2019 book "Bitten: The Secret History of Lyme Disease and Biological Weapons").

Generally, for obvious reasons, any pathogen that is extremely virulent will not also be extremely contagious. There are billions of years of cumulative evolutionary pressures against the existence of any such pathogen, and that result will be deeply encoded into all lifeforms.

Furthermore, it would be suicidal for any regime to vehemently seek to create such a pathogen. Bioweapons are intended to be delivered to specific target areas, except in the science fiction wherein immunity from a bioweapon that is both extremely virulent and extremely contagious can be reliably delivered to one's own population and soldiers.

In my view, if anything COVID is close to being a bioweapon, it is the military capacity to massively, and repeatedly, rollout individual injections, which are physical vectors for whichever substances the regime wishes to selectively inject into chosen populations, while imposing complete compliance down to one's own body, under the cover of protecting public health.

This is the same regime that practices wars of complete nation destruction and societal annihilation, under the cover of spreading democracy and women's rights. And I do not mean China.

Fifth, again, since our conclusion is that there is no evidence that there was any particularly virulent pathogen causing excess mortality, there was no need for any special treatment protocols, beyond the usual thoughtful, case-by-case, diagnostics followed by the clinician's chosen best approach.

Instead, vicious new protocols killed patients in hotspots that applied those protocols in the first months of the declared pandemic.

This was followed in many states by imposed coercive societal measures, which were contrary to individual health: fear, panic, paranoia, induced psychological stress, social isolation, self-victimization, loss of work and volunteer activity, loss of social status, loss of employment, business bankruptcy, loss of usefulness, loss of caretakers, loss of venues and mobility, suppression of freedom of expression, etc.

Only the professional class did better, comfortably working from home, close to family, while being catered to by an army of specialised home-delivery services.

Unfortunately, the medical establishment did not limit itself to assaulting and isolating vulnerable patients in hospitals and care facilities. It also systematically withdrew normal care, and attacked physicians who refused to do so.

In virtually the entire Western World, antibiotic prescriptions were cut and maintained low by approximately 50% of the pre-COVID rates. This would have had devastating effects in the USA, in particular, where:

- the CDC's own statistics, based on death certificates, has approximately 50% of the million or so deaths associated with COVID having bacterial pneumonia as a listed comorbidity (there was a massive epidemic of bacterial pneumonia in the USA, which no one talked about)
- the Southern poor states historically have much higher antibiotic prescription rates (this implies high susceptibility to bacterial pneumonia)
- excess mortality during the COVID period is very strongly correlated ($r = +0.86$) — in fact proportional to — state-wise poverty

Sixth, since our conclusion is that there is no evidence that there was any particularly virulent pathogen causing excess mortality, there was no public-health reason to develop and deploy vaccines; not even if one accepted the tenuous proposition that any vaccine has ever been effective against a presumed viral respiratory disease.

Add to this that all vaccines are intrinsically dangerous and our above-described vaccine-dose fatality rate quantifications, and we must recognize that the vaccines contributed significantly to excess mortality everywhere that they were imposed.

In conclusion, the excess mortality was not caused by any particularly virulent new pathogen. COVID so-called response in-effect was a massive multi-pronged state and iatrogenic attack against populations, and against societal support structures, which caused all the excess mortality, in every jurisdiction.

It is only natural now to ask "what drove this?", "who benefited?" and "which groups sustained permanent structural disadvantages?"

In my view, the COVID assault can only be understood in the symbiotic contexts of geopolitics and large-scale social-class transformations. Dominance and exploitation are the drivers. The failing USA-centered global hegemony and its machinations create dangerous conditions for virtually everyone.

***

Did you find this book informative? If so, we would be interested to hear from you. Please share your thoughts by rating and reviewing this book on Amazon and share your knowledge with others who may benefit.

Follow us on Substack: https://canaryinacovidworld.substack.com and Twitter/X https://twitter.com/canary_covid